Research
in
Psychophysiology

Research in Psychophysiology

Edited by

PETER H. VENABLES

Psychology Department, University of York

and

MARGARET J. CHRISTIE

*St. Mary's Hospital Medical School
and Bedford College, University of London*

JOHN WILEY & SONS
London · New York · Sydney · Toronto

Library of Congress Cataloging in Publication Data:

Venables, Peter H.
  Research in psychophysiology.

  1. Psychology, Physiological. I. Christie, Margaret J., joint
author. II. Title. [DNLM: 1. Psychophysiology. 2. Research.
WL102 V448r] QP360.V46 1975   612′.8   74–18266
ISBN 0 471 90555 0

Photosetting by Thomson Press (India) Limited, New Delhi and
printed by J. W. Arrowsmith Ltd., Bristol, England.

Preface

This collection of invited chapters represents the fulfilment of the editors' plans to compile a book which would provide a sample of approaches which are representative of the field of psychophysiology in 1975. It is intended that the book should provide interest for all psychologists and not only those who label themselves as psychophysiologists. It was felt, when the plan for the book was first mooted, that there were insights which the field of psychophysiology could offer and which could be incorporated within the corpus of general psychological knowledge. The plan of the book and particularly the last section bears this in mind. Inevitably, the book does not conform to the tidy schema originally intended. For instance, like our distinguished predecessors, Greenfield & Sternbach (1972) we had difficulty in persuading workers in the field of developmental and life-span psychophysiology to write for us. It may be that no-one really covers, in their own research, more than patchy periods of our life span and this inhibits the reviewing of data from a more longitudinal point of view.

Nevertheless, we hope that we have generally succeeded in our original plan. This plan had three main divisions. Firstly, we wanted some discussion of methodological problems, not from a comprehensive point of view, but rather with the aim of alerting readers to some of the wide variety of factors that face workers in this field. Secondly, we wanted to present a wide variety of coverage in a section which we thought of as including 'states'. These were states brought about by situations, and those resulting from conditions of the individual. In selecting our authors to write chapters in this section we interpreted psychophysiology in the widest sense, not confining attention only to polygraphically measured variables. We have, however, invited our authors to write under the definition of psychophysiology which includes the psychological state of the subject or his behaviour as the independent variable and the physiological state as the dependent variable. This section includes some chapters where the material is not of the kind that has appeared in the pages of such traditional journals as *Psychophysiology*, and this provides a variety of viewpoints which we hope the reader will find stimulating.

Finally, in the third section, the authors have been specifically invited to write about the links which they see between what a few years ago was thought of as 'main stream' experimental psychology and that presumptuous outsider— psychophysiology. We suspect, however, that the view that psychophysiology is not quite respectable has already disappeared and psychophysiology itself may be part of the 'mainstream'. No longer is psychophysiology an aspect of psychology receiving no formal teaching in universities; Johnson & May (1973) provide data on the number of courses in the U.S. which specifically cover this area. Nevertheless, there is still a gulf between some of the traditional aspects of psychology and psychophysiology. For that reason we view the third section of this book as being particularly important. Ways in which perceptual, attentional, conditioning and memory processes may receive some illumination from work in psychophysiology have been outlined. Also, conversely, how some of the procedures of the psychophysiologist need to take into account the expertise of those in other field has been pointed out. If this section does no more than suggest ways in which we need to peer out of our cocoons occasionally it will have achieved what the editors intended.

The book does not aspire to be comprehensive, indeed, we took some deliberate decisions to omit areas, particularly those which have received recent extensive coverage elsewhere. A whole topic which we have not included is that of bio-feedback; a lot of material is available on this controversial area which lies between solid work which unfortunately seems to have been not wholly repeatable, and a fashionable quackery with less than desirable ethical connotations. Perhaps the recent paper by Blanchard & Young (1973) puts all the points we would wish to make.

While there will be some who find that their favourite topic is not covered we feel sure that what is presented provides a valuable sample of what is going on in the field today, and a flavour of the enthusiasm which this area of psychology engenders in its practitioners.

We would like to thank our different classes of authors. We would especially like to thank those who provided their chapters on time fully in accordance with editorial requirements; we apologize for the delays which they have had to suffer before seeing their work in print. We would like to thank those who filled last minute gaps and who provided stimulating material under time pressure. We would also like to thank those who eventually made it, we feel that their contributions were worth waiting for. Additionally, we should like to apologize to our readers for those chapters where in one position or another the editors' names appear where this inclusion was not originally intended. There were aspects of the subject which we did not wish to see omitted and in our somewhat inexpert ways we attempted to fill the gap.

Finally, we would like to acknowledge our indebtedness to Verner Knott for his invaluable editorial assistance, and to Patricia Caple for her work in coping with the secretarial background to launching the book.

PETER H. VENABLES
MARGARET J. CHRISTIE

Blanchard, E. B. & Young, L. D. Self-control of cardiac functioning: A promise as yet unfulfilled. *Psychological Bulletin*, 1973, **79**, 145–163.

Greenfield, N. S. & Sternbach, R. A. *Handbook of Psychophysiology*, New York: Holt, Rinehart & Winston, 1972.

Johnson, H. J. & May, J. R. The educational process in psychophysiology. *Psychophysiology*, 1973, **10**, 215–217.

List of Contributors

Brian Bell
Psykologisk Institut, Kommunehospitalet, Oster Farimagsgade 5, 1399 Copenhagen, Denmark

Kirk Blankstein
Department of Psychology, Erindale College, University of Toronto, 3359 Mississauga Road, Clarkson, Ontario, Canada

F. I. M. Craik
Department of Psychology, Erindale College, University of Toronto, 3359 Mississauga Road, Clarkson, Ontario, Canada.

Margaret J. Christie
*Department of Psychiatry, St. Mary's Hospital Medical School, Woodfield Wing, Harrow Road, London W9 and
Department of Psychology, Bedford College, Regent's Park, London NW1 4NS, U.K.*

Jo-Ann H. Farr
Department of Psychology, Pennsylvania State University, University Park, Pennsylvania 16802, U.S.A.

Marianne Frankenhaeuser
Psychological Laboratories, University of Stockholm, Box 6706 5–113 85 Stockholm, Sweden.

Robert D. Hare
Department of Psychology, The University of British Columbia, Vancouver 8, Canada.

Laverne C. Johnson
Neuropsychiatric Research, Building 36–4, Department of the Navy, Naval Regional Medical Center, San Diego, California 92134, U.S.A.

Malcolm Lader
Institute of Psychiatry, De Crespigny Park, Denmark Hill, London SE5 8AF, U.K.

David T. Lykken
Department of Psychiatry, Research Unit, Medical School, Box 392, Mayo Memorial Building, Minneapolis, Minnesota 55455, U.S.A.

Irene Martin

Department of Psychology, Institute of Psychiatry, De Crespigny Park, Denmark Hill, London SE5 8AF, U.K.

Roy B. Mefferd Jr.

Psychiatric and Psychosomatic Research Laboratory, Veterans Administration Hospital, 2002 Holcombe Boulevard, Houston, Texas 77031, U.S.A.

Paul Naitoh

Neuropsychiatric Research, Building 36–4, Department of the Navy, Naval Regional Medical Center, San Diego, California 92134, U.S.A.

Peter Noble

Institute of Psychiatry, De Crespigny Park, Denmark Hill, London SE5 8AF, U.K.

William J. Ray

Department of Psychology, Pennsylvania State University, University Park, Pennsylvania 16802, U.S.A.

B. McA. Sayers

Engineering in Medicine Laboratory, Department of Electrical Engineering, Imperial College, London SW7, U.K.

Robert M. Stein

Department of Psychology, Pennsylvania State University, University Park, Pennsylvania 16802, U.S.A.

Samuel Sutton

Biometrics Research, 722 West 168th Street, New York, N. Y. 10032, U.S.A.

Judy L. Todd

Kennedy Child Study Center, Santa Monica, California, U.S.A.

Patricia Tueting

Biometrics Research, 722 West 168th Street, New York, N. Y. 10032, U.S.A.

Peter H. Venables

Department of Psychology, University of York, Heslington, York, YO1 5DD, U.K.

Contents

x

SECTION 1

Methodological Problems

Chapter 1

The Role of Individual Differences in Psychophysiological Research

DAVID T. LYKKEN

University of Minnesota

1.1. INTRODUCTION

All ships within a given class of naval vessels, say destroyers, are built in accordance with the same general set of blueprints, the same 'species plan'. Any navy man, however, will testify that each ship is an individual, that no two destroyers handle just the same way, that each has its crochets and idiosyncracies. These idiographic deviations from the nomothetic rule come about as a result of two kinds of causes. Firstly, all varieties of mechanisms—nautical, electronic, organismic—show *parametric variation*, i.e. deviation from whatever value is specified for each component part in the blueprint, wiring diagram or species plan. The particular behaviour of each mechanism, while generally similar to that of other members of the class, will vary from the norm in consequence of such deviations. Secondly, the actual structure of a complex mechanism may differ in small ways from other members of the same class, either because of differences in the original blueprint or due to changes made *later*, by design or by the accidents of experience. One class of man-made mechanisms, the digital computer, is uniquely susceptible to structural modification. Each new computer program modifies or elaborates the essential structure of the computer, making it into a new and different special-purpose machine which will operate in a unique manner upon the data input. It is, of course, precisely this extraordinary modifiability of structure which impels the familiar analogy between the computer and the brain. The human nervous system is a mechanism which, while it conforms generally to a common species plan, (i) shows great individuality, due to (ii) nomothetic, parametric variation, i.e. relatively fixed or stable differences between individuals, resulting largely from genetic factors; and (iii) idiographic structural variation, due primarily to the effects of learning.

Psychologists, by long tradition, tend to focus their research efforts more or less exclusively on one of the three categories of problems suggested above. Physiological and what are called 'experimental' psychologists focus on the species plan; their objective is to elaborate a nomothetic account of the 'generalized mind' or the average or typical case. At the other extreme, the clinician may attempt a psychodynamic, idiographic understanding of the individual case. Somewhere in the middle are the psychometrists or differential psychologists, the students of ability and temperament and behaviour genetics, whose interest is in nomothetic trait variables, definable across individuals but with a focus on parametric variation rather than on structural regularities. For the traditional experimental psychologist, parametric variations—individual differences—are nuisance variables, a source of noise. For psychologists trained in the psychometric tradition, individual differences are the data base itself.

Psychophysiology, with origins that antedate both Galton and Wundt but only lately emerging from its chrysalis, is an interface between these two traditions. Experimentalists, often with a physiological perspective, move into psychophysiology on the hunt for general laws while others, renegade clinicians perhaps or refugees from the swamps of personality research, seek more modestly for objective measures of (important) dimensions of individual differences. This chapter will not be the first place where a plea will have been offered for a more effective, a more calculated and deliberate blending of the two points of view. For the radical experimentalist, science is the job of weaving the nomological net, the discovery of nomothetic laws relating the basic variables of a discipline. For the radical psychometrist, science rather is the business of discovering what these basic variables *are*; for some, e.g. some factor analysts, there is even a Skinnerian disinterest in intra-organismic inter-relationships, based upon a simple faith in transfer functions, in the idea that one can predict as accurately as one might wish if one merely includes the right factor scores in one's specification equation.

The truth is, however, that the identification of the 'basic' variables and the study of the laws relating them are the two legs on which science moves forward; to try to hop along on one is to stumble and even a creature with two legs will be ambi-sinister if the two are driven by separate, uncoordinated brains. Galileo, the 'father of modern physics', showed us the power of mathematical laws derived from quantitative experiments but one must not forget that laws state relations between variables and that, even in simple mechanics, it required the insight of genius of identify the *right* variables—the concept of mass, for example, which did not come easily to a 16th-Century mind. In the behaviour sciences, the problem of identifying 'basic' variables is particularly acute, not because of a shortage of candidates but rather the reverse—we are drowning in them. Each new test or measure, nearly every new experiment, defines one or more new variable; the dictionary offers names for more than 50,000 candidates for the field of personality alone. Considering only laws relating three variables at a time ($x = F(y, z)$), these 50,000 trait terms imply the empirical study of more than 10^{13} separate nomologicals. An experimentalist who would advocate forging ahead without prior winnowing of such a list would be more than radical, he would be mad.

But the task of identifying the 'short list' of basic variables—'basic' in the sense that they might figure in the most orderly set of laws, deriving from a parsimonious and manageable theory—typically requires the study of individual differences. Even a task like choosing amongst competing methods of expressing the GSR (e.g. SRR, SCR, $SCR/SCR_{max,}$ log SCR, the Autonomic Lability Score, etc.) requires the technology of the differential psychologist. An issue of considerable contemporary interest is the Lacey hypothesis (Lacey, 1967) to the effect that cardiac activity may be involved in the modulation of external stimulus input. The existence and nature of such an alleged mechanism in the mammalian nervous system is a fairly typical problem area for the experimentalist but the concerns and the techniques of the differential psychologist become immediately relevant also. To determine whether cardiac activity tends to increase when attention is deployed inward, for example, one must decide whether to use, as one measure of the level of cardiac activity, heart *rate* of heart *period*. Although these two indices are perfectly reciprocally related, it is not a matter of indifference which one is used in experimental work. For example, imagine a test of the Lacey hypothesis based on the expectation that some measure of the degree of effectiveness of the internal deployment of attention ought to be correlated with the amount of increase in cardiac activity. It is easy to invent imaginary, but possible, data which would show a positive correlation, supporting the hypothesis, when cardiac activity is measured in terms of heart rate but a correlation of *zero*, refuting the same hypothesis, if the scientist chooses to measure activity in terms of heart period instead. As in the problem of the choice of electrodermal units, this methodological issue must be approached with the help of both experimental and individual differences techniques.

The same experiment illustrates the use of the individual differences approach to theoretical as well as to methodological issues. Of the many conceivable corollaries of the Lacey hypothesis, some lead to traditional experimental tests in which an independent variable (e.g. direction of attention) is manipulated while one observes the effect of this on an appropriate dependent variable (e.g. heart rate). However many other tests, like the one suggested above, depend for their existence and utility on the facts of individual differences. Even under the same conditions of measurement (i.e. with no attempt at manipulation), different *S*s will show a range of degree of attention deployment inward as well as variation in cardiac response and it is of course this variation in both variables, related *ex hypothesi*, which makes possible a testable deduction from the theory.

This idea can be stated more generally along the following lines. Most theories in psychology are hypotheses concerning some portion of the species plan, conjectures about the nomothetic structure of the nervous system (this account assumes, of course, that all psychological theories are 'about' the CNS in the sense that it is the CNS which mediates between input and output, between stimulus and behaviour). An elementary theoretical proposition would be of the form $y = f(x)$, where x and y may be either observable or theoretical variables. A direct experimental test of this bit of theory would be to vary x and observe y, but such experimental manipulation is often difficult. However, most biological variables naturally vary from one organism to another and many variables change in value over time, due to a variety of reasons. This natural variation, within or between individuals, will often provide a substitute—or at least a supplementary—method for testing theories.

1.2. IMPROVING METHODS OF MEASUREMENT USING INDIVIDUAL DIFFERENCE DATA

If $X = $ a judge's estimate of Jones' weight, $Y = $ a prediction of weight based on Jones' height and girth, and $Z = $ the reading obtained when Jones steps on a scale, then X, Y and Z are three potential variables of, say, physiology. Here we know that they are actually all measures of the same, underlying variable but this is not always so easy to see. Our problem, then, might be to determine, first, whether X, Y and Z represent three different dimensions or only one and, having answered this first question, to decide, second, which of these three is the *best* measure (i.e. of body weight).

1.2.1. Dimensional analysis

A way to determine whether X, Y and Z all measure the same thing—albeit unequally well—would be to examine their intercorrelations. One must be careful about the linearity assumption, e.g. one should look at the bivariate scatter plots, since we know, for example, that SCR and SRR measure more-or-less the same thing but their product-moment correlation is attenuated since they are reciprocally rather than linearly related. Where the bivariate regressions are linear, the magnitude of intercorrelations should be evaluated in terms of the reliabilities of the individual variables. Body height and weight, for example, correlate about 0·80 yet, since we know that the reliability of these two variables is 0·95 or better, it is sensible to treat them as separate dimensions. On the other hand, the Taylor Manifest Anxiety Scale, the Repression–Sensitization Scale, and the Neuroticism subscale of the Eysenck Personality Inventory all intercorrelate between 0·7 and 0·8 while their reliabilities are in the same range; hence, we can conclude that all three are essentially measures of the same personality dimension, *viz.* stability *vs* neuroticism or what Block (1965) calls 'ego resiliency'.

While it is important to avoid treating such measures as separate entities when virtually all their reliable variance is common variance (merely, e.g. because their inventors have given them romantically individual names), an equally serious sin is to assume that some other set of measures which are claimed to relate to a common underlying variable really do so. Dimensional analysis provides protection from this danger also. Some years ago, for example, psychologists were busily turning out a spate of studies of the personality trait known as 'rigidity', each author employing his favourite from among five or six tests alleged to measure this trait. When several investigators finally tried to intercorrelate these measures on the same *S*s (Jenkins & Lykken, 1957, p. 99), with results ranging about zero, research interest in 'rigidity' tailed off precipitously.

Western psychophysiologists have become increasingly interested in the Pavlovian concept of 'strength of nervous system' (SNS), as developed by Nebylitsyn and others of the school of Teplov (Nebylitsyn & Gray, 1972). A number of alternative methods have been advanced for measuring this basic nervous parameter, rate of extinction with reinforcement of the photochemical reflex, slope of the function relating reaction time to stimulus intensity, susceptibility to photic driving of the EEG, etc. Studies are appearing in which the correlates of some one of these measures are interpreted as correlates of SNS (*ibid*, Chaps. 2, 4, 6, 18–21). Because the several putative indices of SNS are apparently only weakly correlated with each other (*ibid*, Chap. 10), such interpretations seem premature. A more efficient research strategy would seem to be to concentrate first on increasing the common factor variance by trying to improve the measures, i.e. to find ways of reducing the extent to which each variable is affected by measurement error or by irrelevant factors. As discussed in the next section, such an increase in common variance can in fact be employed as a criterion in choosing among alternative methods of measurement.

Another example of dimensional analysis in psychophysiology concerns the problem of partitioning the frequency spectrum of the EEG. There is a well-established convention of calling waves of less than 3 Hz 'Delta' waves, frequencies from 3 to 7 Hz 'Theta', 8 to 13 Hz 'Alpha', and frequencies higher than 13 Hz 'Beta' activity. It is clear that this conventional partition is not intended to be just an arbitrary convenience; Delta and Theta waves are believed to have different psychophysiological significance and activity at 13 Hz is thought to have less in common with 14 Hz activity than it does with activity at 8 Hz. The warrant for these rather surprising claims lies in an accumulation of years of rather informal, 'clinical' observations of patterns of co-variation of the spectrum components. An increase in 11–13 Hz activity is in fact likely to be accompanied by an increase from 8–10 Hz (e.g. when the eyes are closed) and not by an increase in the Beta band.

With a view toward corroborating these now classical assumptions in a somewhat more systematic fashion, Auke Tellegen and the author analysed 3-minute samples of EEG obtained from 70 pairs of same sex, adult twins. Each sample was spectrum-analysed, yielding a magnitude spectrum of 40 ordinates at 0·5 Hz intervals from 0·25 to 19·75 Hz. The spectra were then 'standardized', i.e. reduced to unit area, a process which eliminates differences due to average EEG amplitude. The 40 spectrum ordinates were then inter-correlated across the 140 Ss and these data were factor analysed. After rotation (Varimax), there appeared to be five—possibly six—significant factors which accounted for from 80 to 84 per cent of the variance in these spectra. Three of the rotated factors were immediately identifiable with three of the classical frequency bands, Delta, Theta, and Beta; total activity in these bands corre-lated 0·92, 0·94 and 0·91 with Factors V, II and I, respectively. Factor III was positively loaded by activity from 7·25 to 8·75 Hz and negatively by activity from 10·25 to 12·25 Hz. Factor IV was positively loaded by spectrum activity from 11·75 to 14·25 Hz and negatively by activity from 9·25 to 10·25. Factor VI, although very weak, also showed this bipolar contrast between higher and lower portions of the Alpha band (9·25–9·75 vs 10·75–11·25 Hz). From a study of the original spectra themselves, we believed that three dimensions would be required to describe activity within the Alpha band, viz. the median frequency of the 'Alpha bump', which we call 'Rho', the amount of activity in a 3-Hz band centered on Rho (i.e. on each S's own median Alpha frequency), and an index of the constancy of Alpha frequency, measured in terms of the kurtosis of the Alpha 'bump', a parameter that we call 'Kappa'. As a test of this inference, we intercorrelated our six a priori parameters (Delta, Theta, Beta, Rho, Alpha and Kappa) with the scores for the same 140 Ss on the six orthogonal Varimax factors, finding that the six factors accounted for from 92 to 100 per cent of the variance in the first five parameters and 72 per cent of the variance in Kappa. Obversely, from the multiple regressions of the factors on the parameters, we found that our six rational parameters accounted for 91, 95, 53, 49, and 94 per cent of the variance in the first five factors, respectively.

To summarize, the factor analysis tells us that nearly all of the linear common variance in the EEG spectra can be contained within a factor space of only five orthogonal dimensions (Factor VI being very weak and ill-defined). Six (non-orthogonal) parameters (Delta, Theta, Alpha, Beta, Rho and Kappa), more easily translated into standard EEG parlance than the factor scores themselves, were able to account in their turn for about two-thirds of the total spectrum variance. Thus, the analysis both corroborates and extends the traditional practice. It provides an objective, quantitative basis for the definition of Delta, Theta and Beta. It also suggests, however, that Alpha and Rho should not be· defined in terms of the entire classical alpha band but, rather, in terms of the alpha 'bump' only. That is to say that not all of the spectrum from 8 to 13 Hz represents alpha activity in a dynamic sense but only that portion within an elevation or 'bump', seldom more than 3 Hz wide, whose centre frequency, Rho, is characteristic of the subject and the situation and may vary at least from 8 to 12 Hz.

1.2.2. The 'orderliness' criterion

Since science is a search for an orderly description of nature, 'good' scientific variables are those which tend to behave in an orderly fashion. Measures of relatively stable properties should not vary greatly over time; thus, retest reliability is a common test of the goodness of a measure, one example of a test based on the orderliness criterion. Identical twins provide a less widely recognized opportunity for the application of the same criterion to the improvement of methods of measurement. Genetically identical and having usually shared very similar environments, a pair of monozygotic (MZ) twins can be thought of as 'parallel forms' of the same individual. As the error variance is reduced in some psychological or physiological measure, the intra-class correlation of that measure within pairs of MZ twins should correspondingly increase. In the case of traits or properties that are thought to be genetically determined, an additional 'orderliness' criterion can be specified, namely that the ratio of the DZ to MZ intro-class correlations will tend toward 0·5.

As an illustration of this use of twin data in methodological research, the six EEG spectrum parameters referred to in the previous section were found to have intra-class correlations ranging above 0·80 in a sample of 40 pairs of MZ twins. While obviously not a *necessary* criterion of a 'good' measure, such a finding is *sufficient* evidence that the parameters in question are reliable and at least potentially meaningful.

More generally, when any variable, x, is known to be related to some other variable, y, then that measure, $f_i(x)$, which shows the most orderly relationship to y, thereby recommends itself as the best among competing methods of measuring x. For example, tonic skin conductance level (SCL) is known to increase generally with CNS arousal; the two-flash threshold (TFT) is known to *decrease* with arousal. In the set of studies reviewed by Lykken, Rose, Luther & Maley (1966), the average correlation between SCL and TFT was only $-0·44$. When a range-corrected index was substituted for raw SCL as the measure of 'electrodermal arousal', this correlation increased sharply to $-0·67$. In a later study (Lykken, 1972), evidence in favour of range correcting measures of tonic SCL and heart rate, as well as phasic SCRs, was provided by showing that experimental manipulations which were expected to produce differences in all three variables gave substantially larger F-ratios (i.e. smaller residual error) when the range-corrected measures were employed. By a similar test, the phasic heart rate response (HRR) variable was shown not to be improved by range correction.

1.2.3. Individual differences in range of responses

Having mentioned the range correction procedure in the examples above, it may be appropriate here to explain the concept on which that procedure is based, since it is pertinent to the topic of this chapter. Suppose one were to ask *S*s to indicate the subjective strength of a set of stimuli by squeezing a hand dynamometer, gently for weak stimuli and fiercely for strong ones. Analysing such data, the most inexperienced investigator would quickly realize that a 20 kg squeeze by an amateur wrestler (who can do 100 kg without even trying) should not be considered equivalent to the same response from a dainty female *S* (for whom 25 kg is a supreme effort). Instead, one should express each response from a given *S* as a proportion of the maximum response of which he is capable. Symbolically, if R_{ij} is the response produced by the *i*th subject to indicate the intensity of the *j*th stimulus, and if $R_{i(max)}$ is the largest response that *S* can emit, then the proper statistic to express his response to *this* stimulus, independently of individual differences in the range of possible variation of response amplitude, will be:

$$RC_{ij} = \frac{R_{ij}}{R_{i(max)}}$$

By substituting these *RC* values for the original raw scores, one can immediately eliminate a large component of error variance, i.e. that portion of the variance across *S*s in the raw scores, R_j, which is due to the variation in $R_{(max)}$.
(Note that an ANOVA would separate this component of raw score variance as 'variance due to individuals', assuming that we had repeated measures on each *S*. However, if we wanted to *correlate*, say, stimulus intensity with squeeze-rated subjective intensity we should use the range-corrected scores. Similarly, if we have only a single measure from each *S*, then one should be sure to obtain the $R_{(max)}$ also and compute *RC* even when using ANOVA.)

It may be less obvious—but it is equally true—that the same situation obtains with a great many of the dependent variables used by psychologists, including psychophysiologists. One *S*, for example, will nonchalantly emit SCRs of $5\mu\Omega^{-1}$ each time he clears his throat or someone speaks his name while another, with identical electrode arrangements, could not deliver more than a $3\mu\Omega^{-1}$ response falling out of an airplane. Therefore, obviously, an SCR of, say, $1\mu\Omega^{-1}$ produced in an experiment is most unlikely to have the same psychological meaning for both individuals. Thus, it behooves an experimenter using the GSR to deliver one strong, standard stimulus, preferably near the start of each experimental session, which will provide an estimate of $R_{(max)}$ that can be used to range-correct all subsequent GSRs recorded during that session. The maximum SCR of which an *S* is capable depends upon the density of sweat glands at the electrode site, the ambient temperature, the thickness and condition of the palmar epidermis, and other such factors which vary from person to person but normally have no relation whatever to the psychological processes one is using the GSR to measure; it is this irrelevant variance which the range-correction methods is designed to reduce or eliminate.

Some dependent variables show 'irrelevant' variation not only in $R_{(max)}$ but also in $R_{(min)}$ (the minimum possible GSR is of course zero for all *S*s). Rating scale data, for example, show that some *S*s frequently make use of the most extreme rating categories while others almost never do. If one is studying attitudes with an 11-point rating scale ranging from 'Utterly Disagree' (1) to 'Absolutely Agree' (11), a rating of '8' from an *S* who rates many other times '9', '10' or '11' cannot have the same meaning as an '8' from a more cautious *S* who never uses higher than a '9'. Such data can be range-corrected by expressing each raw score as a proportion of the range between that *S*'s $R_{(max)}$ and his $R_{(min)}$:

$$RC_{ij} = \frac{R_{ij}}{R_{(max)} - R_{(min)}}.$$

Tonic levels of heart rate and SCL are variables of this kind. In an experiment in which the *S* is severely stressed during one part of the session and allowed to relax to drowsiness during another part, one *S* may show an SCL while relaxed that is higher than another shows when he is most excited. Individual differences in range of heart rate variation are perhaps not quite so extreme but they are great enough so that range-correction of tonic heart rate scores will usually prove to reduce error variance also (Lykken, 1972). If the experiment already includes enough variation in demand characteristics so that each *S* will be caused to display SCL or HRL values near both his minimum and his maximum capability, then one can merely take the smallest and largest values produced as estimates of $R_{(min)}$ and $R_{(max)}$, respectively. In other experiments it may be necessary to modify the plan of the session so as to ensure that reasonable estimates will be available. I have found, for example, that one can conveniently elicit adequate estimates of $SCL_{(max)}$ by asking *S* to blow up a small balloon until it bursts. Since *S*s are generally more reactive when they are first hooked up to the apparatus, it is wise to plan to estimate $R_{(max)}$ near the start of any session. Similarly, the only time one can be reasonably sure that most *S*s will follow instructions to relax is at the end of the session when they can be assured that 'we're almost finished now, there'll be no more tasks or stimuli, so just relax for a few minutes and when I wake you up you can leave'.

1.3. INDIVIDUAL DIFFERENCES AND PSYCHOLOGICAL THEORY

Individual difference data are useful not only for methodological purposes—identifying 'basic' variables, improving experimental measures—but also more generally in the testing of scientific generalizations and hypotheses.

1.3.1. Function fluctuation

Every experimentalist should be alert to the possibility that his *S*s may differ not only in their parametric values for *x* and *y* but also even in the nature of the function relating x to y; i.e. some 'laws' may hold for only certain sub-groups of the population. Thus, Venables (1963) reported moderate positive correlations ($+0·45$ and $+0·61$) between palmar skin potential (SPL) and the two-flash fusion threshold in two samples of normal Ss together with strong *negative* correlations ($-0·79$ and $-0·72$) in two groups of non-paranoid schizophrenics. Clearly (assuming that these results are replicable facts of nature, although *cf.* Lykken & Maley, 1968) a similar study based on unselected psychiatric patients might have suggested that these putative measures of cortical and autonomic arousal were in fact unrelated altogether. More recently, Gruzelier & Venables (1972) have found that while some schizophrenics show greater than normal GSR reactivity to non-signal stimuli, coupled with poor habituation, others are grossly hypo-responsive, either habituating too fast or not responding at all. These two types of abnormal response are thought to be related to the psychiatric status or degree of decompensation of the patient. Again, a failure to be alert to the possibility of function fluctuation within the population studied might have prevented the discovery of this potentially important finding. Therefore, it is plain that one should always be careful to scrutinize the univariate and bivariate plots of the data, to determine whether there seem to be systematic differences between those Ss who fall on the positive and the negative diagonals, and the like—always keeping in mind, of course, that with this additional 'massaging' of the data goes the obligation to test in separate studies any serendipitous findings that may seem to emerge. The worst procedure, on the other hand, is to run the usual mechanical correlations and ANOVAs and then ignore the actual data altogether, under the delusion that one has squeezed it dry.

1.3.2. Correlation *vs* manipulation

As already mentioned, it is often possible to study the dependency of y on x in a correlational design, employing the natural variation in x across Ss as a substitute for manipulating x in the experiment. Where x is a fixed structural or constitutional trait variable, this approach may be the only one available. Since it is doubtful that many experimentalists are so moss-backed as to be unaware of this possibility, the emphasis here will be on the limitations and potential dangers of the correlational approach. As an example, imagine a study in which y is some biochemical measure, x is a self-report measure of, say, anxiety, and x and y are found to be correlated. The usual conclusion would be that plasma-formaldehyde (y) is either a cause or a manifestation of fear; this suggests, in turn, that longitudinal or repeated-measures study of individual Ss would show x and y varying nicely together. But one has only to articulate this corollary to see that it is not necessarily so. In fact, the only time when the R-type or between-subject correlation will properly estimate the P-type or within-subject covariation is when both parameters of the within-subject regression line are quite constant across individuals. Thus, for example, assuming that the range of y can vary considerably across Ss, it is possible for x and y to be perfectly correlated within each individual over time and yet for the usual between-subject correlation to be zero! Alternatively, a high R-type correlation can be associated with P-type correlations ranging about zero. It is probable that most psychological and psychophysiological variables show both 'trait' (between-S) and 'state' variation; the two trait components may be correlated and the state components not, or the state components may co-vary and not the trait components, or both of these, or neither. Therefore it follows that a complete study of the relationship of x and y will require *both* an R-type correlational design and either a P-type longitudinal study or else an experimental manipulation of either x or y (followed, of course, by a repetition of both, preferably in another laboratory, on the principle that the probability that a psychological finding will replicate seems to be inversely related to the intrinsic interest of that finding.)

Those of us who, like myself, are delighted to contemplate the extraordinary and manifold differences between people would be well advised to cultivate the acquaintance of our dour colleagues for whom these differences are just a nuisance and a source of irritation, for the experimentalist is like the trout fisherman who keeps catching tasty bass and bream and throwing them away. Although he knows a great deal about his favourite variables and has ingenious and precise (and borrowable) methods for measuring and controlling them, it seldom occurs to him to wonder why it is that some Ss consistently score so differently from others, i.e. in what other ways these extremes might differ from each other (indeed, he commonly discards the deviates and forgets about them!). Needless to say, he would be most unlikely to speculate on how his variables might be related to stress or fatigue or extraversion or schizophrenia. Since he doesn't care for bass or individual differences there seems to be nothing immoral about using his methods or his discards for one's own (to him incomprehensible) purposes.

A recent and elegant example of successful poaching of this sort can be found in Sutton (1971) who made a foray into the very heartland of experimental psychology to seize upon the venerable Bunsen–Roscoe Law which states that, below some critical duration, the effect of a stimulus depends upon its total energy without regard to how that energy may be distributed in time; e.g., a 4 msec. light pulse of intensity 5 will be equivalent to a 2-msec pulse of intensity 10. Sutton quite properly realized that the length of this critical duration, within which this time-intensity reciprocity holds, must like any other biological parameter show variation from one individual to another, the only question being whether the degree of such variation is sufficient to be of any interest. Specifically, he proposed that schizophrenics might have shorter critical durations than do non-schizophrenics and this hypothesis, which seems now to have been correct, led to the development of an ingenious test, perhaps the only test yet found on which the schizophrenic can be shown to perform 'better' than the normal. Briefly, the test requires S to attempt to discriminate between two light flashes, one consisting of a single pulse of 4 msec and the other a 'package' of two 2-msec pulses separated by 2 msec. Discrimination is measured through reaction time (RT) which, since RT decreases with increased stimulus intensity, allows one to determine whether the '2 + 2' package is being fully integrated so that it is equivalent to the single 4-msec pulse. If the normal critical duration allows full integration while the shorter duration for schizophrenics does not, then the schizophrenics will be able to respond consistently differently to the two stimuli while the normals will be unable to do so. In fact (Collins, 1971), all 10 schizophrenics performed 'better' on this test than any of the normals or non-schizophrenic patients used as controls, seven of the 10 scoring more than 3 SD's above the normal mean.

1.3.3. A concluding caveat

We have attempted to show that individual differences are by no means just a nuisance, that they constitute a considerable part of the very *raison d'être* of psychological science, and to illustrate a few of the ways in which the methods of the differential psychologist can be of value to the experimentalist. But it must be admitted, I think, that research employing correlations and the study of group differences (where the groups are segregated by their scores on some other variable and are not differently treated) seems to be more chancy and less reliable than that based on the traditional methods of experimental manipulation. I have not attempted an actual survey of the relevant literature but it seems a safe bet that, if one took a random sample of 100 recent articles from Journal of Experimental Psychology or Journal of Comparative and Physiological Psychology and another 100 purporting to show that variables X and Y are correlated or that Groups A and B have different mean values of Z, and then replicated each study (preferably by means of *constructive replication*, cf. Lykken, 1968), one would find strong evidence that traditional experimental methods lead to more dependable conclusions about the state of Nature. Indeed, one way of distinguishing the experienced researcher from the neophyte (apart from counting gray hairs) is to show them a recent paper reporting high correlations between cortical evoked response latency and IQ or that schizophrenics have less blood-turpentine than normals, and then observe how excited they get. Experience in this field leads (or should lead) to an attitude of open-minded scepticism and one learns not to invest heavily in even the most provocative finding until one has seen it in one's own laboratory (or seen it twice, if the finding is one's own). In respect to one's own research strategy, an approach which recommends itself is the two stage process that begins with a 'pilot' study. It is important to remember that the only intended consumer of the results of this first stage is the researcher himself. The only purpose of the pilot study is to inform and to convince one's self and most of the cumbersome controls and precautions which have become rituals in the field can be set aside except for those which seem essential to uncover the truth of the matter. Then, if the pilot study shows something interesting, one can design the formal study, observing all the rituals, for the purpose of demonstrating to one's colleagues what one has already learned in Stage I. The benefits of this manner of proceeding include (i) that, having invested less time and effort in the rough-and-dirty Stage I, one is better able to accept a negative finding in the pilot study for what it is rather than to twist and torture those data until they emit a publishable squeak; and (ii) the elegant confirming findings of Stage II are more likely to be true since they are already a kind of replication of the previous result.

1.4. REFERENCES

Block, J. *The challenge of response sets*. New York: Appleton-Century-Crofts, 1965.

Collins, P. Reaction time measures in time intensity reciprocity between psychiatric patients and normals. Paper presented at meetings of the Eastern Psychological Association, 1971, New York.

Gruzelier, J. H. & Venables, P. H. Skin conductance orienting activity in a heterogeneous sample of schizophrenics. *Journal of Nervous and Mental Disease*, 1972, **155**, 277–287.

Jenkins, J. J. & Lykken, D. T. Individual differences. In P. Farnsworth & Q. McNemar (Eds), *Annual review of psychology*, Vol. 8. Palo Alto, Calif.: Annual Reviews, Inc., 1957.

Lacey, J. I. Somatic response patterning and stress: Some revisions of activation theory. In M. H. Appley & R. Trumbull (Eds), *Psychological stress: Issues in Research*. New York: Appleton, 1967.

Lykken, D. T. Statistical significance in psychological research. *Psychological Bulletin*, 1968, **70**, 151–159.

Lykken, D. T. Range correction applied to heart rate and to GSR data. *Psychophysiology*, 1972, **9**, 373–379.

Lykken, D. T. & Maley, M. Autonomic versus cortical arousal in schizophrenics and non-psychotics. *Journal of Psychiatric Research*, 1968, **6**, 21–32.

Lykken, D. T., Rose, R., Luther, B. & Maley, M. Correcting psychophysiological measures for individual differences in range. *Psychological Bulletin*, 1966, **66**, 481–484.

Nebylitsyn, V. D. & Gray, J. A. (Eds) *Biological bases of individual behaviour*. New York: Academic, 1972.

Sutton, S. Fact and artifact in the psychology of schizophrenia. In M. Hammer, K. Salzinger & S. Sutton (Eds), *Psychopathology: Contributions from the biological, behavioral, and social sciences*. New York: John Wiley, 1971.

Venables, P. H. The relationship between level of skin potential and fusion of paired light flashes in schizophrenic and normal subjects. *Journal of Psychiatric Research*, 1963, **1**, 279–291.

Chapter 2

Some Experimental Implications of Change

ROY B. MEFFERD, Jr.

Psychiatric and Psychosomatic Research Laboratory
Veterans Administration Hospital
Houston, Texas
and
Baylor College of Medicine
Houston, Texas
and
University of Houston
Houston, Texas

2.1. INTRODUCTION

A major source of unwanted variance arises from the somewhat mysterious periodic changes that occur in all biological systems. The unwary researcher who fails to sample in synchrony with these oscillations has programmed himself to obtain noisy and confusing results. One purpose of this chapter is to show just how important it is to plan and conduct experiments with an eye held squarely on the biological clock.

Another purpose here is to explore systematic change itself—its complexity and irregularity, its possible source, its interactions with other changes. This is the province of the longitudinal experiment, and of the analysis of curves, trends and cycles. We shall make a case that control of superfluous variance is merely a first objective of research—that the investigator can increase the power of his experiment by knowledgeable selection of the sampling period. It is not merely a matter of noise—inappropriate sampling can generate strange new data completely unrelated to the real situation. The cross-sectional experiment is peculiarly sensitive to these pervasive, continuous changes among the Ss. If, for example, testing of the S is done one after the other throughout the day, the effects of the ever-present circadian rhythms are defied. If the testing is done only in the fore-noon, it usually must be spread over weeks or months. In this case the rhythms are again defied, since biological time changes constantly from day-to-day relative to any clock hour except perhaps noon and midnight. If the waves of the circadian rhythms are ignored, as, for example, is done in throughout-the-day testing, the exaggerated differences between the Ss tested at the crest and at the nadir of the daily wave may obscure the quest. Not only does this increase the unwanted variance, but the effect of this error on apparent responsiveness due to the operation of the Law of Initial Values is far from negligible. If the testing is spread across seasons, surprising differences may be observed between Ss tested in the summer and those tested in the winter.

Skilful control of variance entails knowledge of the underlying 'naturally' occurring changes in the floating platform on which the S stands. Unfortunately, there is no adequate model for the analysis of longitudinal data. We are stuck with trying to bend existing models to fit the requirement. In this chapter we can provide no model, but we shall summarize some of our explorations using existing models. We add our plea to Cattell's (1966a) that mathematical statisticians interest themselves in such a model!

2.1.1. The 'average man' philosophy

The innate instability of biological systems led to the development of influential concepts to account for some of the more evident variability—homeostatic balance, autonomic balance, adaptation, acclimatization, conditioning. Unusual departures from the hypothesized 'balance' also were conceptualized—activation, orientation, alarm, stress.

The large observed intra-individual variability of uncertain origin also led to the concept of the 'normal range' which made the practice of modern medicine possible. So long as each of a person's multitude of variables, processes or functions remains within the 'normal range', he can be assumed in most cases to be in satisfactory health. The situation where an apparently healthy person has values outside the normal range is of little concern so long as he is un-complaining. For the busy practitioner this use of a statistical property—the range about a mean—made his life more productive and pleasant. For the busy researcher, faced with the same dilemma of extreme differences between individuals at any given time, statistics also provided a practical way to proceed—*most* Ss will cluster around a central value for any given variable.

Accordingly, the researcher can zero-in on this mean position, and simply ignore the relatively scarce outriders far removed from the mean. He gains increasing security in his conclusions about his synthesized 'average man' merely by adding more and more 'for example'. In the process, of course, he also discovers more and more outriders (exceptions). However, he usually does not perceive this peculiarity, since the thrust of experimental designers has been to 'average out' these exceptions in order to focus on the important generalizable truths.

In the real world, individual variability was explained with the concept of individual differences. Long-continued use, however, tends to restrict the range of this concept—there is a strong tendency to relegate an individual to a fixed position on the continuum of a dimension of individual differences which then is viewed to be as constant as his fingerprints. Even casual observation refutes this state-of-mind. Improved measurement technology makes it apparent that variation cannot be explained away as merely resulting from poor technique and random errors (Mefferd & Pokorny, 1967). Fortunately, the concept is again broadening to account for *real* movement of an individual about his mean position—the momentary state level that is constantly varying about a stable trait (individual mean) level (e.g., Cattell, 1966a).

The 'average man' is now known to change with the seasons (Wenger, 1943; Brody, 1945; Mefferd, LaBrosse, Gawienowski, & Williams, 1958; Mefferd, 1959; Hale, Ellis, & Van Fossan, 1960; Holtzman, 1963). While these mean changes are not negligible *per se*, just suppose that one group of the Ss are peculiarly sensitive to the ambient temperature, another to the humidity, another to the geomagnetic activity. The means might reflect only a small influence of any environment, and these effects probably would be averaged out across environmental variables. Yet different individuals might be grossly influenced by a particular variable. What difference does it make to a man to know that vitamin X is not 'significantly' related to condition Z, if vitamin X does in fact reverse his own brand of condition Z?

The relatively scarce individual data show that the changes across weeks and months within a S are very large (for discussions of this see Mefferd & Pokorny, 1967; Wieland & Mefferd, 1969, 1970). Differences of 2- to 10-fold are not uncommon between summer and winter, even in an air-conditioned society. Such systematic variation is not limited to biochemical and physiological processes—perceptual processes that are directly dependent on chemical systems, such as taste, also vary systematically (e.g., Mefferd & Wieland, 1968). In fact similar systematic variation occurs with most variables—parameters of the autokinetic effect (Wieland & Mefferd, 1966), performance on word association tests (Mefferd & Wieland, 1965), perspective reversal rates with various ambiguous figures, performance on paper-and-pencil tests, and more than 500 other variables studied in this laboratory (unpublished; and see Fiske & Rice, 1955).

We shall now depart from the 'average man' and will peer intently at the individual. The vehicle primarily used for this discussion will be a longitudinal study of three young male volunteers who were pursuing active careers. A large battery of measurements was made on each of these for 120 consecutive days (see Mefferd & Wieland, 1965; Wieland & Mefferd, 1970, for a more detailed description of the physiological aspects of the experiment). The daily 2-hour testing sessions were held at the same time throughout—1000–1200, 1100–1300, 1200–1400 hrs, respectively for the three Ss. Testing was done around the noon hour in an effort to obtain as constant an anchor point in biological time as possible (*viz.*, for all practical purposes noon splits the daylight hours equally in any season).

2.2. DAY-TO-DAY CHANGE

2.2.1. What is the nature of day-to-day change in biological systems?

The apparent stability of biological systems is deceiving. Constancy of almost all systems is only a mean position between the extreme of a constantly varying position. Even when measurements are made at the same biological time each day, the day-to-day variations in most of these measures are surprisingly large. Much of the variation is saw-toothed in nature with a high value on one occasion being followed by a low value on the next one or two occasions. This alteration is far too systematic to be due to mere measurement error. Superimposed on this daily variation are long-term trends and oscillations that not only are different for different variables, but also are not the same from one individual to another within the same time-frame.

In some cases the oscillations are regular, with the uniform rates of change characteristic of positive equalized-bucking control systems. In other cases the oscillation results from a single control where a rise (or a fall) is due to the action of a positive control, but the recovery occurs passively as the degree of control is lessened. Or, the rate of change may be variable—systematic or erratic. The oscillations may be perceptible only by means of sophisticated procedures, as with the dynamic equilibria of enzyme systems, or they may be as obvious as the wakeful-sleep cycle. The oscillations may have a high frequency, measured in cycles per second, or they may have an extremely low frequency measured in months or years. The amplitude of the oscillations may be large or small, regular or erratic. The oscillations may be simple, reflecting the operation of a single control system, or they may result from complex mixtures of several systems, often of different frequencies requiring Fourier analyses to unravel.

2.2.2. Randomness

Some investigation into the degree of randomness of the 'noise' in longitudinal data is warranted before it is arbitrarily eliminated as random error. It may be noise only by definition, e.g. because it is only of 'minor' importance or magnitude. Actually the amount of variance involved may be relatively quite large. Furthermore, a jagged, random-appearing curve may result from the interaction of two or more out-of-phase smooth oscillations sampled discretely. The components of such variance may be separated with analysis of variance techniques, although this requires considerable data manipulation. The correlogram (see 2.2.4.4) is also quite useful for this purpose. To illustrate, a correlogram of the daily suicides in Texas for a 3-year period had no discernible pattern even with lags up to 40 days, and there was not a single significant correlation coefficient at any lag (Pokorny & Mefferd, 1966). This is the result to be expected with a set of random numbers.

Typically in longitudinal experiments, several measurements are made of a given variable on each occasion—often before, during, and after a stimulation of some sort. These individual measurements provide another means to estimate the degree of randomness of erratic-appearing longitudinal data. The occasion-to-occasion variation of a single of these measurements is compared with that of the mean of all such measures made on one occasion. To illustrate, a single blood pressure measurement made on successive days before some stimulus is applied, inevitably yields a jagged and erratic appearing curve across time. So will another measurement made during or after the stimulation. If this occasion-to-occasion variation is due to random error, it should 'average out' when all the individual daily measures are averaged, and the jagged nature of the curve should decrease greatly in the graph of these means relative to that of the individual blood pressure measurements. Actually, in such an example, the amplitudes of the saw-teeth decreased, but the jagged nature of the curve remained (Wieland & Mefferd, 1970).

Often, repeated measurements of the same variable are averaged for each occasion to create a more accurate occasion-measure. This procedure often inflates the correlations of such occasion-means with those of other averaged-variables where both have longitudinal trends or cycles. This inflation due to the long range concomitant changes may be serious enough to lead the unwary to make incorrect conclusions (Pokorny & Mefferd, 1966). A factor analytic technique for managing the within-occasion variance will be discussed below.

2.2.3. Experimenter-generated noise

Many factors conspire to impart to longitudinal experiments their own experiment-generated curves: novelty at the outset; increasing boredom with the repetition in the later stages and anticipatory exhilaration at the finish; establishment of unintentional conditioned and related responses to aspects of the testing situation; unintentional changes in the attitude of the experimenter and in the situation; and uncontrolled events in the life and environment of the S (Wieland & Mefferd, 1970). If most of the intra-individual variability between occasions were of a random nature, it could be handled by the use of adequate sampling procedures, the imposition of experimental controls, and the use of suitable statistical techniques. However, if much of the variability actually is systematic, experimental control becomes imperative. This consideration is almost as important with cross-sectional as longitudinal designs. The pervasive influence of situational or environmental processes that introduce systematic intra-individual variation in some or all of the Ss is of particular concern in experiments designed to investigate individual differences or in those in which the same S is measured on more than one occasion (e.g., in pre-post designs).

Here we shall explore the consequences of the complicated multitude of interactions in longitudinal data on the interpretation of psychophysiological research. Failure to allow for this real-world situation in an experiment can lead to un-interpretable results caused by the confounding of effects or by the incorporation of large blocks of noisy, unintentional variance. Worse, it can lead to erroneous conclusions. Two functionally unrelated oscillating variables may be correlated statistically solely as a result of the *fact* of their simultaneous change—its direction, rate, magnitude, uniformity—rather than as a result of a common cause. Any variance that is shared by two variables regardless of the reasons for its commonality contributes to the computed correlation. For example, several of man's afflictions that are changing in incidence or severity or diagnosis can be shown to be correlated with the increased incidence of the use of electric refrigerators, or of automobiles, or of miles travelled in space. Even supposedly random numbers will correlate under certain circumstances (e.g., when they are grouped, Pokorny & Mefferd, 1966). The investigator can generate a new man-made oscillation merely by out-of-phase 24-h repeated sampling of a 25-h circadian cycle, or by any other out-of-phase sampling, and this new curve may correlate spuriously with an otherwise unrelated variable. Manipulations of the data also may result in the generation of entirely new curves. For example, in 'smoothing' a curve, the selection of a base for computation of either moving or stationary means that does not correspond with the actual cycling period of the variable may yield curves that are significantly different from the original curve (the Slutsky-Yule effect, see Holtzman, 1963; Wieland & Mefferd, 1969). Averaging across group longitudinal data may impose on it an artificial regularity which may obscure extreme intra-individual variability so completely that the group means actually may *falsely* appear to support a steady-state threshold-dependent satiation hypothesis (Sadler & Mefferd, 1970, 1971). Any blind averaging procedure runs the grave risk of reducing or eliminating the variance that is of greatest interest to the investigator—of throwing the baby out with the wash-water.

2.2.4. Longitudinal analytical methodology

Analytical techniques are as poorly developed for individual response data as they are well developed for that of the 'average man'. The longitudinal investigator is quickly inundated in waves, cycles, curves, and trends. If he is to unravel the real-world, and determine what influences what, he must concern himself with geometric methodology. Unfortunately, as mentioned in the introduction, there is at present no model adequate for the task. Frequencies of complex curves may be examined by means of Fourier or spectral analyses. However, such possibilities are restricted since there seldom are sufficient data points available, many variables exhibit strong linear trends, and, anyway, frequencies are only one parameter of an oscillating curve. The curves may be analysed into geometric components, but usually the curves are so variable in all aspects as to render such an analysis meaningless. Polar plots—the period clock—excellent for use with single, or a few variables, are inadequate for associational analyses. Correlational techniques have been the primary tool used to date, yet all such procedures entail serious problems, some of which we will discuss below. Even so, we are pretty well stuck with correlational techniques until a more adequate analytical model is developed.

2.2.4.1. General analytical strategy

It is well to digress momentarily to remember that in a typical group comparison study, every S is riding along his own pattern of curves at the moment that his photograph is snapped. If the next S is photographed at a different time, the common temporal denominator is lost, and the variance is inexorably increased. The curve problem exists just as surely in cross-sectional as longitudinal data—we just ignore it!

One can proceed along two lines of analytical strategy with longitudinal experiments: (i) study the periodic and trending curves *qua* curves without regard to associational patterns, and (ii) study the associational patterns within the maze of curves without special regard to the individual natures of the curves. The first approach involves questions such as short- and long-term periodicities and/or trends; variabilities, uniformities, and reliabilities; dependencies within and between variables and their influence on the available degrees of freedom; and the like. The second approach involves a search for co-variation—patterns, clusters, factors, discriminators, predictors, validities.

2.2.4.2. Correlograms

Serial correlations—*auto* (the product moment correlation coefficients of a sequential array of values versus the same array lagged one or more periods) and *cross* (the correlations between pairs of differently lagged variables)—provide a major tool for the analysis of various dependencies (Kendall, 1948; Holtzman, 1963; Sollberger, 1965; Wieland & Mefferd, 1969). The techniques have also been used widely in the analysis of seismographic and earthquake data (e.g., involutional analysis), but there the geophysicists' concern is with the responses of a fixed, static system to a momentary disturbance rather than so much with dynamic interactions.

An autocorrelation with a lag of one is obtained by first pairing the initial value of a variable with its value on the second occasion, the second occasion with the third and so on through the entire series. The correlation with a lag of two is obtained in the same manner by pairing successively the value from occasion one with that of occasion three and so on. A single auto-correlation coefficient has some of the characteristics of regular non-serial coefficients. However, a given autocorrelation, within a series of such coefficients determined for increasing lags, takes on special meaning. By plotting these coefficients for successively lagged periods, a correlogram is obtained which shows the degree of dependency throughout the series, but which also reflects the time-pattern of the period-to-period changes. It is this time pattern that is exceedingly useful for developing an understanding of the internal structure of a time-series. The cycles and trends in the data are reflected directly in the correlogram. The autocorrelations of an error-free sine wave at successive lags (i.e., the correlogram) forms a cosine-wave relative to the sine wave. As error variance distorts the sine wave, the magnitude of the coefficients in the correlogram will be depressed, but the pattern remains.

The coefficients of systematically varying events have special properties, since they designate position as well as degree of correlation. When a sine wave is lagged by half its period, the correlation coefficient becomes zero, while it is $1\cdot0$ at no lag and $-1\cdot0$ at the lag of a complete period. In contrast to usual correlation coefficients, the zero coefficient does not suggest un-predictability of occasion y from occasion x. Actually, the correlation at any point within the correlogram has as much meaning in this respect as do coefficients of $1\cdot0$ and $-1\cdot0$ that happen to occur at the inflection points or at arcophase. Thus, the *pattern* of the correlogram is more meaningful than the statistical significance of individual coefficients within it.

Casual observation of a curve formed by longitudinal data does not reveal the true structure of the curve. Many such curves for a single variable are complex resolutions of several schedules—daily, weekly, monthly, seasonal—the schedule often may be resolved by means of the correlogram. A complex curve yields a distinctive set of inflection points in its correlogram for each of its component simple curves. The periods of the succeeding inflection points on the correlogram reflect directly the periods of the oscillations in the original data—inflection points at 7-day, and 10-day lags reflect cycles having these periods. For the investigator who feels compelled to 'smooth' his curve, the base for his averging may be determined directly from this correlogram. Even if he chooses a 7-day base in this example, however, he will generate strange new non-data in his moving average, since his averaging base is out-of-phase with the 10-day cycle also present. No single base is suitable for smoothing most complex curves.

The correlogram is useful with what is perhaps, the key issue with longi-tudinal data—steady increases or decreases in a variable across many occasions. Such trends are usually complicated by being imposed upon one or more cycles. Trends are the source of such large pools of variance that correlational procedures well may reflect only the trend *per se*. Further, trends grossly alter the predictability of one occasion from another and the degrees of freedom available for hypothesis testing may be reduced to a distressing degree. Since a correlogram reflects the nature and extent of a trend directly, it is a useful analytical tool for evaluating the degree of dependency in longitudinal data (Wieland & Mefferd, 1970). If the correlogram oscillates systematically or erratically around a zero correlation, there is no significant linear trend in the data (see Pokorny & Mefferd, 1966).

2.2.4.3. P-technique of factor analysis

A favourite tool for exploring the patterns of inter-relationships within longitudinal data has been the P-technique of factor analysis (Cattell, 1957, 1963, 1966a). We have explored this technique at some length over the years (e.g., Mefferd, Moran, & Kimble, 1958). Recently, we have used it for another purpose—as a powerful tool for averaging and smoothing of data. Two examples, both taken from the longitudinal study under discussion, will be presented to illustrate this application. The first example, using taste judgments as the vehicle (Mefferd & Wieland, 1968), explored the relationships between general structural factors such as those attributable to individual or occasion differences, or to changes in a variable within a given occasion. The second example explores primarily the management of trend variance between occasions. This topic is germane to this discussion, since a great deal of the trend variance in physiological variables is related to seasonal changes.

Five series of taste judgments using the ascending method of limits with no standard were made at the same time each day by each of the three Ss in the experiment under discussion. The subliminal starting point of each series was varied daily and occasional duplicates were inserted. Ten judgments, five 'uncertain' ('I believe I taste salt, but I cannot be certain'), and five 'certain', were obtained each day. Such judgments ordinarily would be averaged to obtain an *occasion* or *subject* mean value for comparison with other variables. However, this is wasteful of the total information available (e.g. of that due to the within-session range of judgments). Much of this information can be preserved in useful form by partialing it into orthogonal linear components of variance by principal axis factoring (Harman, 1960). While the common variance is extracted non-linearly but symmetrically, the error variance is extracted linearly. Therefore, the early components of variance are relatively error-free (Mefferd, 1968), much of the error remaining in the residual matrix. Orthogonal factor scores (i.e. which are computed using the factor loadings of *all* variables and the inverse of the correlation matrix [Overall, 1962]), summarize each of the resulting components. This information so segregated and preserved by factoring all the data points for an occasion may provide significant correlations with other variables that would not have been observed with the mean alone.

Correlograms derived from the individual raw taste judgments for each of the three individuals were very similar. This indicates that interpretation of the factors that emerged in the analysis need not involve the possible effects of confounded curves within the taste judgments *per se*.

The factor scores for the first principal axis component correlated perfectly within rounding error with the daily means of all ten judgments. Thus, this factor contained *all* the variance attributable to systematic trends in the judgments, and the factor scores of the other factors correlated zero with these factor scores. However, when the principal axis factors were rotated, the daily mean now correlated significantly with the factor scores of *all* the varimax factors, though the major variation (and, therefore, correlation) was still that due to occasion-to-occasion variation (in this case, this was the first varimax factor). However, rotation accomplished one objective— a management of trend variance. When a variable has a strong trend, the day-to-day values are not independent, and as a result there may be far fewer degrees of freedom available for hypothesis testing than the investigator may realize. Factoring and the subsequent redistribution of the occasion-to-occasion variance attributable to each of the factors, reduced the dependency materially (e.g., the autocorrelations for the factor scores of the first principal axis factor—and thus also for the daily *mean* judgments—were significantly different from zero [$P < 0.05$, t tests] for all coefficients up to lags of 20, 40, and 10 days, for the three Ss, respectively, while the significant coefficients dropped to lags of 9, 30, and 1 days for the varimax factor scores of the rotated factor that correlated most highly with the daily means [in this case, varimax factor 1]; the correlations of this factor's scores with the mean were only 0·59, 0·72, and 0·46, for the three Ss, respectively, after rotation, as compared to 0·99 for all three before rotation) (Mefferd & Wieland, 1968).

Since all the variance due to the variations in the daily mean was partialled from the residual matrix by the first principal axis factor, subsequent factors involved additional stable effects or dimensions in terms of deviations from the daily means. The second factor was shown to be due to a within-day trend among the five pairs of judgments; the third, to independent changes in the anchor point of the uncertain and certain judgments; and the fourth, to non-trending alternating shifts in anchor points from judgment-to-judgment. Upon rotation, that part of the overall trend variance (i.e., of the occasion mean) that was attributable to each of these effects was distributed to the appropriate factor or dimension.

The quite satisfactory reliabilities of each of these taste effects evidenced by the factors made the sets of orthogonal factor scores derived for each component of variance suitable for use as 'new' variables in further analyses. Where it is desirable to examine trend *per se*, or certain effects independent of trend, the factor scores derived from the principal axis components would be the choice. Where the actual changes are believed to be important (e.g., as where it is hypothesized that increasing daily temperatures in summer are accompanied by increasing sweating rates), the varimax factor scores would be the choice.

For the second example, the factor analysis was of 13 partially automated standard clinical measurements of systolic blood pressure made daily on each of the three Ss in the experiment. These were made as follows: three during an initial resting baseline period, one before and another after a word association test, one before a cold pressor test, and another after a second word association given during the latter part of the cold pressor test, and five during a final recovery period.

As is usually the case with longitudinal data, the day-to-day variability in systolic blood pressure was quite large for all three Ss (Figure 2.1). Although

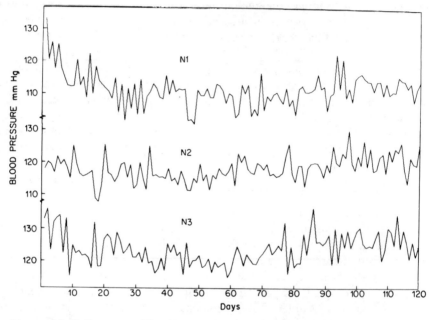

FIGURE 2.1. Daily means ($N = 13$) of systolic blood pressures of three subjects measured for 120 consecutive days

some of the total variability obviously is due to sharp day-to-day changes, systematic changes also are evident in the form of cycles of varying periodicities as well as of long-term trends. It is these systematic changes that introduce the statistical problems discussed above. In spite of these trends and cycles, however, the distributions of the mean daily blood pressures were essentially normal (Figure 2.2). This was also true with individual measurements (Figure 2.3), and with most of the 500 + other variables measured. The total variance of the 120 series of 13 daily measurements was partialled separately for each S into 13 orthogonal linear components. The *skree* test (Cattell, 1966b) (we [Mefferd & Wieland] reported this independently as the *tallus* test at the Washington meeting of the Society for Psychophysiological Research, 1966); was used to select the components to be analysed—in this case, four factors for each S. These four components were rotated by the varimax procedure and the results are presented in Table 2.1. Approximately half the total variance

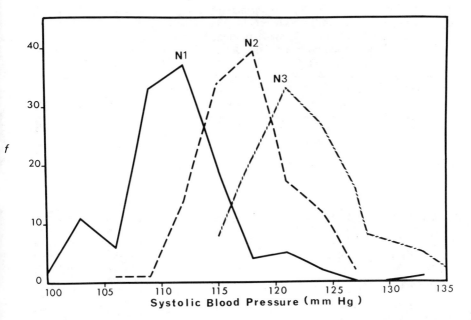

FIGURE 2.2. Distribution of daily means of systolic blood pressures for the three subjects shown in Figure 2.1

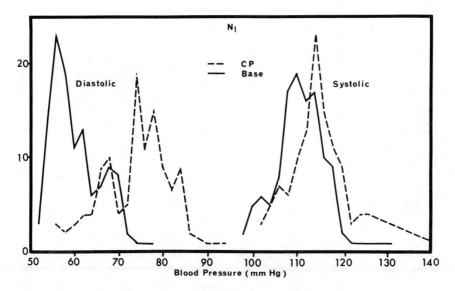

FIGURE 2.3. Distributions of blood pressures made on the first subject, N1, during a quiet baseline period, and during a cold pressor test

TABLE 2.1. Principal axis (PAX) and varimax (VAX) factor loadings on the first four components of variance of three subjects for 13 systolic blood pressures made daily for 120[a] consecutive days (leading decimals omitted; percentages of the variance accounted for by each component are shown at bottom of the Table)

Variable No.	Subject	Components							
		PAX				VAX			
		1	2	3	4	1	2	3	4
	N1	78	−37	10	−24	73	24	47	05
1	N2	65	09	19	43	16	25	58	48
	N3	69	−32	−17	−18	73	17	16	23
	N1	78	−35	16	10	60	09	55	31
2	N2	67	05	36	09	24	37	62	12
	N3	68	−25	16	54	21	12	47	75
	N1	69	−09	63	05	20	29	84	22
3	N2	54	23	47	08	19	16	72	03
	N3	75	−22	−16	−10	67	27	22	28
	N1	84	−05	07	02	52	36	40	38
4	N2	59	57	15	−19	64	08	55	−06
	N3	68	−30	−36	33	50	29	02	68
	N1	80	−09	−14	23	56	19	23	57
5	N2	72	28	−08	−20	70	21	32	08
	N3	71	−27	06	−20	66	11	37	17
	N1	78	−22	−26	05	73	17	14	40
6	N2	76	24	−25	−16	76	24	20	20
	N3	75	−17	−07	−23	69	26	29	14
	N1	84	−20	−11	−01	70	26	28	35
7	N2	74	25	−17	−09	69	21	28	21
	N3	73	−01	45	07	30	16	76	23
	N1	80	−03	−25	−22	70	46	08	24
8	N2	71	−12	−39	−15	63	48	−06	25
	N3	77	−02	11	−23	58	31	48	06
	N1	78	06	−20	−19	60	50	09	27
9	N2	51	05	−42	66	23	11	08	89
	N3	73	09	27	00	33	31	62	17
	N1	74	38	09	−30	29	19	23	20
10	N2	66	−31	−26	−18	46	62	−06	15
	N3	79	31	11	06	26	58	55	18
	N1	76	45	13	−12	20	75	26	37
11	N2	63	−52	13	−07	13	80	17	07
	N3	73	34	11	−06	27	56	52	04
	N1	81	31	−10	24	32	48	15	69
12	N2	63	−44	28	−08	10	75	31	−01
	N3	63	53	−29	13	12	84	16	16

TABLE 2.1. (*Contd.*)

Variable No.	Subject	Components							
		PAX				VAX			
		1	2	3	4	1	2	3	4
13	N1	81	21	01	36	30	35	28	73
	N2	76	−33	08	06	26	70	30	24
	N3	73	31	−28	−05	39	71	18	14
Variance	N1	61·9	6·6	5·2	3·9	23·3	22·8	10·7	20·8
%	N2	44·1	9·8	7·7	6·3	21·8	20·7	15·3	9·8
	N3	52·1	7·7	5·4	4·8	23·3	18·1	18·0	10·5

[a] The variables are the 13 individual systolic blood pressure measurements in the order in which they were made on each of 120 consecutive days.

was extracted by the first principal axis factor for each S. The factor scores from this factor correlated $r = 0.99$ with each S's daily mean of the 13 blood pressures. The factor scores of the other unrotated factors, correlating zero with the daily mean, are equivalent to deviation scores. Therefore, the trend and other systematic day-to-day variance could be removed simply by eliminating the first unrotated factor. This would accomplish what has been suggested by many (*viz.*, to partial-out trend, e.g., Anderson, 1958; Holtzman, 1962, 1963). However, this would also eliminate about half of the total variance! We do not agree that this is the way to manage biological trend (Mefferd, 1966). We feel that a better strategy is that discussed below.

Upon rotation, all but about 20 per cent of the variance due to mean day-to-day differences that was consolidated in the first unrotated factor was distributed to the other three factors. This re-distribution of variance was expected to reduce materially the autocorrelations of the primary factor, while introducing too little mean-difference variance onto the special-effects deviation-score factors to cause a serious dependency problem in these. The correlograms of the unrotated and rotated factor scores for lags up to 40 days for the first S are present in Figure 2.4 (the other two Ss had very similar results). Considering first the correlograms of the sets of unrotated factor scores, 17 of the 40 autocorrelations of the first unrotated factor were significantly different from zero. This represents a significant trend and, therefore, a material reduction in available degrees of freedom. The factor scores for the second factor had only one and those of the third and fourth factors, no significant autocorrelations.

After rotation the correlograms for the varimax factor scores of the first factor had only four significant autocorrelations as compared with 17 of the first unrotated factor. The second, third, and fourth rotated factors now had seven, five, and one significant autocorrelations, respectively, and these were smaller and more scattered than was the case with the first unrotated factor. Thus, rotation distributed the strong trend seen in the first factor approximately equally to all components, thereby reducing materially the sequential depen-

30

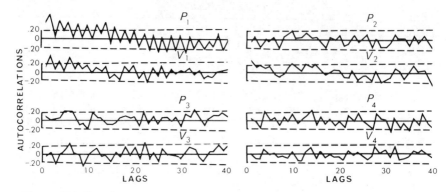

FIGURE 2.4. Correlograms (autocorrelations at various lags from 1–40 days) of systolic blood pressures for the orthogonal (principal axis [P] and varimax [V]) factor scores of the first four components of variance for the first subject (Nl); dashed lines indicate the $P = 0.05$ significance level of the autocorrelations (t tests)

dency seen in the primary factor. In the present case none of the four sets of rotated factor scores exhibited enough sequential dependency to cause worry about a reduction in degrees of freedom.

The correlograms of the first two factors of the other two Ss are shown in Figure 2.5 to illustrate that this spreading upon rotation of the variance due to dependency is a general effect. The other two components for these Ss also yielded correlograms comparable to those of the first S. Each had 15 significant autocorrelations in the unrotated factor scores of the first factor. Rotation of the second S's factor scores reduced these to 12, and these 12 were smaller than before rotation. After rotation, the third S had only two significant autocorrelations in the first factor.

One way of quantitating the re-distribution of variance accomplished by

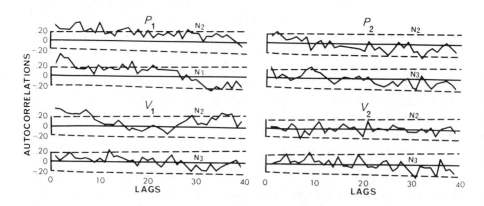

FIGURE 2.5. Correlograms for the second (N2) and the third (N3) subjects for the first two components of variance

rotation is to correlate the unrotated and rotated factor scores. Table 2.2 shows that the patterns of these correlations were very similar for the three Ss. After rotation all the sets of varimax factor scores correlated at moderate levels with those of the first unrotated factor. This indicates that significant amounts of the variance in that unrotated factor were re-distributed to all four rotated factors, yet in this case the pool of variance consolidated originally in each unrotated factor retained its identity upon rotation (see the correlations in the diagonal of the Table).

TABLE 2.2. Correlations of the factor scores of the first four principal axis (PAX) components and the resulting varimax (VAX) components for systolic blood pressures of three subjects (the largest correlations for a row are in italics)

PAX components	Subject	VAX components			
		1	2	3	4
1	N1	*63*	57	44	27
	N2	*62*	57	45	30
	N3	*61*	50	51	33
2	N1	48	*71*	08	52
	N2	46	*80*	38	00
	N3	52	*75*	14	38
3	N1	38	29	*85*	09
	N2	45	11	*77*	44
	N3	27	43	*83*	16
4	N1	46	28	19	*79*
	N2	45	14	24	*85*
	N3	52	06	03	*80*

We have found that this spreading of the occasion-mean variance upon rotation reduces extreme trends to negligible magnitude with many variables (e.g., rate of excretion of various urinary constituents, kinesthetic after-effect judgments, performance on paper-and-pencil tasks, etc., unpublished), and it hedges quite well against large statistical complications. The procedure seems to be applicable to any variable in which there are systematic changes. It also may be used to modulate extreme drift in continuous recordings made in a single session.

This application of the P-technique works well with a group of different, though tightly inter-correlated measures of the same process so long as they all change at least somewhat in unison. However, interpretation rapidly becomes more complex as additional variables with different cycles of variation are added to the analysis. It soon becomes meaningless simply to reify a factor with the name of its leading variable. Unravelling the variance from a maze of varying curves which are only sometimes in phase, in an effort to cast light upon the *raison d'être* for the pool of common variance that has been consolidated in a factor becomes a detective job—a search for clues and a prayer for insight. Where heavy trends or cycles are present in much of a data set (e.g., that due to learning, fatigue, age, seasonal changes, etc.), the major factors consolidate so much variance due to these pervasive effects that lesser effects may be obscured. Yet, these massive trend-effects may be of only minor interest in themselves.

Regardless of the difficulties enumerated, factor analysis is a perfectly legitimate device for the analysis of longitudinal data. The technique segregates components of variance just as it does with cross-sectional data where dependencies among the data are less evident and are rationalized in other ways. In the cross-sectional design the primary dependencies are between variables whose quantities or rates are correlated because of direct, indirect, or fortuitous relationships. The resulting factors reflect these relationships. In the longitudinal design the same relationships occur within one individual, but an additional dependency arises as a result of the trends and periodicities within a given variable *per se*. Two variables that change together for any reason contribute common variance to the total pool. At first glance it might appear that the primary concern lies in the inflation of correlations in 'trend' factors. However, of equal concern is the fact that very real relationships may disappear in the computations. For example, a variable that increases steadily throughout the period of the experiment may have a negative relationship with another variable for half this time period as the second variable decreases, but then have a positive relationship for the other half as the variable now also increases (as for example, occurs in various compensatory mechanisms). The computed correlation is zero regardless of whether the observed changes are the result of the direct operation of a control of one variable on the other, or whether they are entirely fortuitous. However, the same pair of variables would exhibit a range of non-zero correlations depending entirely on the duration of the time periods chosen for analysis. Were the period reduced to the half-way point, the correlation would have been perfect, positive in one experiment, but negative were the other half used! Various intermediate selected durations would yield the full range of correlations. This illustrates the fundamental arbitrariness of the longitudinal experiment—the investigator's decision as to the duration and sampling regimen may yield a family of results that have no apparent relation to one another (Mefferd, Moran & Kimble, 1960). This poses a dilemma to the investigator which is resolvable only if he attends the duality of the problem: the time-course curves *per se*, and the traditional inter-variable relationships. The first factor may inflate or obscure the second, and it *usually* does. Is the answer to this curve-confounding effect the separation of the trend and cycle information from the deviation scores for separate analysis as the traditions of economic statistics suggest?

In our opinion at the present time, if factor analysis is to be used in the exploration of longitudinal data, the analysis should be of the raw, unaltered data (i.e., rather than of grouped, smoothed, or partialled data). The whole point of factoring is to locate and segregate pools of common variance. Use of the factoring techniques will permit this to be achieved far more objectively than the investigator can accomplish by any means of arbitrary, and possibly biased, interventions of his own invention. Interpretation of the resulting factors may be advanced by sub-analyses of several contiguous segments from the entire time-frame (e.g., of the first half and last half, separately), of odd and even occasions separately, of some variables lagged relative to others (e.g., of weather and physiological variables), of variables exhibiting linear and oscillating characteristics separately; analyses with criterion marker variables included (e.g., a synthesized trending or oscillating curve) and so on. Such procedures are expensive, time-consuming and discouraging to the investigator.

2.2.4.4. Multiple regression techniques

Another technique offers some respite to the impatient explorer—multiple regression analysis (Williams, 1959; Draper & Smith, 1966). While all the problems inherent in the use of factor analysis also apply here, and though the processes of interpretation of *why* particular variables clustered is just as difficult, the technique has three advantages. First, the investigator may delineate and examine a specific relationship by his selection of the dependent variable. This variable may be one of the raw data variables, an exterior variable (e.g., occasion number, day-of-week, barometric pressure), or a set of orthogonal factor scores from some factor of special interest, such as one of the taste factors discussed above. Second, the technique consolidates *all* the variance that is common with the dependent variable rather than distributing it to several factors (i.e., the individual regression scores obtained for occasion or for S in the cross-sectional analysis will usually correlate to varying degrees with *several* sets of orthogonal factor scores from the same data). Furthermore, traditional factor loadings for the factor represented may be readily computed from the regression equation. Third, unlike the format of canonical correlation, the multiple regression format permits the investigator conveniently to predict future expectations. Cross-validation of results is thereby facilitated.

There are no unique solutions with multivariate techniques. All are a function of the number and kind of variables analysed. Add another variable and the solution changes. Regression techniques are particularly sensitive to the inter-correlation patterns among the independent variables. If a new independent variable is added to a group with which it is highly correlated, little new variance in common with the dependent variable is added. While redundancy may 'build a factor' in factor analysis, it does not contribute to predictability of a given dependent variable. However, the addition of a new independent variable that is not highly correlated with the others, but still is correlated with the dependent variable will yield a material increase in the predictability of the later. By a like token, the addition of a variable may 'suppress' a relationship, and its inclusion may actually reduce predictability.

A procedure that permits the investigator to control objectively for the factors of redundancy and suppression is the step-up, step-down multiple regression procedure available at most computer centres (Draper & Smith, 1966, p. 171). The step-up feature in which one variable is added at a time, permits him to find without equivocation, for example, that combination of variables that is maximally influenced (i.e., predicted) by daily maxima in temperature. The step-down feature guards against the inclusion of suppressor variables. While the results may be circumstantial for a given regression analysis (i.e., they possess only concurrent validity), the investigator can determine if this is the case by means of a simple cross-validation using the regression equation developed in the first analysis on a different sample. He can protect himself against over-optimism (and consequent large 'shrinkage' upon cross-validation) by imposing suitable controls on the analysis (e.g., by setting a limit on the number of steps to be made that is well below the number of variables in the analysis; by choosing, after the fact, a step where the contributions of a newly added variable became so small that the 'F' ratio of the extracted-to-residual variance fell below unity; and so on). This technique will be used in the next section to examine the inter-relationship of environmental and physiological variables.

2.2.5. The influence of environment on physiological variables

We examined rather extensively the relationship of environmental and physiological variables of the longitudinal experiment under discussion by means of factor analytic techniques. These techniques left no doubt that there were important inter-relationships involved. However, these results were so different for each S that it was impossible to generalize beyond the fact that weather and physiological variables definitely are related. We then turned to regression techniques.

From a battery of available environmental variables, 20 were selected for examination. These included indices of temperature, humidity, barometric pressure, wind speed, sunshine, and geomagnetic activity (maxima, range, mean [see Pokorny & Mefferd, 1966, for a description of the geomagnetic measures]). Thunderstorm activity, the passage of cold and warm fronts and the temperature and humidity in the room at the time of testing of each S were also included. In an effort to reduce the data, these 20 variables were factored with the principal axis technique (unities in the diagonal), and the first eight factors were rotated by the varimax procedure (Table 2.3). Orthogonal factor scores for the 120 days were computed for these eight factors to be used *in lieu* of the original 20 variables. For all practical purposes, these factors were the same for all three Ss, since only the room temperatures and humidities varied between Ss, and these were almost identical. The physiological variables were measured with standard clinical procedures by a physician who had rehearsed extensively to achieve constant and accurate techniques: pulse and respiration rates, blood

TABLE 2.3. Varimax factor structure of 20 environmental variables for 120 consecutive days in the autumn and early winter, Houston, Texas

	Components of Variance[a]							
	1 (18·5)[b]	2 (11·9)	3 (5·8)	4 (6·5)	5 (10·3)	6 (5·3)	7 (10·8)	8 (13·5)
Temperature								
Outdoor maximum	77	34	−02		19		22	20
Outdoor range	00	85	−12					
Test room[c]	15	−08	86					
Humidity								
Outdoor maximum	78	−21	−04					
Test room	85	−18	−23				22	
Barometric pressure								
Outdoor maximum	−90		−19					
Test room	−84		−33					
Fronts								
Cold		01	−21	79	03			
Warm		32	28	20	50	−21		−22
Thunderstorm	32	−51		39			−20	
Distant thunder				08		93		
Day of week[d]			−22	−66				22
Wind speed								
Maximum					−95			
Mean					−91			
Sunshine (%)		91						
Geomagnetic activity								
K, Maximum							88	25
K, Sum							88	31
Storms (Number)							55	72
Storms (Cumulative)							18	95
Storms (Cumulative K)							22	95

[a] Decimals omitted
[b] Per cent of total variance
[c] Air conditioned room not based on ambient temperature
[d] Monday = 1

pressures, and oral temperatures. He made a set of the measurements after the *S* had been sitting quietly for 5 min, another (except that oral temperature was not repeated) immediately after he had drawn a blood sample from the *S*'s arm, and a third set 5 min later. Even on the 120th day all three *S*s were still experiencing mild stress responses as a result of the blood taking. While these physiological data might also have been consolidated by factoring techniques as was done with the environmental variables we elected to treat them individually.

A series of step-up, step-down multiple regression analyses were made with the physiological variables taken one-by-one as the dependent variables to be predicted by the eight environmental factors (i.e., sets of factor scores). Every physiological measure in each of the three conditions (i.e., pre-stress, stress, and post-stress) in all three Ss was predictable at a significant level (i.e., $P < 0.05$) by at least one of the sets of environmental factor scores. However, as with the factor analysis of the same date, there was little consistency between Ss or between variables as to which process was predictable by what set of environmental variables. We collided head-on with the curve-confounding effect and succeeded only in compounding the interpretation problem! Therefore, we returned to the 20 original environmental variables themselves to predict each physiological variable. Now the results were much more consistent—for two of the Ss, the daily maximum outdoor temperature had significant regression coefficients in the multiple regression equations for all the physiological variables, and for all three Ss they were significant for pre-stress pulse rate (negative signs), and diatolic blood pressure (positive signs), and for the post-stress systolic and diastolic blood pressures (positive signs). The room humidity was significantly related to all three sets of blood pressures and respiration rates in all three Ss, and it was significant with oral temperatures for two of the Ss.

The individuals were differentially responsive to the environmental variables. Two Ss were especially responsive to temperature fluctuations, another was highly sensitive to changes in humidity. For the variables associated with geomagnetic storms, one S was responsive under any condition, the second was responsive to this influence only in the pre-stress period, while the third was essentially unresponsive. Among the physiological variables, the blood pressures—particularly the diastolic—appeared to be especially responsive to environmental variables. This may be illustrated by considering simultaneously the significant regression weights in the equations of the three Ss, recalling that most of the environmental variables were the same on each day for all three. Thus, for one of the daily periods, such as the pre-stress period, there were 20 variables × 3 Ss yielding 60 possibly significant regression weights. During this pre-stress period there actually were 14 significant regression weights of environmental variables with diastolic pressure as compared with 12 for the pulse rate and 8 for the oral temperature. In the post-stress period these were 17, 11, and 8, respectively.

2.3. WITHIN-DAY CHANGE—CIRCADIAN RHYTHMS

The discovery and description of biological cycles has been a busy and exciting page of recent scientific history. Most oscillations are proving to be complex resolutions of the activities of multiple systems (e.g., Fröberg, Karlson, Levi, & Lidberg, 1972). Early in this discovery stage, it appeared that many variables oscillated systematically within the 24-h daily cycle—the diurnal cycle. This was a very satisfying possibility, neatly tying several phenomena together—the light–dark cycle, the active–inactive cycle, the sleep–

wakeful cycle, etc. However, this simple explanation was soon discredited as it became apparent that most oscillations were only 'about a day'—circadian—in length (Aschoff, 1965; Halberg, 1969; Brown, Hastings, & Palmer, 1970). Longer term oscillations (infradian) were originally thought to be direct reflections of the weather, seasons, moon phases, and other obviously cycling natural phenomena. These simplist explanations are also proving to be founded only partially in truth (Pokorny & Mefferd, 1966).

These fascinating rhythms are intriguing because we feel intuitively that they must reflect answers to many vital questions. The consequences of crossing well-established time schedules in our daily activities are impressive. Jet travel has focused attention onto the problems of sudden disruption of ongoing physiological rhythms (Hale *et al.*, 1972). For generations long-suffering people in some occupations have been subjected to torture with assorted rotating shifts, extra-duty during unusual hours, etc. Traditions and resistance to change in this factor have saddled police and fire departments, the military services, hospitals and the like with employees who are unnecessarily fatigued, physiologically disrupted and inefficient much of the time. A large mass of research reports now attests to the wisdom of having 'regular' work hours scheduled as a constant time, and to the maintenance of established regularity in daily routine schedules as well as during travel (e.g., Hale *et al.*, 1972).

The mounting results of long-term isolation studies (e.g., the cave studies) indicate that while some processes have free-running rhythms, others undergo severe drift in circadian rhythms with concomitant physiological disruptions during the first weeks of isolation (Siffre, 1964). During this unsettled interval, even the subjective time of the isolated individual changes and he underestimates time intervals. Various synchronizers (*Zeitgerber*) can effectively entrain the rhythms of physiological processes. Left to themselves, the rhythms of isolated Ss gradually re-establish but with new periods that are characteristic of an individual.

Why should continual perceptual reduction and isolation be so disruptive, regardless of whether schedules of activity, rest and sleep are maintained? Why should sudden changes in daily schedules be so traumatic? Perhaps the situation may be likened to what happens when two oscillators are operated at different frequencies. The combined output in this case may actually yield quite satisfactory sets of random numbers—the larger the phase shift, the more random the output appears. Perhaps a particular environmental condition that induces a change (e.g., in frequency or regularity) in a particular process leads to disruptions in other systems due to the phase shift (e.g., Klein, Wegmann & Hunt, 1972). Such shifts may change the characteristics of the feedback signals of overlying control systems with resulting changes in the rhythm of the control signals.

From an experimental standpoint, the existence of circadian rhythms makes life difficult for the psychophysiologist whether he is assessing the response to some stimulus or to the passage of time. The magnitude of the differences between the crests and troughs of normal circadian cycles is large, and different conclusions may be made by the unwary depending on the time of day at which the measurements were made. Fröberg, Karlson, Levi, & Lidberg, (1972), for example, reported excretion rates for epinephrine of 3 ng/min at the early morning (0200 hrs) circadian nadir. This rate increased to about 10 ng/min in the early afternoon (1300–1400 hrs) crest. Fitting the cosine functions of the means of these rates and using a 24-h cycle (Halberg, 1969), they computed the mean amplitude of the daily curve to be from 2·0 to 3·4 ng/min. The urine flow rate dropped to less than a ml/min before midnight, but then the rate crested in the forenoon (0900) at more than 2 ml/min.

The large out-of-phase variation between epinephrine and urine flow rate reminds us that impressive experimental problems are involved. What relation does one variable have with the other? If the investigator examines the epinephrine and urine excretion rates at the same point-in-time, only a modest positive correlation is noted (0·31 and 0·34 in the two experiments of the Fröberg *et al.*, 1972, report). Yet, since both variables are cycling systematically, the correlation between the pair increased to 0·82 and 0·76 in their two experiments when the epinephrine rate was lagged three hours behind that of the urine. While this is a pleasing confirmation of the existence of out-of-phase circadian rhythms in both variables, it provides only inferential information on a possible cause-effect relationship between the pair. In the first part of the same experiment the norepinephrine excretion rate had a rhythm that was almost in phase with that of the urine flow rate. Other authors have reported that another component of the total response system—the 17 hydroxycorticosteroids—is also excreted with a circadian rhythm almost in-phase with the urine flow rate (*cf.* Mills, 1966; Halberg, 1969). Since all three of these latter variables are cycling in-phase, the inter-correlations between the three variables will be high positive, and all will be low positive with epinephrine (since the latter was only out-of-phase by about 3 hours).

In fact, the correlations of the three in-phase variables may approach unity where sampling intervals are frequent and analytical procedures are adequate. Conversely, as one of the variables is lagged, the correlations should become zero halfway through the period, and become negative thereafter. Thus, the important question of whether or not these variables are interacting cannot be resolved at one point in time. Longitudinal designs are required for this purpose.

It appears increasingly likely that the evolution of the generalized response system (i.e., all aspects of response control—anticipation, organization, actuation and recovery, starting with the roles played by the hypothalamus and the reticular activation system and extending to those of the autonomic nervous system, the adrenal gland and the cell membranes), progressed in a manner favouring a development of a series of interacting control sub-systems that changed their levels of readiness-activity throughout the day in a staggered sequential manner. Early in the morning darkness the activation level is turned-up as normal upcoming activity-demands are anticipated by the basic system, and the somatic elements are prepared to respond normally on demand via, in part, the anterior hypophysis and its target organs. Later in the day the response system is tuned via the hypothalamus as these demands become more specific and imminent. Surges of demand activity are called directly by the hypothalamus and the sympathetic nervous system, modulated by the parasympathetic system and by the limbic system, sustained for short periods by the norepinephrine released directly in the periphery by the sympathetic impulses, and sustained for longer periods by the adrenal medullary secretion of epinephrine and the operation of the cyclic AMP system in the cell membranes. With continued response activity, the response systems gradually become unresponsive as the levels of essential energy-sources and of mediating and regulating components of the endocrine system become depleted, and parasympathetic predominance appears. Overt warning signals, possibly mediated by the limbic system, appear in guises such as reduced motivation and aspiration levels, increased response errors and pauses, increased irritability and fatigue.

It is gratifying to note the recent increase in the number of experiments designed to permit evaluation of this complicated interacting system. Referring again as an example to the Fröberg, *et al.* (1972) experiment, these authors measured a variable at each of four critical points in the response system: the direct response sustenance—norepinephrine; the prolonged performance sustenance—epinephrine; the quality of the response *per se*—shooting performance; and the system warning of depletion—subjective stress-fatigue ratings. The authors' clearly perceived the over-riding importance of the parameters of the individual circadian rhythms to the interpretation of their results *vis-à-vis* the interactions among these variables. Their design yielded definitive statements about the phases and amplitudes of the four curves. This permitted them to examine the effects of prolonged sleep deprivation not only relative to their specific hypothesis, but also relative to its effect directly on the parameters of the circadian curves *per se* (to wit, the effects of sleeplessness were slight, at least once the sleep deprivation was underway). More significantly to phychophysiological theory, they were able to sharpen Schubert's (1969) view that the rate of response, at least with a simple task, is directly related to the 'diurnal' degree of sympathetic predominance. They concluded more definitively that this rate is a *delayed* function of sympathetic predominance.

2.4. WITHIN-MEASUREMENT CHANGE

Does the initial, pre-response level influence the response level within an individual? The very large variation within an individual across days and weeks, and within a day raises another methodological question. When responsiveness is being measured, how dependent is the observed response magnitude on the initial level on a particular occasion? Few reports have dealt with repetitive measurements of individuals. Unfortunately, most of these few reports have serious limitations. For example, Block and Bridger (1962) measured only GSR, while Bridger and Reiser (1959), and Oken and Heath (1963) dealt only with the heart rates of neonates. To what extent the results obtained using heart rates of neonates can be generalized to adults and further, to what extent heart rate results (or the results from any single variable), can be generalized to those of other variables is questionable (Hord, Johnson, & Lubin, 1964). In several longitudinal studies (e.g., that of Lacey and Smith, 1954), all data were collected within a single session under conditions that may have modified the relationships as a result of habituation or conditioning processes.

We explored this question by examining the responses to the cold pressor test administered daily to the three Ss under discussion (results presented to the Society for Psychophysiological Research, Monterrey, Calif., Oct. 1969). The pulse rates for a quiet minute 2 min prior to the cold pressor test (X) were ranked from low to high for the 120 days, and the corresponding response values (Y) for the first 40-sec (corrected to 1-min) of the cold pressor test (a word association test was commenced at 40-sec) were plotted on the same graph (Figure 2.6). The response values (Y) were ordered within a given initial (X) level. The general convergence of the graphs of the two heart rates, X and Y, across the 120 days is indicative of the operation of the Law of Initial Values (i.e., Y regresses on X; Wilder, 1957, 1958, 1962). This was not a trend effect, since the distribution of day-numbers was extremely varied. However, the range of response values for a given level of X was very large. In Table 2.4, five relevant Pearson product moment correlations ($N = 120$) are presented that involve the initial (X) and response (Y) levels, the change (D) and the autonomic lability scores (ALS, Lacey, 1956) of these periods. In general, the correlations across variables were similar among the three Ss. A negative correlation between the initial level and the change (column 1 of the Table) has been considered to evidence the operation of the Law (Wilder, 1960; Oken & Heath, 1963). On this basis pulse rate and its variability and the blood pressures (pulse pressure had the same pattern as the blood pressures) clearly would be categorized as evidencing the Law within a S. The GSR, baseline skin resistance, and finger temperature, however, would not be so categorized. In this same experiment, the Ss took word association tests under two conditions—one during the quiet baseline period and another during the cold pressor test 40-sec after it commenced. The results of the comparison between a quiet minute 2 min prior to word associations without cold pressor are shown in Table 2.5 (blood pressures could not be obtained during this verbalization). The results were very similar in all three of these response-inducing situations. In fact when the reverse situation was examined, the *recovery* during the second minute following the cold pressor word association section—the Law of Final Values (Heath & Oken, 1962)—was also seen to be operative (Table 2.6). Except for the difference in signs resulting from the direction of the changes, the patterns of correlation were quite similar whether the effect was a response or a recovery.

Much of the concern with the Law of Initial Value has arisen from con-

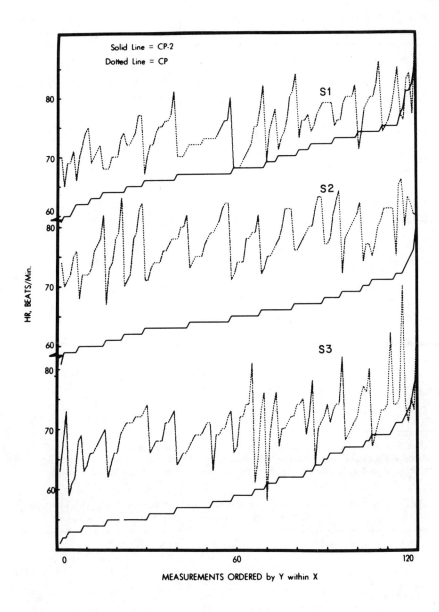

FIGURE 2.6. Regression of pulse rate cold pressor response levels (Y) on pre-stress (X) levels within three individuals across 120 consecutive days. X values were ordered from low to high, then within each set of X values, the Y values were ordered in the same fashion

TABLE 2.4. Inter-correlations of pre-stress (X) and response (cold pressor) (Y) levels, change (D), and autonomic lability scores (ALS) (decimal point omitted)

Variable	Subject	Correlations[a]				
		$X \times D$	$X \times Y$	$Y \times D$	$Y \times$ ALS	$D \times$ ALS
Pulse rate	N1	−55	67	25	74	84
	N2	−38	41	40	65	60
	N3	−34	67	47	74	94
Pulse rate variability	N1	−81	00	59	99	59
	N2	−69	02	71	99	72
	N3	−73	25	42	95	68
Blood pressure: systolic	N1	−33	68	46	73	94
	N2	−40	57	53	82	92
	N3	−45	52	53	85	89
Blood pressure: diastolic	N1	−29	72	46	70	96
	N2	−37	44	67	90	93
	N3	−62	52	34	85	78
Galvanic skin response	N1	−29	29	83	96	96
	N2	−06	22	96	98	99
	N3	−13	16	96	99	99
Baseline skin resistance	N1	21	99	34	21	88
	N2	−14	96	13	27	99
	N3	22	99	32	11	75
Finger temperature	N1	−33	99	−18	16	94
	N2	−22	99	−09	13	97
	N3	19	99	31	13	98

[a] X = level of a quiet 1-min pre-stress period 2 min before the cold pressor; Y = level of a 40-sec cold pressor response period expressed as 1-min; $D = Y - X$ change; ALS = autonomic lability score using X and Y; coefficients significantly different from zero, $P \leq 0.05$ are in italics.

TABLE 2.5. Intercorrelations of baseline and response (word associations) levels, change, and ALS (decimal points omitted)

Variable	Subject	Correlations[a]				
		$X \times D$	$X \times Y$	$Y \times D$	$Y \times$ ALS	$D \times$ ALS
Pulse rate	N1	−54	68	25	75	83
	N2	−43	59	48	80	91
	N3	−32	70	45	71	95
Pulse rate variability	N1	−88	−12	58	99	47
	N2	−71	26	49	96	72
	N3	−88	32	17	95	48
Respiration rate	N1	−36	18	85	98	93
	N2	−03	29	95	96	99
	N3	−51	27	69	96	86

TABLE 2.5. (*Contd.*)

Variable	Subject	Correlations[a]				
		$X \times D$	$X \times Y$	$Y \times D$	$Y \times$ ALS	$D \times$ ALS
Respiration rate	N1	−44	18	81	98	90
variability	N2	−45	−03	91	99	89
	N3	−98	10	16	99	22
Galvanic skin	N1	02	30	96	96	99
response	N2	−18	34	87	94	98
	N3	25	45	98	89	97
Baseline skin	N1	−21	95	12	32	98
resistance	N2	−26	93	12	37	97
	N3	−27	96	01	28	96

[a] See Footnote on Table 2.4 for description of symbols.

TABLE 2.6. Law of final values (LFV) *vs* law of initial values (LIV): comparisons of inter-correlations of levels and changes of LFV where Y is for a quiet, recovery period following an activated state (*X*, cold pressor word associations) and of LIV where Y is the preceding an activated state considered earlier (cold pressor) (decimal points omitted)

Variable	Subject	Correlations[a]					
		LFV $X \times D$	LIV $Y \times D$	LFV $X \times Y$	LIV $X \times Y$	LFV $Y \times D$	LIV $X \times D$
Pulse rate	N1	−57	25	54	67	39	−55
	N2	−34	40	79	41	49	−38
	N3	−31	40	65	67	68	−34
Pulse rate	N1	−64	59	−18	00	84	−81
variability	N2	−42	71	05	02	87	−69
	N3	−16	42	23	25	93	−73
Galvanic skin	N1	−90	96	21	29	22	−29
response	N2	−84	98	04	22	51	−06
	N3	−88	99	10	16	38	−13
Baseline skin	N1	−20	12	99	99	−11	21
resistance	N2	−00	12	99	99	11	−14
	N3	09	01	99	99	16	22

[a] See Footnote on Table 2.4 for description of symbols.

siderations of how to express responsiveness or reactivity (e.g., Lacey, 1956; Benjamin, 1963). The correlations among three of the most popular ways—the response level (*Y*), the change (*D*) value, and the autonomic lability score (ALS)—are shown in the last columns of Tables 2.4 and 2.5. In some cases it is immaterial which measure is used—the correlations were all quite high (e.g., with GSRs). With other variables, however, the difference between the measures was tremendous (e.g., with finger temperature), and the question of the measure that most accurately reports a 'response' is open. The solution depends on the process measured, the duration of the measurement period, etc. Because of this unresolved problem, two basic questions of individual differences in reactivity remain confused.

The first question is whether on a given day an individual has an autonomic responsiveness or a reactivity level which is non-specific, elicited regardless of the particular stimulus. In Table 2.7 the correlations between responses to cold pressor and word associations expressed in each of the three ways discussed above are given for four different variables. With the response expressed as Y, the correlations for the responses to the two stimuli were all

TABLE 2.7. Correlations between response level (Y), change (D), and ALS of two stimuli—word associations (WA) and cold pressor (CP) (decimals omitted)

Variable	Subject	WA × CP correlations using different criteria of response		
		Y	D	ALS
Pulse rate	N1	58	25	20
	N2	40	15	26
	N3	73	08	19
Pulse rate variability	N1	28	16	26
	N2	05	03	03
	N3	28	18	11
Galvanic skin responses	N1	40	20	30
	N2	71	69	70
	N3	35	25	23
Baseline skin resistance	N1	96	13	10
	N2	92	33	33
	N3	94	−06	−09

significantly different from zero except for one (i.e., pulse rate variability for the second S; however, with this S, the correlations were all low with this variable for all three criteria). The magnitudes and patterns of these correlations to two different stimuli suggest that there was considerable stimulus specificity imposed upon the non-specific autonomic response. This is not surprising since the two stimuli elicit a variety of different activities as well as the generalized activating–alerting response. The latter is confounded by the former.

TABLE 2.8. Intra-individual intercorrelations of variables between a minute of a quiet baseline period and of a cold pressor test with the response expressed as Y, D, and ALS (decimals omitted)

Variable	Period or response	PR 1	PR 2	PR 3	PRσ 1	PRσ 2	PRσ 3	BPs 1	BPs 2	BPs 3	BPd 1	BPd 2	BPd 3	PP 1	PP 2	PP 3	GSR 1	GSR 2	GSR 3	BSR 1	BSR 2	BSR 3
Pulse rate variability (PRσ)	X	*18*	−17	−33																		
	Y	−31	−53	−39																		
	D	21	−41	−27																		
	ALS	−15	−46	−27																		
Blood pressure	X	*55*	*30*	*32*	−08	11	−09															
	Y	55	39	17	−05	−14	−02															
	D	11	08	13	−07	03	10															
	ALS	21	26	06	−02	−13	00															
Blood pressure diastolic (BPd)	X	00	−05	−01	−05	−01	01	*27*	08	*28*												
	Y	08	11	−18	−01	−14	12	40	18	47												
	D	04	10	02	00	−14	14	−07	−01	24												
	ALS	03	16	−12	03	−12	16	06	08	39												
Pulse pressure (PP)	X	*42*	*24*	*33*	−02	08	−07	*54*	*60*	*40*	−67	−75	−18									
	Y	39	15	34	−03	03	−14	46	48	42	−63	−78	−40									
	D	07	−04	07	−06	13	−06	71	56	48	−75	−83	−04									
	ALS	13	02	−15	−04	03	−14	61	49	45	−71	−82	04									
Galvanic skin responses (GSR)	X	*37*	*14*	*34*	02	17	05	*20*	−15	*18*	01	−08	*14*	15	−04	01						
	Y	13	04	02	−24	00	−17	06	−19	27	−04	04	15	09	−16	08						
	D	−11	12	02	−08	04	02	−03	09	−01	−06	−02	−02	02	07	01						
	ALS	−09	06	00	−22	−01	−13	−03	−02	12	−07	−00	07	04	−05	06						
Baseline skin resistance (BSR)	X	*−45*	*−34*	*−34*	−12	−02	−03	*−43*	−23	*−17*	−01	−04	−01	−27	−13	−10	−15	−03	−11			
	Y	−47	−10	−40	−05	−08	01	−37	−34	−25	−07	−13	−01	−25	−11	−21	−09	09	01			
	D	27	−19	−06	21	13	−18	03	−19	−10	07	−25	−03	−03	10	−04	−27	−50	−04			
	ALS	07	−23	−04	07	08	−10	−02	−14	−12	08	−26	−17	−12	12	04	−34	−49	−07			
Finger temperature	X	*−36*	*24*	*12*	−16	02	12	*−36*	12	*−21*	−32	−19	−21	24	23	−21	−20	−04	07	24	−19	−21
	Y	−29	−11	33	03	11	−05	−48	02	−19	−22	−23	−19	25	22	−19	−07	−03	−06	25	−14	−19
	D	−05	10	02	03	11	−03	−09	02	05	−03	03	05	06	−01	05	00	−08	−13	06	−13	05
	ALS	00	−14	−04	−05	10	04	−17	−08	06	02	−03	06	−02	−03	06	06	−08	−08	−02	−09	06

The second question is whether a given stimulus elicites a general autonomic responsivity that is reflected in all the physiological processes (Lacey, Bateman, & Van Lehn, 1953). The intercorrelations among seven of the variables expressed as X, Y, D, and ALS are given in Table 2.8. With a few notable exceptions (e.g., for $S1$, pulse rate variability and finger temperature; for $S2$, baseline skin resistance and both diastolic and pulse pressures; and for $S3$, the diastolic and pulse pressures, and the GSR and baseline skin resistance), the three Ss had very similar correlation patterns. Using Y as the criterion of response, 30 of the 84 coefficients were significantly different from zero as compared to 40 with X. However, with either D or ALS used as the response criterion, fewer than half this many coefficients were significant (17 and 15, respectively). Clearly the criterion of response used would influence the decision to this question that is basic to present concepts of psychosomatic medicine.

Two correlations are pertinent in the interpretation of response data whether it is within or between Ss: (i) the initial level (X) by the response level (Y) (to determine whether there was in fact a reliable response), and (ii) the initial level (X) by the response-induced change (D) (to determine whether the degree of response is dependent on the initial level—whether there is in fact a regression of Y on X). If $X \times Y$ is zero, there was either no response, or on half the occasions (or Ss) the response was paradoxical. The correct interpretation of such a correlation requires examination of the paired data-points. If $X \times D$ is zero, and $Y \times D$ is positive, either the change score or Y is an appropriate measure of response (an example of this is seen with GSR where quiet baseline periods have virtually no activity relative to that of the stimulus period). If $X \times D$ is zero but $Y \times D$ is also zero (e.g., as with slowly changing variables that exhibit little evidence of direct neural servo-control such as skin temperature or the related basal skin resistance), the change score itself is an appropriate measure of response. Where the initial level is correlated with the change score as occurs with processes where the action of the neural servo-control is both rapid and evident—heart rate, respiration rate, blood pressure—the change score is an inappropriate response measure. In this case the autonomic lability score (Lacey, 1956) is appropriate.

2.5. CONCLUSIONS

As anyone who has attempted longitudinal experimentation has learned, this is not an enterprise for the faint-hearted. There are few guidelines. Many respected scientists are sceptical of the whole technique—the N of *one* presents an insurmountable barrier in many minds. The conduct of such experiments is arduous and demanding. A new way of life inevitably emerges for the intrepid researcher. The sighs of relief at the termination of an experiment soon turn to groans of anguish when he begins detailed examination of his mountains of data. Little can prepare him for the maze of complications that awaits his analysis. Soon the investigator is tempted simply to report a brief summary of the whole mess, or to present the raw data and let someone else interpret it.

Yet, the potential power of the longitudinal design demands that we persevere. Three advantages alone warrant the effort: the elimination of inter-individual variation, the clarification of cycling and trending phenomena, and the side-stepping of the diagnostic dilemma in many areas of medical uncertainty (i.e., the patient is his own control irrespective of what the true diagnosis later may prove to be). Perhaps the most exciting of the potentialities is that of exploration of a new individual differences concept. The Law of Diminishing Returns is rapidly catching up with us in medical science. The 'normal range' philosophy yielded such exceedingly powerful medical returns that individuality was lost in the shuffle. Few prominent scientific voices are heard espousing this cause (for notable exceptions see Cattell, 1966a; Williams, 1967; Pauling, 1968). In our work we found that among our three Ss, weather variables were correlated with different physiological processes. These correlations would have been obscured by group averaging techniques. If an extrinsic variable does in fact influence some endogenous variable in even one individual, the question then is only pragmatic and economic. If only one ill man in a hundred with similar symptoms is helped by a scientific treatment, the pragmatics of the situation are perfectly clear to him personally. From a scientific standpoint, if the specific treatment reversed a malfunction in any individual, it did so for a discoverable reason. Regardless of how vicarious are the routes leading to a disorder, a supportable goal of science is to discover the low stave in the barrel. With many nutritional, endocrine, and mental disturbances it is probable that we face the formidable task of discovering many low staves in many different individuals. Where group statistics of heroic proportions would be required for this search, the longitudinal exploration of individual cases provides a feasible approach—perhaps the only practical approach!

2.7. ACKNOWLEDGMENTS

The late Dr Betty A. Wieland collaborated in the experiments discussed here, and in the many 'think' sessions that surrounded them. Her many contributions to both the theory and practice of longitudinal experimentation are gratefully acknowledged.

2.7. REFERENCES

Anderson, T. W. *Introduction to multivariate statistical analysis.* New York: Wiley, 1958.

Aschoff, J. (Ed.) *Circadian clocks.* Amsterdam: North Holland Publ. Co. 1965.

Benjamin, L. S. Statistical treatment of the Law of Initial Values (LIV) in autonomic research: A review and recommendation. *Psychosomatic Medicine*, 1963, **25**, 556–566.

Block, J. D. & Bridger, W. H. The law of initial value in psychophysiology: A reformulation in terms of experimental and theoretical considerations. *Annals of New York Academy of Sciences*, 1962, **98**, 1229–1241.

Bridger, W. H. & Reiser, M. F. Psychophysiologic studies of the neonate: An approach toward the methodological and theoretical problems involved. *Psychosomatic Medicine*, 1959, **24**, 265–276.

Brody, S. *Bioenergetics and growth.* New York: Reinhold. 1945.

Brown, F. A., Jr., Hastings, J. W. & Palmer, J. D. *The biological clock*. New York: Academic Press, 1970.

Cattell, R. B. *Personality and motivation structure and measurement*. New York: Harcourt, Brace, & World, 1957.

Cattell, R. B. The structuring of change by P-technique and incremental R-technique. In *Problems in measuring change*, C. W. Harris (Ed), Madison: University of Wisconsin Press, 1963, p. 167–198.

Cattell, R. B. (Ed.) *Handbook of multivariate experimental psychology*. Chicago: Rand McNally, 1966(a).

Cattell, R. B. The skree test for the number of factors. *Multivariate Behavioral Research*, 1966, 1, 245–276(b).

Draper, N. R. & Smith, H. *Applied regression analysis*. New York: John Wiley & Sons. 1966.

Fiske, D. W. & Rice, L. Intra-individual response variability. *Psychological Bulletin*, 1955, 52, 217–250.

Fröberg, J., Karlson, G. S., Levi, L. & Lidberg, L. Circadian variations in performance, psychological ratings, catecholamine excretion, and diuresis during prolonged sleep deprivation. *International Journal Psychobiology*, 1972, 2, 23–26.

Halberg, F. Chronobiology. *Annual Review of Physiology*, 1969, 31, 675–725.

Hale, H. B., Ellis, J. P., Jr. & Van Fossan, D. D. Seasonal variation in human amino acid axcretion. *Journal of Applied Physiology*, 1960, 15, 121–124.

Hale, H. B., Hartman, B. O., Harris, D. A., Williams, E. W., Miranda, R. E. & Hasenfeld, J. M. Time zone entrainment and flight stressors as interactants. *Aerospace Medicine*, 1972, 43, 1089–1094.

Harman, H. H. *Modern factor analysis*. Chicago: University of Chicago Press, 1960.

Heath, H. A. & Oken, D. Change scores as related to initial and final levels. *Annals of New York Academy of Science*, 1962, 98, 1242–1256.

Holtzman, W. H. Methodological issues in P-technique. *Psychological Bulletin*, 1962, 59, 248–256.

Holtzman, W. H. Statistical models for the study of change in the single case. In C. W. Harris (Ed.), in *Problems in measuring change*. Madison: University of Wiscons Press, 1963, p. 202.

Hord, D. J., Johnson, L. C. & Lubin, A. Differential effect of the Law of Initial Value (LIV) on autonomic variables. *Psychophysiology*, 1964. 1, 79.

Kendall, M. G. *The advanced theory of statistics*. London: C. Griffin, Co. 1948.

Klein, K. E., Wegmann, H. M. & Hunt, B. I. Desynchronization of body temperature and performance of circadian rhythm as a result of outgoing and homecoming transmeridian flights. *Aerospace Medicine*, 1972, 43, 119–127.

Lacey, J. I. The evaluation of autonomic responses toward a general solution. *Annals of New York Academy of Science*, 1956, 67, 125–163.

Lacey, J. I., Bateman, D. E. & Van Lehn, R. Autonomic response specificity. *Psychosomatic Medicine*, 1953, 15, 8–21.

Lacey, J. I. & Smith, R. L. Conditioning and generalization of unconscious anxiety. *Science*, 1954, 120, 1045–1052.

Mefferd, R. B., Jr. Adaptative changes to moderate seasonal heat in humans. *Journal of Applied Physiology*, 1959, 14, 995–996.

Mefferd, R. B., Jr. Structuring physiological correlates of mental processes and states: The study of biological correlates of mental processes. In R. B. Cattell (Ed.), *Handbook of multivariate experimental psychology*. Chicago: Rand McNally, 1966, pp. 684–710.

Mefferd, R. B., Jr. Techniques for minimizing the instrumental factor. *Multivariate Behavioral Research*, 1968, 3, 339–354.

Mefferd, R. B., Jr., LaBrosse, E. H., Gawienowski, A. M. & Williams, R. J. Influence of chloropromazine on certain biochemical variables of chronic male schizophrenics. *Journal of Nervous and Mental Disease*, 1958, 127, 167–179.

Mefferd, R. B., Jr., Moran, L. J. & Kimble, J. P., Jr. Use of a factor analytic technique in the analysis of long-term repetitive measurements made upon a single schizophrenic patient. Paper presented at a symposium on Multi-Analysis of Repeated Measurements on the same Individuals. American Psychological Association, 1958.

Mefferd, R. B., Jr., Moran, L. J. & Kimble, J. P., Jr. Methodological considerations in the quest for a physical basis for schizophrenia. *Journal of Nervous and Mental Disease*, 1960, **131**, 354–357.

Mefferd, R. B., Jr. & Pokorny, A. D. Individual variability re-examined with standard clinical measures. *American Journal of Clinical Pathology*, 1967, **48**, 325–331.

Mefferd, R. B., Jr. & Wieland, B. A. Modification in autonomically mediated physiological responses to cold pressor by word associations. *Psychophysiology*, 1965, **2**, 1–9.

Mefferd, R. B., Jr. & Wieland, B. A. Taste thresholds for sodium chloride in longitudinal experiments. *Perceptual and Motor Skills*, 1968, **27**, 295–315.

Mills, J. N. Human circadian rhythms. *Physiological Review*, 1966, **46**, 128.

Oken, D. & Heath, H. A. The law of initial values: some further considerations. *Psychosomatic Medicine*, 1963, **25**, 3–12.

Overall, J. E. Orthogonal factors and uncorrelated factor scores. *Psychological Reports*, 1962, **10**, 651–662.

Pauling, L. Orthomolecular psychiatry. *Science*, 1968, **160**, 265–271.

Pokorny, A. D. & Mefferd, R. B., Jr. Geomagnetic fluctuations and disturbed behavior. *Journal of Nervous and Mental Disease*, 1966, **143**, 140–151.

Sadler, T. G. & Mefferd, R. B., Jr. Fluctuations of perceptual organization and orientation: stochastic (random) or steady state (satiation)? *Perceptual and Motor Skills*, 1970, **31**, 739–749.

Sadler, T. G. & Mefferd, R. B., Jr. Data requirements for satiation theories: A rejoinder to Price. *Perceptual and Motor Skills*, 1971, **33**, 999–1005.

Schubert, D. Simple task rate as a direct function of diurnal sympathetic nervous system predominance. *Journal of Comparative Psychology*, 1969, **68**, 434–436.

Siffre, M. *Beyond time*. New York: McGraw-Hill, 1964.

Sollberger, A. *Biological rhythm research*. New York: Elsevier, Co. 1965.

Wenger, M. A. Seasonal variations in some physiological variables. *Journal of Laboratory and Clinical Medicine*, 1943, **5**, 148–152.

Wieland, B. A. & Mefferd, R. B., Jr. Long-term changes in properties of the autokinetic illusion. *Perceptual and Motor Skills*, 1966, **22**, 367–369.

Wieland, B. A. & Mefferd, R. B., Jr. Identification of periodic components in physiological measurements. *Psychophysiology*, 1969, **6**, 160–165.

Wieland, B. A. & Mefferd, R. B., Jr. Systematic changes in levels of physiological activity during a four-month period. *Psychophysiology*, 1970, **6**, 669–689.

Wilder, J. The law of initial value in neurology and psychiatry: Facts and problems. *Journal of Nervous and Mental Disease*, 1957, **125**, 73–86.

Wilder, J. Modern psychophysiology and the law of initial value. *American Journal of Psychotherapy*, 1958, **12**, 199–221.

Wilder, J. Discussion of: Wagner, H. The significance of the a: (a–b) effect in the problem of Wilder's law of initial value. *Basimetry*, 1960, **3**, 55.

Wilder, J. Basimetric approach (law of initial value) to biological rhythms. *Annals of New York Academy of Science*, 1962, **98**, 1211–1219.

Williams, E. J. *Regression analysis*. New York: John Wiley, 1959.

Williams, R. J. *You are extraordinary*. New York: Random House. 1967.

Chapter 3

Experimenter - Subject - Situational Interactions

MARGARET J. CHRISTIE

St Mary's Hospital Medical School and Bedford College, University of London, Regent's Park, London NW1

and

JUDY L. TODD
Kennedy Child Study Center, Santa Monica, California, U.S.A.

3.1. INTRODUCTION

This chapter represents an attempt to bring together social psychology and psychophysiology in exploration of the extent to which a subject may be influenced by the 'social situation' of an experiment. This combining of disciplines has, of course, been pioneered by Leiderman and Shapiro (1965), Shapiro and Crider (1969), Shapiro and Schwartz (1970), and Schwartz and Shapiro (1973) by whom the term 'social psychophysiology' was coined. With the growth of this field experimental psychologists are being made increasingly aware of the effects of experimenter, instructions, and environment on the physiological characteristics of subjects. Sternbach (1966), for example, reviewed under the heading of 'implicit sets', evidence of non-verbal factors predisposing individuals to perceive and respond in certain ways. Under the heading of 'explicit sets' he considered predisposing influences which are verbalized, and in conclusion he argued the urgent need for further work in the area.

There is a modest literature within social psychology relating to experimenter–situational–subject interaction, associated mainly with the name of Rosenthal (Rosenthal, 1966; Rosenthal & Rosnow, 1969); and some data are available within psychophysiology.

To bring a little order into what could easily become an amorphous collection of citations, topics which appear to be of particular relevance have been selected from the material in Rosenthal and Rosnow (1969), providing a foundation for any psychophysiological evidence which may be available. A brief description of their argument is presented here, and subsequent sections examine specific aspects from the points of view of both social psychology and psychophysiology.

Characteristics of the volunteer subject are reviewed by Rosenthal and Rosnow, who suggest that those who volunteer for research often differ in significant ways from those who do not. Further, they argue that the employment of volunteer samples can lead to seriously biased estimates of various population parameters. In the second chapter of Rosenthal and Rosnow (1969) Lana discusses 'pretest sensitization', and problems associated with use of a subject as his own control, writing, 'Any manipulation of the subject or his environment by the experimenter prior to the advent of the experimental treatment, which is to be followed by some measure of performance, allows for the possibility that the result is due either to the effect of the treatment or to interaction of the treatment with the prior manipulation.' He makes a fascinating jump from Heisenberg's (1958) uncertainty principle to the Hawthorne studies described by Roethlisberger and Dickson (1939), arguing that in both sub-atomic physics and social psychology the process of measurement can influence the material being measured and change its characteristics. Orne describes the area which has become particularly associated with himself, namely, that of the 'demand characteristics' of an experiment. Under this rubric he considers the subject as an active participant in a special form of socially defined interaction which is called 'taking part in an experiment'. He argues that subtle cues may communicate what is expected of him, and that his perception of his role and of the hypothesis being tested may become significant determinants of his behaviour. Rosenthal reviews extensively the 'experimenter effect' literature, and Rosenberg discusses 'evaluation apprehension'. This latter tag refers to subjects' apprehensions about being measured, assessed, tested, and perhaps being found wanting in the experimental laboratory. The concluding paragraph of the book comes from Campbell who directs attention to the techniques and ethics of disguised experiments in natural, non-laboratory settings.

Subsequent material in the present chapter follows some of the pointers suggested in Rosenthal and Rosnow (1969), and is grouped under the section headings of: 2. The experimenter; 3. The subjects and their interactions, and 4. The laboratory. Each section consists of a survey of evidence from social psychology, followed by any available data from psychophysiology.

3.2. THE EXPERIMENTER

In considering influences which an experimenter may have on his data it is useful to retain Rosenthal's distinction between those related to the experimenter's expectations which result from his hypothesis, and those arising from his attributes. Further, the latter influences can be divided, following Rosenthal (1969) into the effects 'in the ... eye or hand of the investigator', and those which are interactional, and affect the response of the subject.

The eye-or-hand errors are usually designated as 'recording errors' and have, for example, been exemplified by Boring (1969) with reference to eighteenth-century astronomy and individual differences in recording of stellar transit times. These errors are not considered further here: it may be the case that the increasing mechanization of psychophysiological methodology makes possible a decreasing probability of recording error. The experimenter expectancy phenomena will be examined in the next section, and some account given of Rosenthal's work in this area.

3.2.1. The experimenter expectancy effect

Rosenthal (1966) labelled that bias which results in an experimenter obtaining different results from comparable subjects simply because he expects them as the 'experimenter expectancy effect'. In an early study (Rosenthal & Fode, 1963), students in a laboratory class used rats for examining T-maze discrimination learning. Half of the students were told that their rats had been bred to be 'maze bright' and half were told theirs were 'maze dull'. Significant learning differences in the expected direction were found, although the rats had been randomly drawn from the same population. A study by Laszlo described by Rosenthal (1966) typifies many of similar studies undertaken with human subjects. College age students were required to rate ten photographs of 'neutral' faces on a scale of -10 to $+10$ for failure–success. Graduate students administered the task individually to subjects; the experimenters had been led to expect some of their subjects to give ratings of $+5$ and some of -5. Experimenters contacted the two 'types' of subject in random order. Significant differences in photo ratings were obtained, and these were in the expected directions.

Although the experimenter expectancy effect has been demonstrated many times in various experimental situations (as summarized in Rosenthal, 1969), it has proved extremely difficult to pinpoint the variables in the experimenter's behaviour that produce it. Experimenters appear to be treating subjects identically and claim to be doing so. Closer analysis, however, of subtle non-verbal and paralinguistic cues, made by trained observers rating audio and visual recordings, tends to show differences in experimenter behaviour. Experimenter rated as behaving more professionally, who appear friendlier and less hyperactive, and who show more head and leg movement, tend to bias their subjects more (Rosenthal, 1966). Duncan, Rosenberg and Finkelstein (1967) were able to identify certain paralinguistic cues which contributed significantly to the experimenter expectancy effect. Adair and Espstein (1968) report similar evidence from subjects' ratings: extent of bias correlated with ratings of the experimenter as relaxed, expressive-voiced, expressive-faced, and using head gestures. Yet the precise behavioural differences mediating the experimenter expectancy effect remain undiscovered, both because of the subtleness of the cues involved, and because the cues which different experimenters use, and which different subjects respond to, probably vary from one experimental situation to another. The use of double blind procedures, removal of the human experimenter from the experimental situation, and certain kinds of control groups have been suggested (see, for example, Campbell, 1969). There is also evidence that forewarning experimenter of the possibility of expectancy effects eliminates bias (Bloom & Tesser, 1971), and even suggestion that the effect does not exist (Barber & Silver, 1968). Barber and Rushton (1974) have argued that the experimenter bias hypothesis lacks detail and generality. Their own studies exemplify the problems of pinpointing experimenter bias effects.

3.2.2. Experimenter attributes

It has been amply demonstrated that different experimenters obtain significantly different results, and such differences may be determined in part by differences in experimenters' age, sex, race, and status, and by such indirectly assessed characteristics as anxiety, warmth, hostility and authoritarianism of the experimenter (summarized in Rosenthal, 1966; 1967). Obviously, there is a measure of overlap between the present consideration of experimenter attribute effects, and the previous examination of experimenter expectancy, but it may, perhaps, be reasonable to suggest that the present discussion brings us closer to ideas of experimenter–subject interaction and a more direct effect on the subject's response. It is likely that differences in experimenters' age, sex, anxiety, etc., are confounded with differences in behaviour toward subjects, and the complexity of interaction might well be examined in Section 3.4, under the rubric of The Subject. However, at this point it becomes possible, after the preliminary overview of The Experimenter as seen by Social Psychology, to examine relevant data from psychophysiology.

3.3. THE EXPERIMENTER IN PSYCHOPHYSIOLOGY

As an introduction to this area of discussion, it may be useful before examining specific findings, to suggest two methodological treatments of the area, namely, Gale (1973) and Venables and Christie (1973, pp. 82–104), and a theoretical exposition by Hicks (1971).

Perhaps one of the most interesting examples of the 'experimenter's' influence is the placebo effect, part of which is undoubtedly due to some communication to the subject of the drug effect which is expected. Claridge (1970) provides a most useful general introduction to this area in which he describes the involvement in a drug effect of the drug itself, the characteristics of the subject taking it, and the attributes and behaviour of the person administering it. Most of Claridge's discussion, however, concerns the subject rather than the 'experimenter', and this aspect of the placebo effect will, therefore, be considered in Section 3.4. Sternbach (1966) writes that placebo effects are due to indirect suggestion. He argues also that as there is evidence of direct suggestion from an experimenter altering physiological responses, it is reasonable to expect indirect suggestions, conveyed in the subtle non-verbal behaviour of an experimenter, to be similarly effective in altering a subject's physiological responses.

Hicks (1970) reported what was described as a demonstration of experimenter effects on subjects' reporting of, and physiological responses to, tachistoscopically presented taboo and neutral words. Hicks (1970) demonstrated that different experimenters obtained different results when a sociable female, a reserved female, and what was described as an 'automated' experimenter, tested male subjects in a 'perceptual defence' study. Electrodermal and cardiovascular data were collected before and after each presentation of a stimulus. Hicks did, however, confound experimenter and situational differences: the 'automated' experimenter worked in an austere laboratory where furniture was draped in sheets, while the other experimenters were in a typical laboratory setting.

Bogdonoff, Brehm and Back (1964) varied the verbal behaviour of an experimenter and examined the effect of this on the subjects' physiological responses, in a laboratory examination of the influence of physician behaviour on patient response. Subjects who had, in preparation for a laboratory study, fasted for 17 hours were asked, on arrival at the laboratory, if they were willing to fast for an additional 8 hours. The question was put by a physician in either a permissive or an authoritarian manner. Subsequent analysis of blood free fatty acid (FFA) values, which may be used as an index of neurohormonal activity and particularly of sympathetic arousal (Back & Bogdonoff, 1965), showed that a rise in FFA level when the subjects were approached in an arbitrary manner, was significantly greater than when the approach was permissive. The studies were reported to have implications for the more general field of the effect of the physician–patient relationship upon the patient response to clinical management. Bogdonoff, Back and co-workers also used FFA analysis as the dependent variable in a study (Back, Wilson, Bogdonoff and Troyer, 1969) where an independent variable was subject race. This study is more appropriately described in Section 3.4 during consideration of subject variables, but the general topic of racial 'experimenter effects' has been recently reviewed by Sattler (1970). He reports that physiological responsiveness is affected more by the subjects' racial attitudes than by the experimenters' race, but comments that measures of physiological reactivity appear to be a promising area for studying experimenter effects.

Electrodermal indices of physiological reactivity have been used in a range of social–biological studies: a recent review has been published by Schwartz and Shapiro (1973), in which they describe a series of experiments performed by Cooper and co-workers which used physiological measures to explore relations between emotion and attitudes. The studies showed a reliable relationship between amplitude of the electrodermal response and prejudice. Further, some studies have examined the effects of using either black or white experimenters (Rankin & Campbell, 1955; Bernstein, 1965; Porier & Lott, 1967). Rankin and Campbell (1955) showed a significant effect in that the average amplitude of the skin conductance response (SCR) was greater with a black than with a white experimenter. However, there were differences between the experimenters in other than skin colour; age, height and weight were not comparable, and a recent study (Fisher & Kotses, 1973) has attempted to remedy this defect. Their subjects and experimenters were Negro or Caucasian, and while there were significant subject–race effects, with Negroes showing higher skin resistance levels (SRL), there were no experimenter–race effects shown for this variable. Such findings are similar to those of Johnson and Corah (1963), Johnson and Landon (1965), and Juniper and Dykman (1967), and may perhaps be determined by mechanisms underlying the production of SCL which are other than a direct effect of autonomic nervous system activity (Venables & Christie, 1973). Kugelmass and Lieblich (1968) have discussed the relation between skin colour and SCL, and Lieblich, Kugelmass and Ben-Shakhar (1973) conclude that there is unlikely to be any simple relation between skin colour and SCL. There were, however, in the Fisher and Kotses study, experimenter–race effects on electrodermal responding which the authors attributed to the novelty, for Caucasian subjects, of having a Negro experimenter. This topic of experimenter–subject interaction is returned to in Section 3.4, but at this point it is relevant to introduce a study of electro-encephalogram (EEG) correlates of variation in the experimenter's intensity of gaze. Gale, Lucas, Nissim and Harpham (1972) have reported that, when transoccipital EEG was continuously monitored while the experimenter either smiled at the subject, looked, or averted his gaze, there was a decrease in EEG abundance with increase in the complexity of gaze. The authors concluded that the degree of social interaction influences arousal as measured by the EEG. In a recent, subsequent study by these workers (Gale, Chapman, Spratts & Smallbone, 1974) EEG was recorded while both intensity of gaze (direct and averted) and distance of experimenter (2, 4, 8, 16 and 32 ft) were systematically varied. There were significant increases in EEG abundance associated with reduction in intensity of gaze ($P < 0.05$) and with increase in distance ($P < 0.005$). Williams, Kimball and Williard (1972) have also reported the influence of interpersonal interaction on blood pressure. They suggest that the process of interpersonal interaction is more important than the content in determining the diastolic blood pressure response during an interview.

In summary of this section it may be said that there is more evidence relating to the experimenter's interactive effect than to his attributes *per se*: the topic is, further examined in Section 3.4.

3.4. THE SUBJECTS AND INTERACTIONS

Rosenthal and Rosnow (1969) wrote somewhat pessimistically that the existing science of human behaviour may be largely the science of those sophomores who enrol in psychology courses, volunteer to participate in behavioural research, and keep their appointments. This may be something of an overstatement, but it directs experimenters' attention from data to subjects, and suggests that a need may exist for psychologists to give greater thought to subject recruitment and behaviour when designing their studies.

One suggestion recently made, and which undoubtedly deserves consideration, is that subjects are becomingly increasingly suspicious of experimenter intent (McGuire, 1969). Schultz (1969) also has argued this point, and both writers question the assumption that the subject must always be kept ignorant of the experimenter's aims. It may be that the psychophysiologist has greater freedom of choice to opt for either eliciting co-operation or maintaining secrecy: it is well worth his consideration of the extent to which a subject may be enlisted as an informed collaborator, and especially so when inconveniences or discomforts (such as a prolonged fast) are essential. Such informed collaborators may form a pool of 'habituated' subjects (Christie & Venables, 1972) who have become wholly familiar with the experimental setting, its personnel and techniques.

3.4.1. The volunteer

Perhaps the logical point at which to begin a consideration of subjects is at the act of volunteering. While it may be the case that some experimenters are able to draw on populations of non-volunteer subjects, Rosenthal and Rosnow (1969) review the field comprehensively, concluding with a summary which lists statements about volunteer characteristics in order of warranted confidence. The greatest confidence is associated with statements which attribute superior education, occupational status and intelligence to volunteers, and describe a greater need for approval, and lesser authoritarianism.

3.4.2. The subjects' view of the experiment

A recent collection of reprints (Wuebben, Straits & Schulman, 1974) has the title of *The experiment as a social occasion*; previously, Riecken (1962) argued that the psychological experiment is a '...social situation in which data are collected', and Orne (1969) has said that subjects' thoughts about an experiment may affect their behaviour in carrying out an experimental task. We may, then, ask how subjects, differing in their individual reactions to social situations, differ in their behaviour *qua* subjects.

Riecken (1962) has suggested that subjects have three main aims: to obtain rewards (whether monetary, in the form of approval, or the satisfaction of some need), to discover the aim of the experiment, and to show up well in the test situation. Orne (1969) has described subjects' vague expectations, and attempts to grasp the nature of the 'demand characteristics' of the situation. There may be sex differences in subject behaviour (Hutt, 1972), and inevitably there are differences in the interactional behaviour of experimenter—subject dyads when these are of similar sex or of a dissimilar pairing. It becomes, therefore, convenient at this point to consider subject behaviour within the general context of experimenter–subject interaction.

3.4.3. Experimenter–subject interactions

While there is little research on the interaction between experimenter and subject attributes, writers have for some time been concerned with the social accommodation and mutual influence that occurs in the experimental situation. We have mentioned Riecken (1962): he argued that the social situation in which data are collected involved a 'process of negotiation between investigator and subject through which they come to understand how to behave in the situation'.

Subject differences may interact with an experimenters' biasing behaviour, to affect experimental results in various ways. For example, in discussing the experimenter expectancy effect, Rosenthal (1966, 1967) reported more effect when experimenters smiled at their subjects: but only 12% of male experimenters smiled at male subjects while 70% smiled at female ones. Further, female subjects are, Rosenthal suggests, more protectively treated by their experimenters (Rosenthal, 1966, 1967). This may, he comments, be heartening socially, and be interesting psychologically, but it is methodologically very disconcerting. Adair and Fenton (1971) found subjects with positive attitudes toward psychology gave more hypothesis-confirming data than those with a negative attitude. Minor (1970) reported that subjects induced to feel evaluation apprehension were more influenced by their experimenters than those who did not feel apprehensive. McFall and Shenkein (1970) reported the importance of subjects' field dependence and achievement-need in determining experimenter influence. Rosenthal (1966) has suggested that there will be greater experimenter effect when experimenter and subject agree and have a smooth relationship in the experimental situation, and that friendly experimenters bias their results more than unfriendly ones, with males being more friendly than females (Rosenthal, 1966, 1967).

In some studies both experimenter and subject variables have been manipulated: White (1962) induced expectancies in a photograph rating task in both experimenters and subjects. He reported the absence of experimenter expectancy effects when expectancies conflicted, though such effects *were* present when these were in agreement. Trattner and Howard (1970) divided hospital orderlies who were serving as experimenters into A and B types on the Whitehorn–Betz scale: A types generally work more successfully with very disturbed, and B types with less disturbed mental patients. More experimenter expectancy effect was demonstrated when A types worked with schizophrenics rated as low in social competence, and when B type orderlies worked with patients rated higher for social competence.

3.5. THE SUBJECT IN PSYCHOPHYSIOLOGY

Inevitably, consideration of 'the subject' in psychophysiological research involves one in consideration of interactions with the experimenter, and differential responses of subjects to the totality of the experimental environment.

3.5.1. 'Habituation'

Perhaps one way of reducing that variance which is attributable to such differences in the initial response to the human and physical aspects of the laboratory is by employing 'habituated' subjects whenever this is feasible. The suggestion was put forward in Section 3.3, and a study which, in some measure, compared 20 habituated and 20 matched but non-habituated subjects showed (Christie & Venables, 1972) a significant ($F = 5.68$, $P = 0.02$) interaction effect of habituation with dominant/non-dominant hand differences in 'basal' SPL; this was attributed to hand differences in ductal reabsorption of sweat sodium (Gibinski, Giec, Zmudzinski, Waclawczyk & Dosiak, 1971) and to the consequent increased negativity of SPL (Fowles & Venables, 1970) in non-habituated subjects who, because of increased arousal at the beginning of, and their slower relaxation (Christie & Venables, 1971; Christie & Venables, 1974) during the recording session, had less quiescence in palmar eccrine sweat glands. Such increased arousal in non-habituated subjects may well reflect their response to the novelty of the situation: repeated exposure to the experimental environment, its personnel, and its procedures would be expected to reduce variance attributable to this cause. Chapman (1973, 1974) has measured forehead muscle tension in studies of 'evaluation apprehension' and social facilitation. His concluding discussion (1974) argues the need for further physiological investigation of social facilitation drive theories (Zajonc, 1972), but puts the case for use of subjects who are familiar with the procedures and apparatus etc., of the laboratory environment. Fisher and Kotses (1974) have recently reported a study of experimenter and subject sex effects on the skin conductance response: one finding was that there were significant reductions in habituation when the experimenter was female. This was interpreted as a stimulus novelty effect, similar to that suggested by Fisher and Kotses (1973) to explain results obtained by a negro experimenter working with white subjects. Kopacz and Smith (1971) examined sex differences in skin conductance measures as a function of shock threat. They reported that males exhibited higher skin conductance levels throughout testing while females displayed greater magnitude of the skin conductance response and more non-specific response: their experimenter was male.

3.5.2. Individual differences

It may be that, even with what is thought to be adequate care about habituation to the experimental environment, there are personality differences in amount of previous exposure needed to reduce 'test arousal'. Venables (1967) described the possible differences in test habituation between psychiatric patients and controls, and in a recent study involving preselected 'stable extraverts' (SEs) and 'unstable introverts (UIs) (as defined by Christie and Venables, 1973) the data suggested that while SEs were reflecting a response to the independent variable (a substantial meal) UIs were reflecting responses to aspects of the testing situation. During this study it became obvious that SEs were those subjects who arrived late, and said cheerfully, 'Hi!', (while symbolically slapping the experimenter on the back). In contrast, UIs were those who tapped tentatively on the door five minutes ahead of schedule saying, 'Am I late?'. Even the most experienced and detached experimenter must inevitably respond somewhat differently to both types of subject, but a greater awareness of the possibility of differential response may reduce the variability of behaviour. One strategy usefully employed, for example, by Gale and co-workers, is the assessment of personality by other than the experimenter who undertakes psychophysiological recording: in such circumstances one has only hunches and not confirmed expectancies about one's early and late arrivals. Gale (1973) indeed has written a most comprehensive general account of problems involved in studying the relation between extraversion and electroencephalogram (EEG) characteristics: his perceptive description of 'being a subject' is essential reading!

Another aspect of methodology which is in urgent need of investigation is that of optimal temporal intervals for experimental sessions, and the relation between personality characteristics and the acceptable length of testing periods. In one unpublished study which examined the effects of prolonged ($1\frac{1}{2}$ h) recording of 'basal' SPL the 10 subjects were subsequently asked about their subjective response to this period of rest in unstimulating conditions (Christie & Venables, 1971). Seven reported that the session was too long, three reported it to be tolerable, and none regarded it as pleasant.

Examination of electrodermal activity from the subjects showed that the three who found the situation tolerable had fewest spontaneous electrodermal responses in their records, and that after 40 minutes' rest there were increases in the 'arousal' of subjects. Again, variance may be reduced by greater care from experimenters in fitting suitable temporal intervals for testing to the characteristics of their subjects and the nature of their experimental manipulations.

Returning to the topic of volunteer subjects, it may be that individual differences in personality and thus (if one accepts biological bases of personality, such as those suggested by Eysenck, 1967) in physiological characteristics, require more attention from the psychophysiologist. This may be especially relevant if the procedures he envisages are particularly demanding: Pasnau, Naitoh, Stier and Kollar (1968) comment on the abnormal personality characteristics of their subjects who had volunteered for 205 hours of sleep deprivation.

Lastly, in this section, there is little known about the effects of aging on the response to being a subject (Brown, 1966), and even less about the interaction of subject–experimenter age differences. There is some evidence on the effects of aging on some psychophysiological parameters in, for example, Venables and Christie (1973). These authors also give some account of psychophysiological approaches to ethnic and racial differences, which are the subject of Section 3.5.3.

3.5.3. Racial and ethnic differences

Yet again, it has to be said that any consideration of racial and ethnic differences involves one in a complex of considerations, with the possible implication of physiological factors, and of differences in attitude both to the experimental variable and to the more general aspects of 'being a subject'.

Examples of a number of studies are given in Schwartz and Shapiro (1973) and Venables and Christie (1973): a selection of topics is examined here.

3.5.3.1. Possible physiological differences

In the electrodermal literature one recurring topic is the possibility that racial or ethnic differences underlie differences in electrodermal phenomena. Johnson and Corah (1963), Johnson and Landon (1965), Bernstein (1965), Juniper and Dykman (1967), and Lieblich, Kugelmass and Ben-Shakhar (1973) have been associated with this topic, and interest has focused on differences in sweat electrolyte concentrations as a possible determinant of differences in skin conductance level.

3.5.3.2. Differences in the response to being tested

Another aspect of the field is that of cultural differences in the response to being a subject of psychological study: Lazarus, Tomita, Opton and Kodama (1966) reported on differences between Japanese and American reactions to viewing stressful material: whereas American subjects reacted to specifically stressful aspects of film material the Japanese appeared to react more generally to the stressful aspect of being a subject.

Sternbach and Tursky (1965) and Tursky and Sternbach (1967) examined responses to painful stimuli in Irish, Italian, Jewish and Yankee subjects, and Tursky (1974) has recently reviewed this field of study.

One particular question which arises in relation to Negro subjects in the American setting is their possible feelings of threat (e.g., to esteem) when tested by white experimenters (Katz & Greenbaum, 1963). This theme has, of course, wider implications, for example for assessment of Negro children by white adults (e.g. Forrester & Klaus, 1964), but consideration here is restricted to examination of a study by Back, Wilson, Bogdonoff and Troyer (1969). This study has been selected, not so much for the clarity and value of its findings, but as a means of introducing a number of points relevant to the present discussion.

3.5.3.3. Racial environment, cohesion, conformity and stress

Back et al. (1969) note the existence of 'evaluation apprehension' (Rosenberg, 1969) and 'experimental stress' (Back & Bogdonoff, 1967), and suggest that some subjects may be more susceptible than others to such aspects. They argue that the Negro may be such a subject, and that in an all-white environment would tend to be defensive, and to regard observation and evaluation of his behaviour as equivalent to his being asked for proof of the adequacy of himself and of Negroes in general. They suggest that previous evidence (Back & Bogdonoff, 1967), which showed that subjects recruited in groups of friends were less aroused throughout an experiment than subjects recruited individually as strangers, is relevant to examination of Negro/white interactions. Further, they suggest that greater conformity (e.g., in Crutchfield, 1955; Gerard, 1961) is found in groups of friends: thus, it might be that the Negro recruited in a group of friends, would have a particular protection in 'experimental stress'. Finally, they describe the variable of prior exposure to some aspects of the experimental environment, citing a study in which subjects so treated subsequently showed less general arousal when tested.

Having these considerations in mind therefore, Back et al. (1969) devised a study in which 95 white and 72 Negro subjects were tested in a conformity situation, half being recruited as groups of friends and half as individual strangers. Previous experience was included as a variable, and the index of arousal used was plasma FFA level (Back & Bogdonoff, 1965). There were some predicted differences in FFA levels for the 'friends/strangers' and 'previous experience' variables, and results suggested that the Negro subjects tended to develop strong group ties in the experiment. Their FFA levels suggested a failure to relax during the rest period, which Back et al. (1969) compare with the previously described (Lazarus et al., 1966) response of Japanese subjects to the general experimental situation rather than to specific events. This may be a characteristic feature of the subject who finds the psychological experiment a stressor. Perhaps the 'unstable introvert' previously mentioned (p. 60) is such a subject: the difficulty experienced in recruiting this subgroup, in contrast to the relative ease with which stable extraverts were obtained supports this suggestion.

Back and co-workers have also examined the response of 'friends' and 'strangers' in psychopharmacological studies: this is described in Section 3.5.4. which provides a brief account of drug responses.

3.5.4. Drug responses

There is a complexity of factors determining the human subjects' response to drugs (Prescott, 1974), one of which is the susceptibility of an individual to the placebo effect. Claridge (1970) has described relevant studies of 'suggestibility', acquiescence, and the effect of group influences on drug response in a chapter on the placebo effect. He reports, for example, that in a study by Knowles and Lucas (1960), where a placebo was administered in both 'individual' and 'group' conditions, there was a significant positive relationship between neuroticism (as measured by the Maudsley Personality Inventory) and the number of placebo side-effects reported, but only in the 'group' condition. Back, Oelfke, Brehm, Bogdonoff and Nowlin (1970) have examined an effect of the tranquillizer chlordiazepoxide hydrochloride (Librium) on subjects grouped as 'friends' or 'strangers'. As in the previously described study of Back *et al.* (1969), dependent measures included the extent of conforming behaviour, and changes in plasma FFA. When subjects were divided into groups with high and low initial anxiety the former, when tested as 'strangers' and given the tranquillizer, showed an *increase* in physiological arousal, and greater conformity. The authors cite earlier work with FFA (Back, Bogdonoff, Shaw & Klein, 1963) and the electrodermal data of Costell and Leiderman (1968) as evidence for their suggestion that conforming behaviour tends to be a way of reducing autonomic arousal, and hence is seen in their anxious subjects.

The influence of the group on drug response, and the individual differences in this interaction, is perhaps common knowledge to any barmaid: Eysenck's (1957) more systematic observation of alcohol/personality interaction is part of a comprehensive account of studies with his dimension of extraversion and neuroticism, and the interaction of personality and drug effect.

3.6. THE LABORATORY ENVIRONMENT

So little material being available for this section, the social psychologists' and psychophysiologists' material have been combined. Most of the psychophysiological material consists of hunches and observations which have accrued from experience with human subjects in the laboratory. A recently published review (Kiritz & Moos, 1974) presents ... a model for conceptualizing social environment, and discusses implications for person–environment interaction.' The 'social environment' of Kiritz and Moos is, of course, broader than that of the laboratory, but this review provides a most useful collection of the somewhat widely dispensed material which is relevant to the topic. The social psychologists' contributions are little better: Reicken wrote in 1962 that little is known about how the physical environment, properties and apparatus in view may affect the subject. Rosenthal (1969), however, describes both direct and indirect effects of the 'scene' in which the experiment takes place: Mintz (1959) reported that subjects judged others to be less happy when judgments were made in an 'ugly' laboratory, and as evidence of the indirect effect Rosenthal describes data collected with Woolsey. Their eight laboratory rooms were varied as to the 'professionalness', 'orderliness', and 'comfortableness' in appearance. Fourteen experimenters were assigned to the eight laboratories and were reported as taking the experiment significantly more seriously if they had been assigned to a laboratory which was both more disordered and less comfortable: they were, however, graduate students in the natural sciences or in law school! In contrast to this the more experienced experimenter, and particularly a psychophysiologist with a demanding testing schedule, may well prefer an orderly and systematic environment in which he may attempt to retain his 'efficiency and serenity' (Venables & Christie, 1973).

These authors provide some general suggestions for the psychophysiologist, and Wenger (1962) reports on the significance of temperature, pressure, and humidity. Experimenters may well profit from consideration of the 'design' of their laboratory in addition to the design of their experiment. At the most simple level of analysis the unfamiliarity of the laboratory and equipment may, for a subject not habituated to such surroundings, elicit a psychophysiological reaction. The intensity of this could vary along the arousal continuum, from orienting to the novelty of the scene to a 'fight and flight' response to its perceived threat. The nature and extent of a subject's reaction might well represent interactions between personality characteristics and previous experience: thus the sight of a multi-channel pen recorder purring away in the laboratory might well elicit quite different responses in a stable, extraverted engineer, to those of a neurotic, introverted classicist.

The comfort of a laboratory, in terms of heat, light and ventilation needs, when the experimenter has control over such variables, to be viewed from the subjects' rather than the experimenters' stance. Thus a temperature comfortable for a researcher busy with his various activities in an adjacent room may be distinctly chilly for a subject attempting to relax for half an hour of immobility. Similarly random noise may be virtually unnoticed by the experimenter to whom it is wholly familiar, but its novelty to the subject intensifies its effects on his psychophysiological state.

A more complex aspect of situational effects on a subject is introduced with Orne's work on the 'demand characteristics' of an experiment. Orne (1962, 1969) has argued that the subject perceives the totality of cues from the experimental environment and generates an hypothesis concerning the nature of the experimenters' aim which significantly determines his, the subject's, behaviour. Orne labels the sum total of such cues the 'demand characteristics' of the experimental situation, in which subjects actively try to figure out how to be 'good subjects' in order to 'validate the experimental hypothesis' and thus 'further science'.

Characteristics of the laboratory may serve as 'demand characteristics' in two ways: they may reflect the personality of the experimenter and reinforce his unintentional cues to the subject, or they may predispose the subject to be influenced by the experimenter. Gale (1973) has suggested a relation between an experimenter's unnecessarily imprecise instructions to a subject, and the latter's need to use cues from the laboratory environment in an attempt to resolve ambiguity. Sternbach (1964) also has related Orne's work to his findings on the effects of instructional sets on autonomic responsivity.

Perhaps a suitable conclusion to this attempt at 'social psychophysiology' is a quotation from Gale (1973): 'Psychophysiology does have its own brand of sophisticated alchemy, of course; there are now several manuals of a very technical nature, which discuss (in what may appear to the outsider as obsessional and excruciating detail) problems of electronic circuitry, electrode preparation and placement, waveform analysis, computer storage of data, and so on. My view is that this sophistication has been misplaced, since technical aspects have often been overemphasized at the expense of the art of experimentation.' And that art necessitates an awareness of all the complexities of social interaction which are involved in 'being an E' and 'being an S'.

3.7. ACKNOWLEDGMENT

This chapter was written during tenure of a grant from the Social Science Research Council, and while the authors were in the Department of Psychology, Birkbeck College, University of London.

3.8. REFERENCES

Adair, J. C. & Epstein, J. S. Verbal cues in the mediation of experimenter bias. *Psychological Reports*, 1968, **22**, 1045–1053.

Adair, J. C. & Fenton, D. P. Subjects' attitudes toward psychology as a determinant of experimental results. *Canadian Journal of Behavioral Science*, 1971, **3**, 268–275.

Back, K. W. & Bogdonoff, M. D. Plasma lipid responses to leadership, conformity and deviation. In P. H. Leiderman & D. Shapiro (Eds), *Psychobiological approaches to social behaviour*. London: Tavistock, 1965.

Back, K. W. & Bogdonoff, M. D. Buffer conditions in experimental stress. *Behavioral Science*, 1967, **12**, 384–390.

Back, K. W., Bogdonoff, M. D., Shaw, D. M. & Klein, R. F. An interpretation of experimental conformity through physiological measures. *Behavioral Science*, 1963, **8**, 34–40.

Back, K. W., Oelfke, S. R., Brehm, M. L., Bogdonoff, M. D. & Nowlin, J. B. Physiological and situational factors in psychopharmacological experiments. *Psychophysiology*, 1970, **6**, 749–760.

Back, K. W., Wilson, S. R., Bogdonoff, M. D. & Troyer, W. G. Racial environment, cohesion, conformity, and stress. *Journal of Psychosomatic Research*, 1969, **13**, 27–36.

Barber, P. J. & Rushton, J. P. Experimenter bias and subliminal perception. In preparation for *British Journal of Psychology*, 1974.

Barber, T. X. & Silver, M. H. Fact, fiction and the experimenter bias effect. *Psychological Bulletin*, 1968, **70**, 1–29.

Bernstein, A. S. Race and examiner as significant influences on basal skin impedance. *Journal of Personality and Social Psychology*, 1965, **1**, 346–349.

Bloom, R. & Tesser, A. On reducing experimenter bias: the affects of forewarning. *Canadian Journal of Behavioral Science*, 1971, **3**, 198–208.

Bogdonoff, M. D., Brehm, L. & Back, K. The effect of the experimenter role upon the subjects' response to an unpleasant task. *Journal of Psychosomatic Research*, 1964, 137–143.

Boring, E. G. Perspective: Artifact and control. In R. Rosenthal & R. L. Rosnow (Eds), *Artifact in behavioural research*. New York: Academic Press, 1969, Chap. 1.

Brown, C. C. Psychophysiology at an interface. *Psychophysiology*, 1966, **3**, 1–7.

Campbell, D. T. Prospective: Artifact and control. In R. Rosenthal & R. L. Rosnow (Eds), *Artifact in behavioural research*. New York: Academic Press, 1969, Chap. 8.

Chapman, A. J. An electromyographic study of apprehension about evaluation. *Psychological Reports*, 1973, **33**, 811–814.

Chapman, A. J. An electromyographic study of social facilitation: A test of the 'mere presence' hypothesis. *British Journal of Psychology*, 1974, **65**, 123–128.

Christie, M. J. & Venables, P. H. Characteristics of palmar skin potential and conductance in relaxed human subjects. *Psychophysiology*, 1971, **8**, 523–532.

Christie, M. J. & Venables, P. H. Site, state, and subject characteristics of resting skin potentials. *Psychophysiology*, 1972, **9**, 645–649.

Christie, M. J. & Venables, P. H. Mood changes in relation to age, EPI scores, time, and day. *British Journal of Social and Clinical Psychology*, 1973, **12**, 61–72.

Christie, M. J. & Venables, P. H. Change in palmar skin potential level during relaxation after stress. *Journal of Psychosomatic Research*, 1974, **18**, 301–306.

Claridge, G. *Drugs and human behaviour*. Harmondsworth: Penguin, 1970.

Costell, R. M. & Leiderman, P. H. Psychological concomitants of social stress: The effects of conformity pressure. *Psychosomatic Medicine*, 1968, **30**, 298–310.

Crutchfield, R. S. Conformity and character, *American Psychologist*, 1955, **10**, 191–198.

Duncan, S., Rosenberg, N. J. & Finkelstein, J. *The social nature of psychological research*. New York: Basic Books, 1967.

Eysenck, H. J. *Dynamics of anxiety and hysteria*. London: Routledge, 1957.

Eysenck, H. J. (Ed.) *Experiments with drugs*. Oxford: Pergamon, 1963.

Eysenck, H. J. *The biological basis of personality*. Springfield, Illinois, Charles C. Thomas, 1967.

Fisher, L. E. & Kotses, H. Race differences and experimenter race effect in galvanic skin response. *Psychophysiology*, 1973, **10**, 578–582.

Fisher, L. E. & Kotses, H. Experimenter and subject sex effects in the skin conductance response. *Psychophysiology*, 1974, **11**, 191–196.

Forrester, B. J. & Klaus, R. A. The effect of race of examiner on intelligence test scores of Negro kindergarten children. *Peabody Papers in Human Development*, 1964, **2**, 1–7.

Fowles, D. C. & Venables, P. H. The effects of epidermal hydration and sodium reabsorption on palmar skin potential. *Psychological Bulletin*, 1970, **73**, 363–378.

Gale, A. The psychophysiology of individual differences: studies of extraversion and EEG. In P. Kline (Ed.), *New approaches in psychological measurements*. London: Wiley, 1973.

Gale, A., Chapman, A. J., Spratt, G. S. & Smallbone, A. EEG correlates of interpersonal distance and eye contact. *Journal of Personality and Social Psychology*, 1974. (In press).

Gale, A., Lucas, B., Nissim, R. & Harpham, B. Some EEG correlates of face-to-face contact. *British Journal of Social and Clinical Psychology*, 1972, **11**, 326–332.

Gerard, H. B. Disagreement with others, their credibility and experienced stress. *Journal of Abnormal and Social Psychology*, 1961, **62**, 554–564.

Gibinski, K., Giec, L., Zmudzinski, J., Waclawczyk, J. & Dosiak, J. Body side related asymmetry in sweat gland function. *Journal of Investigative Dermatology*, 1971, **57**, 190–192.

Heisenberg, W. *Physics and philosophy*. New York: Harper, 1958.

Hicks, R. G. Experimenter effects on the physiological experiment. *Psychophysiology*, 1970, **7**, 10–17.

Hicks, R. G. Converging operations in the psychological experiment. *Psychophysiology*, 1971, **8**, 93–101.

Hutt, C. *Males and females*. Harmondsworth: Penguin, 1972.

Johnson, L. C. & Corah, N. L. Racial differences in skin resistance. *Science*, 1963, **139**, 766–767.

Johnson, L. C. & Landon, M. M. Eccrine sweat gland activity and racial differences in resting skin conductance. *Psychophysiology*, 1965, **1**, 322–329.

Juniper, K. & Dykman, R. A. Skin resistance, sweat-gland counts, salivary flow, and gastric secretion: Age, race, and sex differences, and intercorrelations. *Psychophysiology*, 1967, **4**, 216–222.

Katz, I. & Greenbaum, C. Effects of anxiety, threat, and racial environment task performance of Negro college students. *Journal of Abnormal and Social Psychology*, 1963, **66**, 562–576.

Kiritz, S. & Moos, R. H. Physiological effects of social environments. *Psychosomatic Medicine*, 1974, **36**, 96–114.

Knowles, J. B. & Lucas, C. J. Experimental studies of the placebo response. *Journal of Mental Science*, 1960, **106**, 231–240.

Kopacz, F. M. & Smith, B. D. Sex difference in skin conductance measures as a function of shock threat. *Psychophysiology*, 1971, **8**, 293–303.

Kugelmass, S. & Lieblich, I. Relation between ethnic origin and GSR reactivity in psychophysiological detection. *Journal of Applied Psychology*, 1968, **52**, 158–162.

Lana, R. E. Pretest sensitization. In R. Rosenthal & R. L. Rosnow (Eds), *Artifact in behavioural research*. New York: Academic Press, 1969.

Lazarus, J., Tomita, M., Opton, E. & Kodama, M. A cross-cultural study of stress reaction patterns in Japan. *Journal of Personality and Social Psychology*, 1966, **4**, 622–633.

Leiderman, P. H. & Shapiro, D. (Eds), *Psychobiological approaches to social behaviour*. London: Tavistock, 1965.

Lieblich, I., Kugelmass, S. & Ben-Shakhar, G. Psychobiological baselines as a function of race and ethnic origin. *Psychophysiology*, 1973, **10**, 426–430.

McFall, R. M. & Shenkein, B. Experimenter expectancy effects, need for achievement, and field dependence. *Journal of Experimental Research in Personality*, 1970, **4**, 122–128.

McGuire, W. J. Suspiciousness of experimenters' intent. In: R. Rosenthal & R. L. Rosnow (Eds), 1969, *op. cit.*

Minor, M. W. Experimenter-expectancy effect as a function of evaluation apprehension. *Journal of Personality and Social Psychology*, 1970, **15**, 326–332.

Mintz, N. On the psychology of aesthetics and architecture. Unpublished paper, Brandeis University, 1959.

Orne, M. T. On the social psychology of the psychological experiment: With particular reference to demand characteristics and their implications. *American Psychologist*, 1962, **17**, 776–783.

Orne, M. T. Demand characteristics and the concept of quasi-controls. Chapter 5, In R. Rosenthal & R. L. Rosnow (Eds), *Artifact in behavioral research*. New York: Academic Press, 1969.

Pasnau, R. O., Naitoh, P., Stier, S. & Kollar, E. J. The psychological effects of 205 hours of sleep deprivation. *Archives of General Psychiatry*, 1968, **18**, 496–505.

Porier, G. W. & Lott, A. J. Galvanic skin responses and prejudice. *Journal of Personality and Social Psychology*, 1967, **5**, 253–259.

Prescott, L. F. Variation in the clinical response to drugs. Chapter 62, In R. Passmore & J. S. Robson (Eds), *A companion to medical studies*, Vol. 3, Part 2. Oxford: Blackwell, 1974.

Rankin, R. E. & Campbell, D. T. Galvanic skin responses to Negro and white experimenters. *Journal of Abnormal and Social Psychology*, 1955, **51**, 30–33.

Riecken, H. W. A program for research on experiments in social psychology. In N. F. Washburne (Ed.), *Decisions, values and groups*. Vol. 2. New York: Pergamon Press, 1962, 25–41.

Roethlisberger, F. J. & Dickson, W. J. *Management and the worker*. Cambridge, Massachusetts: Harvard, University, 1939.

Rosenberg, M. J. The conditions and consequences of evaluation apprehension Chapter 7, In R. Rosenthal & R. L. Rosnow (Eds), 1969, *op. cit.*

Rosenthal, R. *Experimenter effects in behavioral research*. New York: Appleton-Century-Crofts, 1966.

Rosenthal, R. covert communciation in the psychological experiment. *Psychological Bulletin*, 1967, **67**, 357–367.

Rosenthal, R. Interpersonal expectations: Effects of the experimenters' hypothesis. In R. Rosenthal and R. L. Rosnow (Eds), 1969, *op. cit.*

Rosenthal, R. & Fode, K. L. The effect of experimenter bias on the performance of the albino rat. *Behavioral Science*, 1963, **8**, 183–189.

Rosenthal, R. & Rosnow, R. L. (Eds), *Artifact in behavioural research*. New York: Academic Press, 1969.

Sattler, J. M. Racial 'experimenter effects' in experimentation, testing, interviewing and psychotherapy. *Psychological Bulletin*, 1970, **73**, 137–160.

Schultz, D. P. The human subject in psychological research. *Psychological Bulletin*, 1969, **72**, 214–228.

Schwartz, G. E. & Shapiro, D. Social psychophysiology. Chapter 8, In W. F. Prokasy & D. C. Raskin (Eds.), *Electrodermal activity in psychological research*. New York: Academic Press, 1973.

Shapiro, D. & Crider, A. Psychophysiological approaches to social psychology. In G. Lindzey & E. Aronson (Eds), *The handbook of social psychology*, Vol. III, (2nd ed.), Reading, Massachusetts: Addison-Wesley, 1969, 1–49.

Shapiro, D. & Schwartz, G. E. Psychophysiological contributions to social psychology, *Annual Review of Psychology*, 1970, **21**, 87–112.

Sternbach, R. A. The effects of instructional sets on autonomic responsivity, *Psychophysiology*, 1964, **1**, 67–72.

Sternbach, R. A. *Principles of Psychophysiology*, 1966, New York: Academic Press.

Sternbach, R. A. & Tursky, B. Ethnic differences among housewives in psychophysical and skin potential responses to electric shock. *Psychophysiology*, 1965, **4**, 67–74.

Trattner, J. H. & Howard, K. I. A preliminary investigation of covert communication of expectancies of schizophrenics. *Journal of Abnormal Psychology*, 1970, **75**, 245–247.

Tursky, B. Physical, physiological and psychological factors that affect pain reaction to electric shock. *Psychophysiology*, 1974, **11**, 95–112.

Tursky, B. & Sternbach, R. A. Further physiological correlates of ethnic differences in responses to shock. *Psychophysiology*, 1967, **4**, 67–74.

Venables, P. H. Partial failure of cortical-subcortical integration as a factor underlying schizophrenic behavior. In J. Romano (Ed.), *The origins of schizophrenia*. Amsterdam: Excerpta Medica Foundation, 1967.

Venables, P. H. & Christie, M. J. Mechanisms, instrumentation, recording, and quantification. In W. F. Prokasy & D. C. Raskin (Eds) *Electrodermal activity in psychological research*. New York: Academic Press, 1973, Chap. 1.

Wenger, M. (with T. D. Cullen). Some problems in psychophysiological research. In R. Roessler & N. S. Greenfield (Eds), *Physiological correlates of psychological disorder*. Madison: University of Wisconsin Press, 1962.

White, C. R. The effect of induced subject expectations on the experimenter bias situation. Unpublished doctoral dissertation, University of North Dakota, 1962.

68

Williams, R. B., Kimball, C. P., & Williard, H. N. The influence of interpersonal interaction on diastolic blood pressure. *Psychosomatic Medicine*, 1972, **34,** 194–198.

Wuebben, P. L., Straits, B. C. & G. I. Schulman (Eds), *The experiment as a social occasion.* Glendessary Press, 1974.

Zajonc, R. B. Compresence (Paper read to the Mid-Western Psychological Association, Cleveland, Ohio, 1972.).

SECTION 2

States

Chapter 4

Sympathetic-Adrenomedullary Activity, Behaviour and the Psychosocial Environment

MARIANNE FRANKENHAEUSER

Psychological Laboratories
University of Stockholm

4.1. INTRODUCTION

The sensitivity of the sympathetic-adrenomedullary system to psychological stimuli was first demonstrated by Walter B. Cannon and his associates at Harvard during the early part of this century. These investigators performed a series of experiments in which cats were exposed to emotionally exciting events, such as barking dogs, and adrenomedullary secretion was determined by bioassay procedures. The results obtained in these experiments led Cannon (1914) to formulate the 'emergency function' theory of adrenomedullary activity, based on the view that many of the physiological effects of adrenaline are 'directly serviceable in making the organism more efficient in the struggle which fear or rage or pain may involve'. (For a review of the early work the reader is referred to Cannon, 1929.)

The work by Euler (1946, 1956) and by Holtz, Credner, & Kroneberg (1947) during the 1940's showed that noradrenaline, the nonmethylated homologue of adrenaline, was the adrenergic neurotransmittor as well as an adrenomedullary hormone. These findings, together with Selye's (1950) important work on pituitary-adrenocortical activity in adaptation to stress, and the concomitant advances in biochemical techniques, inspired new research efforts in the behaviourally-oriented work. New methods became available, which were sufficiently sensitive to permit the measurement of small amounts of hormones in plasma and in urine.

The field was thus opened for new psychoendocrine approaches, and since the beginning of the 1950's interest and knowledge have been steadily growing. This chapter reviews the present state of knowledge about peripheral adrenaline and noradrenaline, as measured by urinary excretion, in relation to psychosocial stimuli.

4.1.1. Adrenomedullary secretion

Histochemical studies (Hillarp & Hökfelt, 1953) have shown that adrenaline and noradrenaline occur in different chromaffine cells in the adrenal medulla. The major part of the catecholamines in the chromaffine cells is located in subcellular granules (Blaschko, 1973; Blaschko & Welch, 1953; Hillarp, Lagerstedt, & Nilson, 1953). The metabolism of the catecholamines proceeds in the chromaffine cell from tyrosine, dopa, and dopamine to noradrenaline and adrenaline.

The secreting cells of the adrenal medulla are intimately connected with preganglionic fibres of the sympathetic nervous system, and their secretory activity is controlled by stimulation through these nervous pathways. Stimulation of the splanchnic nerve induces an increase in secretion, while section of this nerve prevents secretion.

Adrenomedullary secretion can be elicited by electrical stimulation of different parts of the brain, both in the hypothalamic and mesencephalic regions, and in certain cortical areas (cf. review by Euler, 1967). It is particularly interesting that adrenaline and noradrenaline can be selectively released by stimulation of specific areas in the hypothalamus (Folkow & Euler, 1954; Redgate & Gellhorn, 1953).

Among the stimuli known to elicit increased secretion should be mentioned: cold, pain, anoxia, hypoglycemia, hypotension, haemorrhage, burns, and physical exercise. Some of these stimuli (e.g., pain, heat, and cold) presumably induce the adrenomedullary secretion primarily by reflex action. The proportion of adrenaline and noradrenaline released by the different stimuli differs characteristically: hypoglycemia, for example, raises adrenaline secretion only.

Various chemical stimuli, e.g. morphine and ether, influence adrenomedullary secretion. Of special interest in the present context is that moderate doses of drugs in common use, such as caffeine, alcohol, and nicotine, cause a marked rise in adrenaline output (Frankenhaeuser, Myrsten, Post, & Johansson, 1971; Frankenhaeuser, Myrsten, Waszak, Neri, & Post, 1968).

Adrenomedullary secretion varies widely under different psychosocial conditions. Under rest and inactivity secretion is generally low, under ordinary daily activities secretion rises to about twice the resting level, and under moderately stressful conditions secretion rates corresponding to between three and five times the resting level are often noted. Severe stressors may induce a further pronounced increase, to levels indicative of pheochromocytoma. A detailed account of effects of psychosocial stimulation is given in Section 4.2.

4.1.2. Action of adrenomedullary hormones

The hormones of the adrenal medulla act on all organs of the body innervated by the sympathetic nervous system, and generally produce effects similar to sympathetic stimulation. The role of these hormones as specific activators of physiological mechanisms under conditions of emergency has already been pointed out. The stimulating effect on the heart, the dilation of the coronary vessels, the vasodilation in the voluntary muscles, the vasoconstriction in the intestinal tract, the decreased peristalsis of the alimentary canal as well as metabolic actions such as mobilization of glucose and of fat, are examples of functions that may all be regarded as serving the goal of preparing the organism to meet threatening situations.

There are distinct differences between adrenaline and noradrenaline with regard to some circulatory and metabolic actions. In general, noradrenaline is more potent in raising blood pressure, and less potent in its metabolic action and in relaxing smooth muscle. However, as emphasized by Euler (1967), recent observations have brought out important similarities in action: both hormones, for example, mobilize fat and increase oxygen consumption.

When comparing the actions of the adrenomedullary hormones, it should also be kept in mind that the proportions of noradrenaline and adrenaline differ widely in different species. In man, as in most species, noradrenaline constitutes the relatively smaller part of the two hormones. However, adrenomedullary secretion is often combined with increased sympathetic nervous activity in general, in which case the noradrenaline liberated directly at the nerve endings must also be taken into account.

The question of a direct action of the adrenomedullary hormones on the central nervous system is of particular interest in the context of behavioural studies. The evidence now available strongly suggests that adrenaline crosses the blood–brain barrier in the region of the hypothalamus, and acts directly on the mesencephalic reticular formation and the posterior hypothalamus (Euler, 1967; Rothballer, 1959; Schildkraut & Kety, 1967). Intravenously infused adrenaline produces a transient EEG activation. It is interesting, that this effect appears in drowsy and sleeping animals only, while it is not evident in animals which are already aroused (*cf.* Rothballer, 1967).

4.1.3. Urinary and plasma catecholamines as indicators of sympathetic-adrenomedullary activity

The liberated catecholamines are partly metabolized enzymically within the cytoplasm or absorbed from the tissues by adrenergic nerves. A small fraction of the liberated amines is excreted in urine as free adrenaline and noradrenaline. This fraction can be estimated quantitatively by biological assay or by fluorimetry combined with chemical separtation methods.

Under normal conditions most of the adrenaline excreted in urine is derived from the adrenal medulla. With regard to noradrenaline excretion, the greater part presumably comes from the sympathetic nerve endings. The adrenaline excreted in urine represents a rough quantitative estimate of adrenomedullary activity. Urinary noradrenaline probably gives a less reliable estimate of sympathetic activity, since a large part of the noradrenaline released is re-absorbed by the nerve endings or bound to various tissues, and does not enter the blood stream or urine. However, in spite of these methodological difficulties, estimates of urinary adrenaline and noradrenaline obtained by the fluorimetric technique (Euler & Lishajko, 1961) show a relatively high constancy over time provided that the conditions under which urine is sampled are carefully standardized. The reliability of the fluorimetric technique, as determined by the correlation between halved urine samples analysed by a skilled technician, is also satisfactory (Levi, 1972; Pátkai & Frankenhaeuser, 1964). An improved automated procedure has recently been developed (Andersson, Hovmöller, Karlsson & Svensson, 1973).

Additional information can be obtained by measuring the major catecholamine metabolites, i.e. metanephrine, normetanephrine, 3-methoxy-4-hydroxy-phenylglycol, and 3-methoxy-4-hydroxy-phenylglycollic acid. These metabolites constitute a much larger proportion of the total catecholmine release than do the free catecholamines. So far, however, little is known about the constancy of this proportion.

Methods are also available for measuring catecholamines in plasma (e.g., Häggendahl, 1963). One advantage of plasma measurements is that they permit precise timing of transient changes in hormone secretion. However, since the half-life of adrenaline in the blood is very short, approximately 1·5 min, the blood level is extremely sensitive to the rate of disappearance. Trying to compensate for this by drawing serial blood-samples introduces a new stressor, which cannot be ignored in behavioural studies.

Urinary catecholamines represent estimates of sympathetic-adrenomedullary activity integrated over extended time periods, usually 1 to 3 h. Such measurements are particularly well suited for studying psychosocial influences of everyday life. The fact that measurements can be made on unrestricted human beings, adds to the usefulness of the method in behavioural research.

4.2. THE INFLUENCE OF PSYCHOSOCIAL FACTORS ON SYMPATHETIC-ADRENOMEDULLARY ACTIVITY

In this section, the influence exerted by psychosocial factors on the sympathetic-adrenomedullary system will be illustrated by reviewing a series of experimental studies. These studied have been chosen with the aim of emphasizing the importance of the psychological element in the widely different conditions which affect sympathetic-adrenomedullary activity.

4.2.1. Novelty, habituation, and control

Exposure to novel and unfamiliar environments is generally accompanied by increased catecholamine secretion. In fact, the sympathetic-adrenomedullary system is very sensitive to any element of novelty in the environment. Thus, increased adrenaline secretion is not only elicited by unusual and extreme environments, but a rise in adrenaline release may occur in any new environmental setting. This particular aspect of adrenomedullary sensitivity should be taken into account in laboratory experiments, since a subject who pays his first visit to the laboratory and meets the observer for the first time, usually shows a marked elevation in adrenaline excretion, even when he is not exposed to any experimental stressor. Baseline values for adrenomedullary activity therefore cannot be obtained until the subject has become acquainted with the observer and the laboratory setting.

Adrenaline excretion is thus a sensitive indicator of habituation to environmental influences, and the amount of adrenaline excreted closely reflects the intensity of the subjective arousal evoked by the stimulating condition. The human centrifuge provides a suitable tool for studying these relationships, since exposure to gravitational stress, when a novel experience, elicits a strong emotional response which tends to diminish when the experience is repeated. Figure 4.1 shows data from an experiment (Frankenhaeuser, Sterky, & Järpe, 1962), in which a group of university students took part in six sessions, spaced at one week, which were identical with regard to G-load. An important feature of this investigation was that estimates of subjective stress were obtained by the method of ratio estimation, a direct scaling method. At the end of each session the subject estimated the degree of arousal experienced during the session as a percentage of the arousal experienced during the previous session. In Figure 4.1 the estimates of arousal, expressed in relation to the first session, have been plotted against the amount of adrenaline excreted, each point in the diagram corresponding to one session. It is seen that there was a close agreement between adrenaline excretion and subjective arousal. Noradrenaline excretion was markedly increased by gravitational stress but, in contrast to adrenaline excretion, showed no tendency to diminish with repeated exposure. It is important to note that the two hormones serve clearly different functions in this particular situation, where noradrenaline secretion may be regarded as part of the homeostatic cardiovascular mechanism counteracting the fall in blood pressure in the upper parts of the body during exposure to gravitational stress.

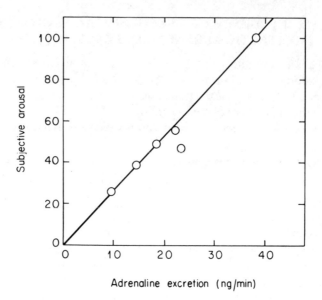

FIGURE 4.1. Mean estimates of subjective stress plotted against mean adrenaline excretion during each of six identical sessions involving exposure to gravitational stress in a human centrifuge. Each point corresponds to one session. Reprinted with permission of publisher: Frankenhaeuser, M., Sterky, K. & Järpe, G., *Perceptual and Motor Skills*, 1962, **15**, 63–72

It should be emphasized that repeated exposure to one and the same physical situation is accompanied by decreased catecholamine secretion only in so far as the repetition is associated with a decrease in the state of subjective arousal. Under conditions where subjective arousal remains at a high level, adrenaline output also stays high. An example is provided by results from an investigation (Bloom, Euler, & Frankenhaeuser, 1963) concerned with physiological reactions to parachute jumping, an activity which retains its stressful and threatening character also after long experience. Figure 4.2 shows the mean catecholamine excretion in a group of trainees performing their first jump, and in a group of officers who had previously performed between 14 and 80 jumps. It is seen that the increase in catecholamine excretion occurring under the condition involving parachute-jumping as compared with a period of ground activity, was of about the same magnitude in officers as in trainees.

Sympathetic-adrenomedullary activity is usually increased under conditions characterized by unpredictability and uncontrollability (Frankenhaeuser & Rissler, 1970a). If the subject is given more control over the situation, and if his feelings of helplessness are thereby reduced, his adrenaline output is likely to be lowered.

The influence of situational control is illustrated in Figure 4.3. by data from an experiment (Frankenhaeuser & Rissler, 1970b) in which the degree

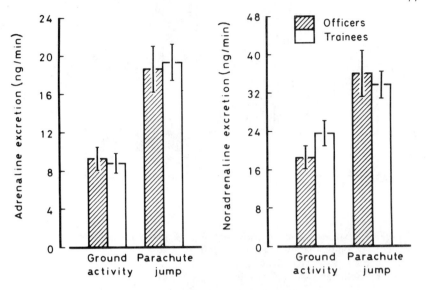

FIGURE 4.2. Means and standard errors for adrenaline and noradrenalinc excretion in a group of officers and a group of paratroop trainees during periods in which either ground activity or parachute jumps were performed. Redrawn and reprinted with permission from Bloom, G., Euler, U.S.v. & Frankenhaeuser, M., *Acta Physiologica Scandinavica*, 1963, **58**, 77–89

of control that the subject was allowed to exert was systematically varied. In Session I the subject was exposed to unpredictable and uncontrollable electric shocks. Under these conditions adrenaline excretion was about three times as high as during a relaxation period (Session IV). Such a rise in adrenaline output can be counteracted by increasing the subject's control over the situation as was done in Sessions II and III where a choice-reaction task was performed. While in Session I the subject had to remain passive and was unable to avoid shock, his ability to cope with the task in the two subsequent sessions influenced the amount of punishment that he received. In Session II the subject was often unjustly punished, while in Session III most shocks could be avoided by rapid performance. As seen in Figure 4.3 adrenaline output (left-hand diagram) decreased successively as the degree of control was varied from a state of helplessness to ability to master the disturbing influences. Noradrenaline excretion (right-hand diagram) was not much affected by degree of control, but remained slightly elevated as long as the subject was engaged in the attention-demanding activity.

4.2.2. Level of stimulation

Individuals living in various extreme environments are likely to become exposed to either stimulus excess or stimulus deprivation, both of which may activate the endocrine response systems. However, also individuals living

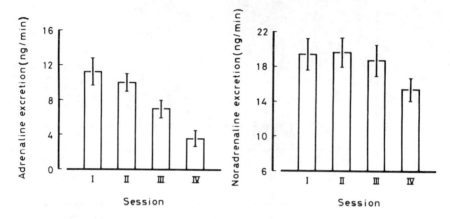

FIGURE 4.3. Means and standard errors for adrenaline and noradrenaline excretion under four conditions. In Sessions I, II and III the subject's control of the situation was successively increased. Session IV was a control condition. Redrawn and reprinted with permission from Frankenhaeuser, M. & Rissler, A., *Psychopharmacologia*, 1970, **17**, 378–390

under ordinary life conditions are subjected to varying levels of stimulation. In fact, stimulus overload and perceptual monotony represent two contrasting environmental influences to which people living in industrialized societies are commonly exposed. It is therefore of interest to find out if sympathetic-adrenomedullary responses are elicited also by relatively minor changes in level of stimulation.

To this end, catecholamine output has been measured in laboratory experiments, in which some aspects of real-life environments have been simulated. Data from an experiment (Frankenhaeuser, Nordheden, Myrsten, & Post, 1971) involving three levels of stimulation are shown in Figure 4.4. During 'understimulation' the subjects performed a prolonged vigilance task while deprived of normal social and sensory inputs. During the condition of 'medium stimulation' they read magazines and listened to the radio, and during 'overstimulation' they performed a complex sensori-motor task. Both understimulation and overstimulation evoked feelings of unpleasantness, while medium stimulation was perceived as emotionally 'neutral'. It is seen that both adrenaline and noradrenaline output increased during understimulation and overstimulation as compared with the condition involving a medium or 'normal' level of stimulation.

A related problem concerns the change in activation level brought about by physical activity. Since muscular and mental strain often occur together in the same situation, for instance in physical contests, it has generally not been possible to distinguish between the relative influence on catecholamine output of these two kinds of stimuli. An interesting study was carried out by Elmadjian, Hope, and Lamson (1957) who measured catecholamine excretion in hockey players, some of whom took part in active competition, while others observed

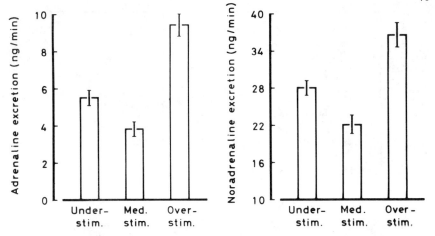

FIGURE 4.4. Means and standard errors for adrenaline and noradrenaline excretion under conditions of understimulation, medium stimulation, and overstimulation. Based on Frankenhaeuser, M., Nordheden, B., Myrsten, A.-L. & Post, B., *Acta Psychologica*, 1971, **35**, 298–308

a game in which they did not participate. The results showed large increases in noradrenaline and smaller increases in adrenaline excretion during active play as compared with increases in adrenaline excretion alone in the physically passive condition.

The same problem was approached in a laboratory study by Frankenhaeuser and her co-workers (Frankenhaeuser, Post, Nordheden, & Sjöberg, 1969) in which a bicycle ergometer was chosen as a suitable tool for varying systematically the physical work load in a 'psychologically neutral' situation. Figure 4.5 shows results obtained in a group of healthy male subjects who participated in a control condition and in three experimental sessions in each of which five successive 6-minute tests, involving different work loads, were performed on a bicycle ergometer. It is seen (Diagram A) that excretion rates of both adrenaline and noradrenaline remained close to control levels at the lower work loads, while the highest work load induced an increase in both catecholamines. Diagram B shows that subjective effort increased consistently with increasing work load. When Diagrams A and B are compared, it is seen that catecholamine excretion remained close to baseline level at the lower work loads, where the subjective effort was judged as 'extremely light', 'very light', or 'fairly light'. When, however, in the condition involving the highest load, the subjective estimate passed the midpoint of the rating scale and approached the point defined as 'laborious', a pronounced increase of both adrenaline and noradrenaline output occurred.

The increased noradrenaline output is readily identified as part of the cardiovascular-response system regulating reactions to muscular work (Diagrams C and D), while the rise in adrenaline output appears to be related to the discomfort perceived during heavy physical strain.

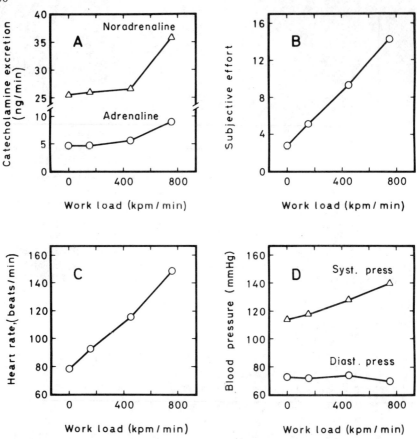

FIGURE 4.5. Mean values for adrenaline and noradrenaline excretion (diagram A), estimates of subjective effort (diagram B), heart rate (diagram C), and blood pressure (diagram D) in a control session and in three sessions involving intermittent work of different loads on a bicycle ergometer. Reprinted with permission of publisher: Frankenhaeuser, M., Post, B., Nordheden, B. & Sjöberg, H., *Perceptual and Motor Skills*, 1969, **28**, 343–349

4.2.3. Affective tone

The investigations cited above suggest that any deviation from the habitual level of stimulation, which is perceived as unpleasant, serves as a stimulus for sympathetic-adrenomedullary activity. The next question is, whether these responses are evoked regardless of the affective quality of the subjective experience accompanying the change in stimulation. In the examples given so far, only negative affects have been involved. A series of investigations will now be described in which the affective quality has been systematically manipulated by varying the stimulus content.

The fact that two different substances, adrenaline and noradrenaline, are involved in mediating the effects of the sympathetic-adrenomedullary system has raised the question of whether these two hormones are selectively released in different affective states. Support for the idea of a differential release of adrenaline and noradrenaline came from several lines of research in the early 1950's.

Among investigations concerned with emotional states in human subjects, Funkenstein's work (1956) aroused particular interest. On the basis of studies concerned with changes in blood pressure induced by injection of mecholyl or adrenaline it was suggested that adrenaline secretion was the predominant response of individuals who tended to direct their anger 'inwardly' when confronted with stressful situations. Noradrenaline secretion, on the other hand, seemed associated with anger directed 'outwardly'. This idea appeared consistent with the results reported by Ax (1953) who, using a variety of polygraphic measurements, found that laboratory situations designed to elicit fear versus anger gave rise to different patterns of cardiovascular responses, i.e. 'adrenaline-like' versus 'noradrenaline-like' responses. Further support was obtained from some of the early studied of catecholamine excretion (Elmadjian *et al.*, 1957; Silverman & Cohen, 1960), which suggested that adrenaline secretion was associated with anxious reactions and noradrenaline secretion with aggressive reactions.

Later studies, however, lend no support to the assumption that adrenaline and noradrenaline would be selectively released in different emotional states. Instead, the general picture indicates that adrenaline is secreted in a variety of affective states, including both anger and fear. Similarly, a rise in noradrenaline secretion may occur in different affective states, but the threshold for noradrenaline release in response to psychosocial stimulation is generally much higher than for adrenaline secretion.

These conclusions are based on a series of studies from the laboratories of Frankenhaeuser (reviewed by Frankenhaeuser, 1971a, 1971b) and Levi (reviewed by Levi, 1972) during the 1960's, in which catecholamine-excretion rates in different experimental situations were related to self-estimates of the intensity and the quality of affect in the acute situation (e.g., Frankenhaeuser & Kåreby, 1962; Levi, 1965) as well as to ratings of more enduring personality characteristics including aggressive and anxious response tendencies (Frankenhaeuser & Pátkai, 1965; Frankenhaeuser, Mellis, Rissler, Björkvall & Pátkai, 1968).

Of special interest in this connection are studies (Levi, 1965, 1972) showing that sympathetic-adrenormedullary stimulation does not occur solely under conditions perceived as unpleasant or agitating, but that amusing situations, which evoke pleasant emotional states, may also be accompanied by increased catecholamine output. A further important finding is that emotionally 'neutral' situations, which evoke feelings of equanimity and tranquillity, may be accompanied by a decrease in sympathetic-adrenomedullary activity.

This is illustrated in Figure 4.6 which shows the mean catecholamine-excretion rates in subjects who were shown four different films, selected with the aim of evoking feelings of either equanimity, amusement, aggressiveness, and fright. Ratings of subjective reactions showed that each film did, in fact, induce the expected emotional reaction. Measurements of catecholamine excretion before, during, and after each film session showed that all the 'arousing' films produced a rise in catecholamine output, irrespective of the specific quality of the emotions evoked. In contrast, the non-arousing film was accompanied by a decrease in catecholamine excretion.

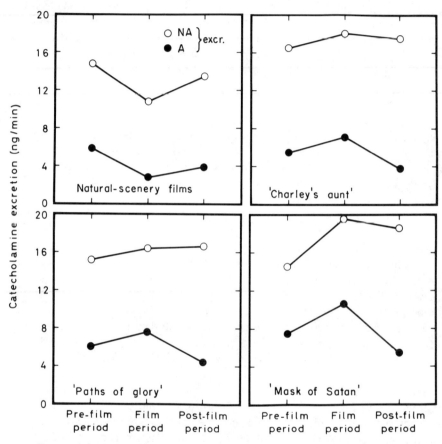

FIGURE 4.6. Mean adrenaline and noradrenaline excretion before, during, and after four film sessions. Based on Levi, L. *Acta Medica Scandinavica*, 1972, Suppl. No. 528, Table 3:2, with the author's permission

Similar results were obtained in a study (Pátkai, 1971) where laboratory situations were designed so as to evoke either pleasant or unpleasant affective states. The pleasant situation involved playing a game of chance, a modified Bingo-game, while in one unpleasant situation the subjects watched medico-surgical films and in another they performed tedious paper-and-pencil tests. One session was spent in neutral inactivity. The highest catecholamine excretion occurred in the game session, which was the session judged by the subjects as the most pleasant.

These results are in complete agreement with the view, based on studies of effects produced by adrenaline infusions, that an increase in circulating adrenaline is accompanied by a rise in non-specific subjective arousal, and that the individual's cognitive appraisal of the situation determines the affective tone. Convincing support for this view has been provided by Schachter and Singer (1962) who showed that adrenaline injections made the subjects feel either euphoric or angry depending upon how the experimental situation was manipulated.

4.3. INTERINDIVIDUAL DIFFERENCES IN SYMPATHETIC-ADRENOMEDULLARY ACTIVITY

While we have a fair knowledge about the nature of the psychological factors which act as stimuli for catecholamine secretion, large gaps remain in our understanding of the mechanisms by which circulating catecholamines influence behaviour.

A promising line of approach has been opened through the study of inter-individual differences in the catecholamine output of normal, healthy individuals in relation to psychological variables. Results from a series of investigations (see reviews by Frankenhaeuser, 1971a, 1971b) show that while there are large differences between individuals in catecholamine output, there is a considerable intraindividual constancy, each individual tending to remain at a fairly constant level of secretion under ordinary life conditions.

There are also large differences between individuals with regard to the change in catecholamine output which takes place in response to a particular stimulus situation. Some individuals respond to psychosocial stressors by a large increase, while others show a moderate or small increase, or even a decrease. Such differences in response, when not of a pathological origin, may be associated with either genetic or psychological factors. Among the former, differences in adrenomedullary sensitivity to afferent stimuli may play a role. Among the latter, the individual's 'coping style' is likely to be of importance. When, for instance, a 'paradoxical' reaction occurs (i.e., decreased adrenomedullary secretion during stress exposure) it is likely that psychological defence mechanisms influence the mode of response.

In this section, interindividual differences in sympathetic-adrenomedullary activity as related to behaviour will be considered on the basis of data obtained in experiments on healthy human subjects.

4.3.1. Efficiency and adjustment

Experimental analysis of relations between human performance and catecholamine output have given interesting results. Among normal, healthy individuals those who have relatively higher catecholamine-excretion levels tend to perform better in terms of speed, accuracy, and endurance than those

84

who have lower levels. This relationship is particularly marked in the case of adrenaline excretion, but seems to hold also for noradrenaline. An example is given in Figure 4.7, which shows that choice–reaction time was consistently shorter in a group of high-catecholamine subjects than in a group of low-catecholamine subjects (i.e., subjects above and below the medium catecholamine-excretion value). Similarly, the number of errors was consistently smaller in the high-catecholamine groups.

Another example is provided in Figure 4.8, which shows that high-catecholamine subjects were superior to low-catecholamine subjects in learning nonsense syllables by the anticipation method (Frankenhaeuser & Andersson: in preparation).

Figure 4.9 shows data from an investigation (Johansson, Frankenhaeuser & Magnusson, 1973) on 12-year-old boys and girls whose catecholamine excretion was determined during an inactivity period, and during a subsequent period in which they performed mental arithmetic. It is seen that those boys

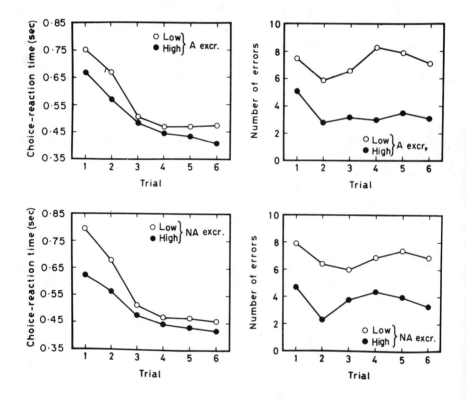

FIGURE 4.7. Mean choice–reaction time and number of errors of subjects with high (above median value) and subjects with low (below median value) excretion rates of adrenaline (A) and noradrenaline (NA). Redrawn and reprinted with permission from Frankenhaeuser, M. & Rissler, A., *Psychopharmacologia*, 1970, **17**, 378–390

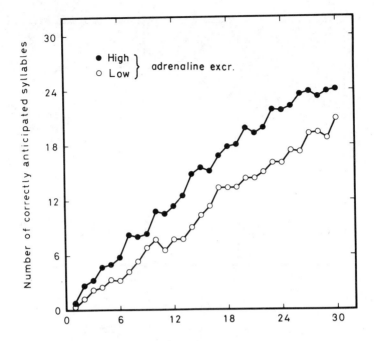

FIGURE 4.8. Mean performance in a verbal rote learning task in subjects with high (above median value) and subjects with low (below median value) excretion rates of adrenaline. (Frankenhaeuser, M., & Andersson, K.: in preparation.)

and girls whose adrenaline output increased while they were engaged in mental arithmetic as compared with a preceding inactivity period, performed consistently better than those whose adrenaline output decreased during mental work. Differences between 'increasers' and 'decreasers' were particularly marked in the group of boys toward the end of the 45-minute work period. Noradrenaline output did not appear to be related to psychological efficiency.

While individuals who secrete relatively more adrenaline tend to perform better when working under conditions of low or moderate activation, the opposite tendency has been noted under conditions of high activation (Frankenhaeuser, Nordheden, Myrsten, & Post, 1971). This is illustrated in Figure 4.10, which shows performance in a vigilance task representing 'understimulation' (left-hand diagram) and in a complex sensorimotor task representing 'overstimulation' (right-hand diagram). When performance efficiency under these two contrasting conditions of work were compared in subjects differing with regard to their catecholamine-excretion rates, it was found that subjects who excreted relatively more adrenaline performed better under conditions of understimulation, while subjects with relatively lower excretion rates of adrenaline tended to perform better under overstimulation. With regard to noradrenaline the relationships were not consistent.

These results may be interpreted in terms of the inverted-U relation between

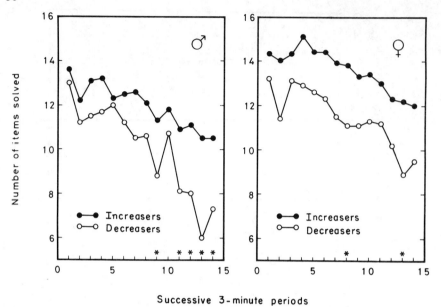

FIGURE 4.9. Successive mean performance scores for subjects whose adrenaline excretion increased, and for subjects whose adrenaline excretion decreased during an arithmetic task as compared with a preceding passive period. (*indicates that the *t*-value for the mean difference between 'increasers' and 'decreasers' was statistically significant.) Reprinted with permission from Johansson, G., Frankenhaeuser, M. & Magnusson, D. *Scandinavian Journal of Psychology*, 1973, **14**, 20–28

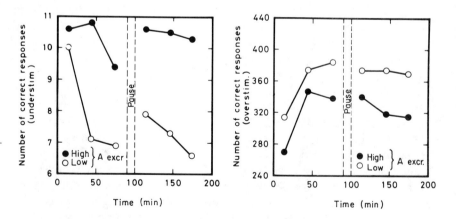

FIGURE 4.10. Mean performance of subjects with high (above median value) and subjects with low (below median value) excretion rates of adrenaline (A) during understimulation (left-hand diagram) and overstimulation (right-hand diagram). Frankenhaeuser, M., Nordheden, B., Myrsten, A.-L. & Post, B. *Acta Psychologica*, 1971, **35**, 298–308

behavioural efficiency and physiological arousal. The data also point to the influence of the nature and difficulty of the task on the relationship between catecholamine release and performance. In this connection it should be noted that the results from catecholamine-excretion studies are consistent with data obtained in experiments with catecholamine infusions (Frankenhaeuser & Järpe, 1963) which show that the infusion of small or moderate doses of adrenaline may have a beneficial effect on performance in cognitive tasks requiring sustained concentration.

In addition to the studies concerned with the relationship between cognitive efficiency and sympathetic-adrenomedullary activity in acute situations, other investigations show that consistent relationships also exist between catecholamine secretion and some enduring psychological characteristics of the individual. For example, a positive correlation has been found in children between adrenaline excretion and intelligence quotient as well as school performance (Johansson et al., 1973; Lambert, Johansson, Frankenhaeuser & Klackenberg–Larsson, 1969). These findings indicate that relations between adrenaline and psychological functions are not restricted to efficiency in acute situations, but involve cognitive functions in general.

In this connection it should be noted that significant correlations have been found between adrenaline excretion and 'positive' personality characteristics such as 'ego strength' (Roessler, Burch & Mefferd, 1967) and different indices of 'emotional stability' (Johansson et al., 1973; Lambert et al., 1969). The relation of noradrenaline secretion to both acute behavioural efficiency and enduring personality characteristics is similar to that of adrenaline secretion, but the data are on the whole less consistent.

Other important questions are associated with the temporal pattern of sympathetic-adrenomedullary activation following exposure to acute environmental pressure. There are large interindividual differences in the time taken for adrenaline secretion to return to baseline level after a brief period of exposure to environmental stress. The time course may be a significant factor in determining the relative potency of harmful versus beneficial adrenaline effects.

Recent data (Johansson & Frankenhaeuser, 1973) suggest that a rapid return to sympathetic-adrenomedullary baselines is indicative of good adjustment. This is illustrated in Figure 4.11, which shows adrenaline excretion, performance scores, and neuroticism scores in two groups of subjects, classified as rapid or slow 'decreasers' depending upon the time taken for adrenaline excretion to return to baseline level after short-term exposure to a heavy mental load. The rapid 'decreasers' differed significantly from the slow 'decreasers' in that they had higher adrenaline output during inactivity, better performance scores in a sensorimotor task, and lower neuroticism scores as measured by the Swedish version of Eysenck's Personality Inventory. These results are in general agreement with those by Eysenck (1967) and other investigators suggesting a relationship between the speed at which autonomic equilibrium is regained and personality traits indicative of emotional stability.

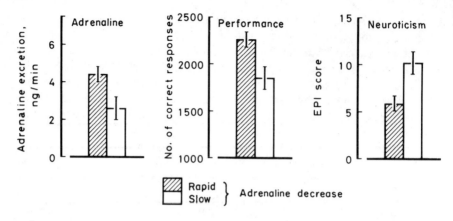

FIGURE 4.11. Means and standard errors for adrenaline excretion during inactivity, performance scores in a sensorimotor task, and neuroticism scores obtained by Eysenck's personality inventory. Redrawn and reprinted with permission from Johansson, G. & Frankenhaeuser, M., *Biological Psychology*, 1973, **1**, 63–73

Thus, the experimental data indicate that good adjustment may require efficient mechanisms both for 'mobilizing' and for 'demobilizing' physiological resources. A rapid decrease in sympathetic-adrenomedullary activation after cessation of the stimulus probably implies an 'economic' way of responding, while a slow decrease may indicate poor adjustment in the sense that the organism 'over-responds' by mobilizing resources that are no longer needed.

4.3.2. Sex differences

The greater part of the investigations concerned with relationships between sympathetic-adrenomedullary activity and behaviour has been carried out on male subjects. It has generally been assumed that when catecholamine excretion is expressed in relation to body weight, no difference remains in excretion rate between the sexes (e.g., Kärki, 1956). This assumption, however, has been based on data from resting and inactivity conditions, and recent investigations by Frankenhaeuser and her associates (Frankenhaeuser, 1973; Johansson, 1972; Johansson & Post, 1972) show that a somewhat different picture is obtained, at least with regard to adrenaline excretion, when the sexes are compared under psychosocial pressure. In Figure 4.12 adrenaline excretion in a male and a female group are compared under a non-stressful condition, i.e. when the subjects carried out their daily routine activities, and under psychological stress, i.e. when they performed an intelligence test under time pressure. In the group of women adrenaline excretion was about the same during intelligence testing as during daily routine activity. In contrast, the male subjects increased their adrenaline output significantly when they were required to perform the intelligence test.

FIGURE 4.12. Means and standard errors for adrenaline excretion, expressed in relation to body weight, in adult male and female subjects during daily routine activities and during intelligence testing. Based on Johansson, G. & Post, B., *Rep. Psychol. Lab.*, University of Stockholm, 1972, No. 379

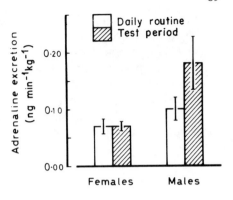

FIGURE 4.13. Means and standard errors for adrenaline excretion, expressed in relation to body weight, in 12-year-old boys and girls during a passive and an active period. Redrawn and reprinted with permission from Johansson, G. *Acta Physiologica Scandinavica*, 1972, **85**, 569–572

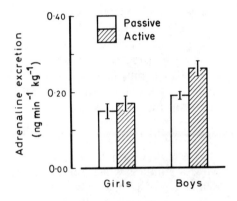

Similar results were obtained when 12-year-old boys and girls were compared (Figure 4.13) under a 'passive' condition, i.e. watching a non-engaging motion picture, and under an 'active' condition, i.e. performing an attention-demanding arithmetic task. In the group of girls adrenaline excretion was only slightly higher during the active as compared with the passive period, while the boys excreted significantly more adrenaline when performing the task.

In this case, as among adult males and females, there was a slight difference in performance between the sexes, in favour of the female group. Hence, a sex-linked difference in motivation does not appear to be a likely explanation of the endocrine sex difference.

Another interesting example of low sympathetic-adrenomedullary reactivity in females is provided in a study by Levi (1972) which showed that male students increased their adrenaline excretion significantly during film-induced sexual arousal, while the excretion rate remained relatively unchanged in female students. In this case, however, the sex difference in hormone excretion was probably associated with a difference between the sexes in the intensity of the sexual arousal evoked by the film, males feeling sexually more aroused than females.

It is also interesting to note that pre-menstrual disturbances do not appear to be accompanied by increased adrenaline excretion (Pátkai, Johansson, & Post, 1971; Silbergeld, Brast, & Noble, 1971) as might be expected in view of the sensitivity to subtle changes in emotional arousal demonstrated in studies of male subjects.

The overall picture obtained from these studies may be tentatively interpreted as indicating that adrenomedullary activity is a less sensitive indicator of behavioural arousal in females than in males.

4.4. DISCUSSION

4.4.1. The influence of cognitive factors

It is an interesting task to search for a common element among the apparently diverse stimuli which elicit a sympathetic-adrenomedullary response. The empirical evidence clearly shows that an event which is perceived as emotionally arousing, regardless of whether the experience is a pleasant or an unpleasant one, will generally be accompanied by increased adrenaline output. Conversely, under conditions which are perceived as relaxing, adrenaline secretion will fall below the 'baseline' level, i.e. the secretion rate typical for a given individual under conditions of 'ordinary' stimulus input. Furthermore, repeated exposure to one and the same arousing stimulus is accompanied by a decrease in adrenaline secretion only if there is a concomitant decrease in subjective arousal, while a stimulus which retains its stressful character will continue to induce a high rate of adrenaline secretion.

We may thus conclude that those psychosocial stimuli which are perceived as deviating from the 'ordinary' input level, or which are in some other way incongruous with a person's expectancies based on his previous experience, are likely to induce changes in sympathetic-adrenomedullary activity. Conversely, stimuli which are perceived as part of the familiar environment, will generally not affect the activity of this endocrine system.

These examples clearly illustrate the part played by cognitive processes in catecholamine secretion: the brain exerts a continuous influence on sympathetic-adrenomedullary activity, and by measuring catecholamine excretion we can monitor the arousing and relaxing influences of the psychosocial environment. At present we have a fairly good understanding of these relationships, which enables us to predict how the sympathetic-adrenomedullary system will respond to specific changes in the environment. However, the mechanisms underlying individual differences in catecholamine secretion, for example the 'paradoxical' reactions (cf. p. 91), are not yet understood.

It should be pointed out that the pituitary-adrenocortical activity also reflects changes in the psychosocial environment (cf. Mason, 1968, 1971). However, it is generally agreed that this system reacts more slowly, and requires higher levels of stimulation before responding than does the sympathetic-adrenomedullary system (cf. Levi, 1972).

4.4.2. Mechanisms of action

Our knowledge about the mechanisms by which the adrenomedullary hormones exert their influence on behaviour is still incomplete. Some of the currently debated problems are associated with the provocative ideas put forward by William James (1890) concerning the causal role of sympathomimetic reactions in the development of emotional states. While studies of effects produced by adrenaline infusions show that sympathomimetic symptoms may contribute to the development of emotions such as fear and anxiety (cf. p. 81), it has also been clearly shown that adrenaline may act directly on the brain (cf. p. 73). Although adrenaline presumably crosses the blood-brain barrier only in some regions, empirical evidence suggests that it can penetrate sufficiently to exert some central effects. Little is known about the intracerebral concentration of adrenaline needed to achieve these effects, but it may well be that very small amounts are required (Rothballer, 1959).

While small doses of catecholamines administered intracerebrally or intravenously usually produce brief arousal, larger doses may produce long-term sedation. The possible significance of these sedative effects has been discussed by Breggin (1964) who suggests that 'adrenaline depression' may underlie the fatigue and exhaustion following excitement and anxiety states.

In this connection the important part played by brain-noradrenaline in affective states should be recalled: drugs and other treatments which increase the amount of functional noradrenaline available in the brain cause behavioural activation and tend to counteract depression, while, in contrast, those which reduce brain-noradrenaline produce sedation and depression (Schildkraut & Kety, 1967).

The experimental results (Frankenhaeuser, 1971a, 1971b) showing that among healthy individuals, those who secrete relatively more adrenaline tend to cope better with both cognitive and emotional stressed, leads to the question of possible long-term effects of adrenaline-mediated adjustment to the psychosocial environment. There is a growing awareness, that although human beings are able to adjust to a wide range of conditions, such adjustments may have after-effects. This means that the adaptive efforts may leave the individual less able to cope with subsequent demands and frustrations. The after-effects may manifest themselves as emotional maladjustments, as impairments of performance efficiency, or as somatic disturbances (cf. Glass & Singer, 1972).

In this connection it is interesting to recall the work by Rahe and his associates (reviewed by Rahe, 1972) which indicates that adjustment to life-changes, whether of a pleasant or an unpleasant nature, adds to the wear-and-tear of the organism and therefore increases susceptibility to illness. It is not yet clear which role the catecholamines play under these conditions, but recent investigations concerning life-change and myocardial infarction suggest that high-adrenaline secreters may be individuals at risk (Theorell, 1970).

There is now a great need for longitudinal field studies of psychoendocrine relationships. Such studies will eventually increase our understanding about possible long-term risks associated with cumulative effects of repeated sympathetic-adrenomedullary stimulation.

4.5. ACKNOWLEDGMENT

Financial support from the Swedish Medical Research Council (Project No. 40Y–2371) is gratefully acknowledged.

This chapter is a review article and contains some findings and conclusions which have appeared in previous papers by the author. For other general surveys of similar topics see the attached bibliography.

4.6. REFERENCES

Andersson, B., Hovmöller, S., Karlsson, C.-G. & Svensson, S. Analysis of urinary catecholamines. An improved auto-analyzer fluorescence method. *Reports from the Laboratory for Clinical Stress Research*, Stockholm, 1973, No. 32.

Ax, A. F. The physiological differentiation between fear and anger in humans. *Psychosomatic Medicine*, 1953, **15**, 433–442.

Blaschko, H. Catecholamine biosynthesis. In L. L. Iversen (Ed.), *Catecholamines. British Medical Bulletin*, 1973, **29**, 105–109.

Blaschko, H. & Welch, A. D. Localization of adrenaline in cytoplasmic particles of the bovine adrenal medulla. *Naunyn-Schmiedebergs Archiv für experimentelle Pathologie und Pharmakologie*, 1953, **219**, 17–22.

Bloom, G., Euler, U.S.v. & Frankenhaeuser, M. Catecholamine excretion and personality traits in paratroop trainees. *Acta Physiologica Scandinavica*, 1963, **58**, 77–89.

Breggin, P. R. The psychophysiology of anxiety. *Journal of Nervous and Mental Diseases*, 1964, **139**, 558–568.

Cannon, W. B. The emergency function of the adrenal medulla in pain and the major emotions. *American Journal of Physiology*, 1914, **33**, 356–372.

Cannon, W. B. *Bodily changes in pain, hunger, fear and rage*. Boston: Branford, 1929.

Elmadjian, F. J., Hope, J., & Lamson, E. T. Excretion of epinephrine and norepinephrine in various emotional states. *Journal of Clinical Endocrinology*, 1957, **17**, 608–620.

Euler, U.S.v. A specific sympathomimetic ergone in adrenergic nerve fibers (sympathin) and its relation to adrenaline and noradrenaline. *Acta Physiologica Scandinavica*, 1946, **12**, 73–97.

Euler, U.S.v. *Noradrenaline: Chemistry, physiology, pharmacology and clinical aspects*. Springfield, Ill.: Charles C. Thomas, 1956.

Euler, U.S.v. Adrenal medullary secretion and its neural control. In L. Martini & W. F. Ganong (Eds), *Neuroendocrinology*. Vol. 2. New York: Academic Press, 1967, pp. 283–333.

Euler, U.S.v. & Lishajko, F. Improved technique for the fluorimetric estimation of catecholamines. *Acta Physiologica Scandinavica*, 1961, **51**, 348–355.

Eysenck, H. J. *The biological basis of personality*. Springfield, Ill.: Charles C. Thomas, 1967.

Folkow, B. & Euler, U.S.v. Selective activation of noradrenaline and adrenaline producing cells in the suprarenal gland of the cat by hypothalamic stimulation. *Circulation Research*, 1954, **2**, 191–195.

Frankenhaeuser, M. Experimental approaches to the study of human behaviour as related to neuroendocrine functions. In L. Levi (Ed.), *Society, stress and disease*. Vol. I. *The psychosocial environment and psychosomatic diseases*. London: Oxford University Press, 1971, pp. 22–35(a).

Frankenhaeuser, M. Behavior and circulating catecholamines. *Brain Research*, 1971, **31**, 241–262(b).

Frankenhaeuser, M. Sex differences in reactions to psychosocial stressors and psychoactive drugs. In L. Levi (Ed.), *Society, stress and disease*. Vol. III. *Problems specific to the relationship between woman and man, and to family life*. London: Oxford University Press, 1973. (In press)

Frankenhaeuser, M. Experimental approaches to the study of catecholamines and emotion. In L. Levi (Ed.), *Parameters of emotion*. New York: Raven Press, 1973. (In press)

Frankenhaeuser, M. & Järpe, G. Psychophysiological changes during infusions of adrenaline in various doses. *Psychopharmacologia*, 1963, **4**, 424–432.

Frankenhaeuser, M. & Kåreby, S. Effect of meprobamate on catecholamine excretion during mental stress. *Perceptual and Motor Skills*, 1962, **15**, 571–577.

Frankenhaeuser, M., Mellis, I., Rissler, A., Björkvall, C. & Pátkai, P. Catecholamine excretion as related to cognitive and emotional reaction patterns. *Psychosomatic Medicine*, 1968, **30**, 109–120.

Frankenhaeuser, M., Myrsten, A.-L., Post, B. & Johansson, G. Behavioral and physiological effects of cigarette smoking in a monotonous situation. *Psychopharmacologia*, 1971, **22**, 1–7.

Frankenhaeuser, M., Myrsten, A.-L., Waszak, M., Neri, A. & Post, B. Dosage and time effects of cigarette smoking. *Psychopharmacologia*, 1968, **13**, 311–319.

Frankenhaeuser, M., Northeden, B., Myrsten, A.-L. & Post, B. Psychophysiological reactions to understimulation and overstimulation. *Acta Psychologica*, 1971, **35**, 298–308.

Frankenhaeuser, M. & Pátkai, P. Interindividual differences in catecholamine excretion during stress. *Scandinavian Journal of Psychology*, 1965, **6**, 117–123.

Frankenhaeuser, M., Post, B., Nordheden, B. & Sjöberg, H. Physiological and subjective reactions to different physical work loads. *Perceptual and Motor Skills*, 1969, **28**, 343–349.

Frankenhaeuser, M. & Rissler, A. Effects of punishment on catecholamine release and efficiency of performance. *Psychopharmacologia*, 1970, **17**, 378–390(a).

Frankenhaeuser, M. & Rissler, A. Catecholamine output during relaxation and anticipation. *Perceptual and Motor Skills*, 1970, **30**, 745–746(b).

Frankenhaeuser, M., Sterky, K. & Järpe, G. Psychophysiological relations in habituation to gravitational stress. *Perceptual and Motor Skills*, 1962, **15**, 63–72.

Funkenstein, D. H. Nor-epinephrine-like and epinephrine-like substances in relation to human behavior. *Journal of Mental Disease*, 1956, **124**, 58–68.

Glass, D. C. & Singer, J. E. *Urban stress. Experiments on noise and social stressors*. New York: Academic Press, 1972.

Häggendahl, J. An improved method for fluorimetric determination of small amounts of adrenaline and noradrenaline in plasma and tissues. *Acta Physiologica Scandinavica*, 1963, **59**, 242–254.

Hillarp, N. Å. & Hökfelt, B. Evidence of adrenaline and noradrenaline in separate adrenal medullary cells. *Acta Physiologica Scandinavica*, 1953, **30**, 55–68.

Hillarp, N. A., Lagerstedt, S., & Nilson, B. The isolation of a granular fraction from the suprarenal medulla, containing the sympathomimetic catecholamines. *Acta Physiologica Scandinavica*, 1953, **29**, 251–263.

Holtz, P., Credner, K., & Kroneberg, G. Über das sympathicomimetische pressorische Prinzip des Harns ('Urosympathin'). *Naunyn-Schmiedebergs Archiv für experimentelle Pathologie und Pharmakologie*, 1947, **204**, 228–243.

James, W. *Principles of psychology*. London: MacMillan, 1890.

Johansson, G. Sex differences in the catecholamine output of children. *Acta Physiologica Scandinavica*, 1972, **85**, 569–572.

Johansson, G. & Frankenhaeuser, M. Temporal factors in sympatho-adrenomedullary activity following acute behavioral activation. *Biological Psychology*, 1973, **1**, 63–73.

Johansson, G., Frankenhaeuser, M. & Magnusson, D. Catecholamine output in school children as related to performance and adjustment. *Scandinavian Journal of Psychology*, 1973, **14**, 20–28.

Johansson, G. & Post, B. Catecholamine output of males and females over a one-year period. Reports from the Psychological Laboratories, University of Stockholm, 1972, No. 379.

Kärki, N. T. The urinary excretion of noradrenaline and adrenaline in different age groups, its diurnal variation and the effect of muscular work on it. *Acta Physiologica Scandinavica*, 1956, **39**, Suppl. 132.

Lambert, W. W., Johansson, G., Frankenhaeuser, M. & Klackenberg-Larsson, I. Catecholamine excretion in young children and their parents as related to behavior. *Scandinavian Journal of Psychology*, 1969, **10**, 306–318.

Levi, L. The urinary output of adrenaline and noradrenaline during pleasant and unpleasant emotional states. *Psychosomatic Medicine*, 1965, **27**, 80–85.

Levi, L. (Ed.) Stress and distress in response to psychosocial stimuli. Laboratory and real life studies on sympathoadrenomedullary and related reactions. *Acta Medica Scandinavica*, 1972, Suppl. 528.

Mason, J. W. A review of psychoendocrine research on the sympathetic-adrenal medullary system. *Psychosomatic Medicine*, 1968, **30**, 631–653.

Mason, J. W. A re-evaluation of the concept of 'non-specificity' in stress theory. *Journal of Psychiatric Research*, 1971, **8**, 323–333.

Pátkai, P. Catecholamine excretion in pleasant and unpleasant situations. *Acta Psychologica*, 1971, **35**, 352–363.

Pátkai, P. & Frankenhaeuser, M. Constancy of urinary catecholamine excretion. *Perceptual and Motor Skills*, 1964, **19**, 789–790.

Pátkai, P., Johansson, G. & Post, B. Variations in physiological and psychological functions during the menstrual cycle. Reports from the Psychological Laboratories, University of Stockholm, 1971, No. 340.

Rahe, R. H. Subjects' recent life changes and their near-future illness susceptibility. *Advances in Psychosomatic Medicine*, 1972, **8**, 2–19.

Redgate, E. S. & Gellhorn, E. Nature of sympatheticoadrenal discharge under conditions of excitation of central autonomic structures. *American Journal of Physiology*, 1953, **174**, 475–480.

Roessler, R., Burch, N. R. & Mefferd, R. B., Jr. Personality correlates of catecholamine excretion under stress. *Journal of Psychosomatic Research*, 1967, **11**, 181–185.

Rothballer, A. B. The effects of catecholamines on the central nervous system. *Pharmacological Review*, 1959, **11**, 494–547.

Rothballer, A. B. Aggression, defense and neurohumors. In C. D. Clemente & D. B. Lindsley (Eds), *Aggression and defense: Neural mechanisms and social patterns*. (Brain Function, Vol. V). UCLA Forum Med. Sci, No. 7. Los Angeles: University of California Press, 1967, pp. 135–170.

Schachter, S. & Singer, J. E. Cognitive, social, and physiological determinants of emotional state. *Psychological Review*, 1962, **69**, 379–399.

Schildkraut, J. J. & Kety, S. S. Biogenic amines and emotion. *Science*, 1967, **156**, 21–30.

Selye, H. *Stress*. ACTA, Montreal, 1950.

Silbergeld, S., Brast, N., & Noble, E. B. The menstrual cycle: a double-blind study of symptoms, mood and behavior, and biochemical variables using Enovid and placebo. *Psychosomatic Medicine*, 1971, **33**, 411–428.

Silverman, A. J. & Cohen, S. I. Affect and vascular correlates to catecholamines. *Psychiatric Research Reports*, 1960, **12**, 16–30.

Theorell, T. Psychosocial factors in relation to the onset of myocardial infarction and to some metabolic variables—a pilot study. *Doctoral Dissertation*. Stockholm: Department of Medicine, Seraphimer Hospital, 1970.

Chapter 5

Physiological Consequences of Informational Load and Overload

B. McA. SAYERS

Engineering in Medicine Laboratory,
Imperial College of Science and Technology
London SW7 2BT

5.1. INTRODUCTION

Physiological variables reflect physical effort when a subject undertakes a physical task. When a mental task is involved, requiring the subject to make judgments and come to decisions on the basis of information presented, certain readily-recorded physiological variables are known to be influenced; however, the effects are secondary and require careful examination to separate the ephemeral from the explicit. This section will explore certain physiological concomitants of judgment and decision-making tasks, both in laboratory and industrial conditions in which no significant physical effort is required. The concept of information load involved is treated here in a semantic sense; information is presented to the subject and the difficulty of the task is regulated by increasing the rate at which relevant information is presented or at which decisions are required. No attempt will be made to quantify the load beyond ensuring operational uniformity, since the aim is to demonstrate the nature and origin of effects in some physiological variables when the subject undertakes such a task. Attention will be focused on these changes that take place quite generally in a variety of experimental situations which are operationally similar.

The main relevant physiological variables to be considered here are useful largely because they are easily measured: heart rate, peripheral blood flow and respiratory movements. These variables are influenced by activity of the sympathetic nervous system but are of course also subject to other influences. For both reasons considerable spontaneous variability must be expected, but it is possible to elucidate the origins of various major factors that contribute to some of the main variables and, using this information, greatly to clarify the significant content of these signals for the present purposes. It will be argued that a detailed scrutiny and analysis of the fluctuations in these signals is required and that due account must be taken of the structure and behaviour of several underlying control systems that regulate variables related to those being studied. A recent symposium (Ergonomics Research Society, 1973) can be consulted for the spectrum of current views on one of the variables (heart rate) to be considered here, but it is argued below that before a single variable like heart rate can be considered alone, a very careful scrutiny of each of several related variables is vital. That detailed scrutiny is attempted here and it will be seen that the emphasis is on dynamic behaviour of variables and the underlying systems that influence them.

5.2. MEASUREMENT AND FEATURES OF THE RELEVANT VARIABLES

5.2.1. Heart rate

The intervals between successive R-waves of the electrocardiographic QRS waveform invariably fluctuate around a short-term mean value. The mean value certainly reflects the physical needs of the cardiovascular system since, in conjunction with stroke volume, heart rate mediates the increased blood flow required when physical effort increases. But both mental load and physical demand achieve an effect on heart rate through autonomic pathways that influence the sino-atrial (SA) nodal pacemaker region of atrial cardiac tissue, and broadly speaking both vagal and sympathetic pathways are involved. It is often implicitly presumed that the mean level of heart rate results from a balance between net sympathetic and para-sympathetic influences acting on the spontaneous pacemaking behaviour of the SA nodal cells. However, this may not be completely realistic. For one reason, the SA nodal region comprises a multiplicity of cells which are spontaneously active and, in isolation, discharge rhythmically; this means that many cells must compete for the initial regenerative depolarization which in turn synchronizes the firing of many of the other cells and initiates the complete atrial contraction leading to the ventricular beat. As a result, since many cells are involved, with different properties and states, an appreciable variability in firing interval from cycle-to-cycle must be expected. The extent of this variability has been investigated both in cell-cultured tissue, and by modelling multiple interacting nodal cells by computer methods that express the physiological facts concerning membrane properties, ion movements and intercellular interactions in mathematical form. Models of individual cells produce cellular-membrane-potential patterns with a time-course closely comparable with those measured in real cells and that alter in a realistic way with the simulated effects of changing autonomic tone. When such cells are allowed to interact, the variability of firing-rate of the bulk of cells is closely similar to that of isolated tissue-cultured preparations and not greatly influenced by altering levels of simulated sympathetic or parasympathetic tone. However, in both tissue-cultured cell groups and in the modelled cells, the variability of firing-rate is appreciably greater than that of heart rate as seen in resting man, thus suggesting a different influence operative in the intact physiological system. Indeed, another possible mechanism, whereby heart rate may be controlled, is available that would account for these observations.

The ventricular contraction leads to a pulsatile increase of pressure in the great vessels of the circulation and thus provides a phasic baro-receptor stimulus; the baro-receptor afferent flow to the brain-stem is also thus phasic, and autonomic outflow to affect the SA node and influence the heart beat then completes a feedback loop. Indirect evidence now accumulating suggests that the passage of the neural signal through the brain-stem is associated with a concomitant time-delay, of the order of 1 sec but greatly variable. A time-delay in a feedback system pathway like this creates a phase-shift, such as is always involved when sustained cyclic behaviour occurs. It is known in other oscillatory systems that when the necessary phase-shift originates mainly in a time-delay, the frequency of the sustained cyclic fluctuation is directly related to delay; a change of delay magnitude then alters the frequency almost proportionally. In the present case, the existence of a time-delay as between signals that traverse different pathways in the brain-stem, can be demonstrated and this time-delay is found to alter according to the observed frequency of oscillation exhibited by the signal. It therefore seems likely that the closed loop system has sufficient phase shift because of the time delay, (and adequate loop-gain) to oscillate for this reason alone, at a rate dominated by the time-delay magnitude. This mechanism has been worked out for the blood pressure control system as discussed below, but it now emerges that a similar mechanism may operate in controlling mean heart rate also.

This possibility indicates three separate mechanisms whereby mean heart rate could be altered; first adjustment of brain-stem characteristics leading to alteration of transmission time-delay and consequent alteration of oscillatory rate, second, adjustment of sympathetic tone, and third, adjustment of vagal tone. It is currently considered likely that any control of time delay for pathways through the brain-stem must be mainly of hypothalamic origin; consequently it is quite feasible that the three possible mechanisms would in some instances act synergistically and in other instances, not. In short, mean heart rate should be regarded as a measure that may sometimes exhibit a change due to one kind of influence, sometimes exhibit a similar or a different kind of change because of some other influence, and sometimes show no effect at all; there is nothing in mean heart rate as a physiological measure that could distinguish these separate origins, or indicate unequivocally when or which underlying factors were altering.

For this reason, mean heart rate seems unlikely to be reliably instructive for indicating effects due to a mental task, for example. What is clearly required instead, is a variable that has a waveshape, the changes of which indicate, more or less explicitly, their origins. With such an indicator a more satisfactory insight could be expected into physiological effects following an increase in the level of perceptual stimulus. In fact, two such indicators are available: transient effects in heart rate, and oscillatory, quasi-oscillatory, or otherwise strongly-phasic fluctuations in heart rate. Transient effects are certainly present but cannot often be interpreted; but as will be seen, phasic effects of a more regular or more periodic kind can be used for the present purpose. Specifically, three separate effects produce recognizable and defined waveform contributions to the heart rate signal, on the basis of which responses to mental tasks can be investigated.

One other introductory point: heart rate is a variable that is subject to adjustment for purposes of a biological control activity intended to ensure adequate blood flow for the current needs of the body. However increased blood flow can also be achieved by increasing stroke volume. Thus there are many possible combinations of heart rate and stroke volume that will meet the need for a specific blood flow rate, although some of these combinations are certainly more costly than others in terms of energy dissipation; consequently some basis must exist in the control system to make the choice possible. It is now thought likely that the choice is made in such a way as to effect the desired control while minimizing the 'cost' to the system in some appropriate sense (perhaps in terms of myocardial oxygen consumption). The existence of such an optimal control would further complicate the interpretation of mean heart rate changes because the different effects of the optimal strategy under different circumstances cannot be discriminated. This also supports the desirability of studying components of the heart rate signals that have specific origins, provided, of course, that these components can be isolated unequivocally and also that they do reflect alterations of interest.

5.2.1.1. Acquisition of the heart rate signal

A cycle-by-cycle value of heart rate is needed for the reasons discussed above. This value must be derived from primary measurements of the interval between successive QRS complexes of the electrocardiogram (ECG) and since there is no reason to do otherwise, it is convenient to utilize the direct measure itself, i.e. the interbeat interval. Hence analysis proceeds on the basis of the sequence of intervals between successive beats—referred to as the interval signal. The independent variable is, of course, interval number, and this reflects real time elapsed since the start of the record only in a somewhat irregular way; however, over a convenient individual signal length of say 256 intervals, the elapsed time = 256 × mean interval duration, so that a transformation to real time is possible if necessary. No advantage of real weight seems to result from converting the interval signal to a heart rate signal, and the former is the measure used here.

Typical interval variations in a resting adult are in the order of 25 msec so for investigational purposes, a resolution of 1–2 msec is sufficient. Consequently, the start of the QRS, or the peak of the R-wave, can reasonably be used to indicate the individual heart-beat for timing purposes. Since the operations to be described are preferably computer-based, digital processing will be assumed; a resolution of 2 msec implies a sampling-rate of 500 per second on the original ECG signal which should therefore be permitted to retain no significant sinusoidal components above 500/2 = 250 Hz. (However low-pass filtering is rarely needed with this signal unless significant electromyographic interference is present on the ECG record, in which event re-recording would be indicated with a different choice of electrode positions.) More serious difficulties are created by missed beats and extrasystoles since these result in substantial transients in the signal which, in subsequent operations, can masquerade as significant signal components. Most missed beats, or premature beats followed by compensatory pauses, can be detected automatically in the interval sequence and corrected, but visual inspection of the final interval signal as a waveform is necessary to confirm that the signal is satisfactory. An editing procedure of the kind described by Vahl, Vickery, Monro & Tinker (1971) is suitable; this uses a computer programmed automatically to mark the occurrence of each QRS maximum, using criteria of maximum rate-of-change of signal slope, absolute magnitude, and time since the last QRS. Using an oscilloscope display, the waveform (together with markers that brighten the trace at each detected QRS peak) is scanned visually; this can be carried out at high speed and erroneously placed or missed markers are readily detectable and can be manually corrected.

The sequence of interbeat interval signals shown in Figure 5.1 is typical. Attending only to variations of the signal around the mean-value, the first task is to characterize the signal in a quantitative and informative way. Several procedures are available: autocorrelation of the signal, or calculation of its power spectrum or of its amplitude spectrum; the first two are often used but for most purposes, are poor choices, but the last is quite satisfactory, Sayers (1970, 1973). The amplitude spectrum is determined from the Fourier series analysis of the interval signal; the basic concept is that a repetitive waveform of whatever complexity can be represented as the sum of a series of sinusoids (Fourier components) each harmonically related in frequency to the fundamental sinusoid (having a period equal to the record length). Suitable choice of Fourier coefficients, i.e. the amplitude of each component, and its phase (relative to the start of the record) is necessary, and the process of Fourier analysis determines the correct choice of amplitude and phase of each sinusoidal

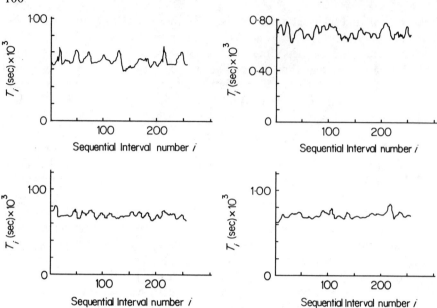

FIGURE 5.1. Four sequences each of 256 cardiac interbeat intervals with a mean interval of about 700 milliseconds

component. The amplitude spectrum is then the (graphical) representation of the Fourier component amplitude as a function of harmonic number; it is utilized mainly on the grounds that the size of the individual Fourier components should be the first focus of interest since small amplitude components clearly contribute little to the overall signal. However, it must be recognized that the phases of the individual Fourier components are vital in specifying the precise waveshape of the signal concerned. The power spectrum is obtained by squaring the amplitudes of individual components, and has the disadvantage of militating against components of relatively small amplitudes (because squaring numerically favours large magnitudes at the expense of small). However, when questions of signal variability are in question, the statistical estimations required are more conveniently handled in terms of signal power or the distribution of the signal power amongst the different spectral components (the power spectrum) rather than signal amplitude or amplitude spectrum.

The notion of signal power is now ubiquitous; it originates from treating a signal $[e(t)]$ conceptually as a voltage appearing across a 1-ohm resistor, in which case the instantaneous power dissipated in the resistor $[e(t)]^2$ is formed of two elements—the power due to the steady part of the signal (the dc term), and the power due to the alternating (ac) component (the instantaneous deviation from the mean). The average value of the power due to the ac component of the signal is simply the sample variance of the signal, but the term a.c. power is commonly employed in place of variance: because of the conceptual simplicity of regarding the total power in a signal as contributed by the power of the individual Fourier components that make up the signal; then the notion and meaning of power spectrum (as the distribution of the power amongst the various Fourier components) follows immediately.

Some workers have attempted to describe the signal in terms of its auto-correlation function. This function portrays the conventional product–moment correlation between the signal and the same signal delayed, as a function of the delay time (Sayers 1970). The main interest is in the shape of the function, which fluctuates periodically if strong periodic components exist in the original signal, but a frequency analysis is often needed to determine if significant components are indeed present; however, the result of such an analysis is precisely the power spectrum of the signal. With the advent of digital computer processing, it turns out to be much faster to compute the amplitude, or power, spectrum of a signal than its autocorrelation function; consequently the spectral description is usually to be preferred.

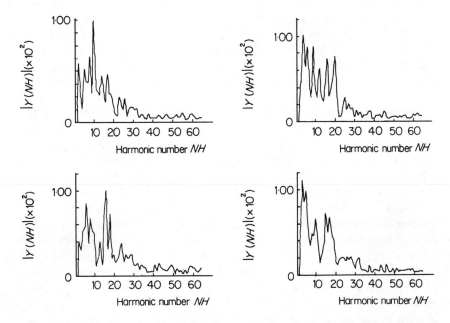

FIGURE 5.2. Amplitude spectra showing the magnitude of the first 64 Fourier harmonics of the fundamental (1 cycle per 256 intervals) for the four cardiac interval sequences in Figure 1. Two main spectral regions can be identified in these particular records: the band 1–12 harmonics and 12–22 harmonics

Figure 5.2 shows some amplitude spectra for the interval signal. The cardiac interval signal is not repetitive; however, the Fourier coefficients calculated as above are sufficient precisely to represent the signal over its total duration, and it can be established that these coefficients can be treated as statistical estimates of the coefficients representing an infinite 'parent' signal of which the given length is a single sample. If successive, equal duration, lengths of the signal are obtained, the Fourier coefficients will in general vary for statistical reasons, and the sampling variability of the coefficients, from sample-length to sample-length of the signal, must be known, so that any effects due to extraneous influences can be detected and quantitated. The sampling variability of the coefficients can be estimated provided it can be assumed that the source remains stable, and this of course forms the basis of a null-hypothesis that can be employed to compare different sample lengths of signal.

Before adopting any specific quantitative measure for assessing a subject's responses to altered external conditions it is therefore important to establish the typical variability of the measure under resting conditions; in the first instance, signal sample variance might be considered as a measure and so its variability must be considered. Dividing the signal into 256 interval sections, and using the full available band of 1–128 harmonics (of 1 cycle per 256 intervals; typically 0·007 Hz or so) the variability of signal variance (the term: alternating component (ac) power will now be used as a better synonym for variance) can be considered. The variable exhibits a coefficient of variation (CV, the ratio of standard deviation to mean) of about 0·25 in a typical individual carrying out a very undemanding industrial task of a decision-making kind but involving no significant physical effort. This typical figure indicates the variability of ac power during a 1-h period, and gives the ratio of standard deviation to mean of the ac power in say, 25 sequential sections each of 256 intervals. On repetition with that individual, the CV itself shows a standard deviation (SD) of 0·11. (These figures are typical of a single group of 25 individuals drawn from the same population of air-traffic-control operators). Intersubject variability of CV is slightly larger, with SD = 0·18. A group of 25 railway traffic regulators on the other hand exhibit somewhat larger average CV = 0·33, with an intersubject SD = 0·24. The power values thus assessed are theoretically distributed according to a χ^2 distribution and this accords moderately well with the observations; however the predicted and observed degrees of freedom in the data do not always match. In a theoretical analysis, it is possible to assume that the variability of the signal power corresponds to that of a random white noise (flat Fourier spectrum) signal, normally distributed in amplitude, but modified by filtering to have the same spectral content as the actual signal, i.e. the same profile of Fourier coefficient versus harmonic number as the actual signal. Filtering in this way reduces the number of independent observations contained in the signal length and so the number of degrees of freedom (DF) is diminished. Hence a length of 256 intervals, showing the usual non-white, non-constant spectrum, will have perhaps as few as 30 rather than 256 DF, and consequently will show much greater variability in power than the corresponding white noise signal. Typically about 40 DF are calculated from the interval signal for the first group above, and from this an estimate of theoretical CV = $\sqrt{(2/\mathrm{DF})} = 0\cdot22$ follows: this estimate approximates the observed value of 0·25, but even this degree of rough agreement is not always achieved. (Incidentally, while a χ^2 distribution with 40 DF is not very different from Normal, the χ^2 distribution is more obviously appropriate when the power due to a restricted range of signal Fourier components is being considered.) The 95 per cent confidence limits for actual mean signal power should correspond approximately to the range [0·6 P, 1·5 P] where P is the sample estimate of power; in the absence of artifacts and isolated transient events (e.g. a burst of speech utterance), this range matches the observations.

Several different effects may be shown by a subject when undertaking a mental workload task; one common claim that is somewhat more commonly accepted than not, is that total ac signal power in the heart rate or interval signal tends to diminish with informational load. Unfortunately, different observers using different measures sometimes inadvertently assess rather different fractions of the total signal power. Some workers measure successive differences or successive signed-differences in rate and summate these over several intervals, thus first emphasizing fast components by differencing and then low-pass filtering, by summating, in a way that somewhat suppresses medium-rate changes; others concentrate on interval durations between reversals of direction of the signal, again emphasizing the faster fluctuations but this time at the expense of slow components. These, and numerous other measures that have been devised, cannot be put on a common basis. However, when data is handled in a standardized way, it now seems probable that heart rate or interval ac power sometimes, but not always, diminishes when a subject undertakes a mental task. On the other hand, it has been suggested that a rearrangement of signal ac power amongst available spectral components can occur under these circumstances (Parin and Baevsky, 1967, Sayers 1971), and now it appears that this is probably the major effect, that relegates changes in total ac power to a secondary, and indeed often incidental role. Hence it is important to consider more closely the nature of these effects and their precise physiological origin, and the procedures of spectral analysis and manipulation that are central to the task.

The actual technique of calculating Fourier coefficients to determine the amplitude spectrum of a signal is well established (Lynn 1973, Bendat and Piersol 1971); the methods discussed here are conveniently based on digital computer analysis of data. Digital computer operations require data to be available as discrete numbers. When the signals are continuous, like blood flow or pressure or respiration, the magnitude of the signal must be measured at sufficiently frequent regularly spaced instants of time (Sayers 1970). In the case of the interval signal, the data is directly available as a series of sequential numbers and the Fourier analysis can proceed immediately by Fast Fourier or Chirp-Z methods. (The Fast Fourier transform is a computer algorithm for calculating efficiently the Fourier coefficients for a set of data values that comprise the signal. This algorithm requires the set of data values to be a power of 2 in total number; if this requirement cannot be met, a procedure known as The Chirp-Z transform [Rabiner, Schafer and Rader (1969); Monro (1973)] allows reasonably speedy calculation of the Fourier coefficients for any number of data points). Whichever procedure is used, once the Fourier coefficients have been computed two further steps are then available. An amplitude spectrum (the amplitude of the sinusoidal contribution at each frequency) can be calculated (as the square root of the sum of squares of the sine and cosine coefficients at that frequency); alternatively a filtering operation can be carried out. In the latter case, the Fourier coefficients of all unwanted components are set to zero and the inverse Fourier operation (to reconstitute the signal from the remaining Fourier coefficients) is then carried out; the result is a waveform of intervals, selectively filtered to eliminate all components except those of interest. Adequate selective emphasis of the different individual contributions due to underlying physiological mechanisms can be achieved in this way.

This is the basic signal processing operation needed in analysing the effects of external factors on the autonomic and cardiovascular systems, and it permits the necessary close investigation of the kinds of alteration imposed by, say, a mental workload task. It is therefore appropriate next to consider the findings of such an analysis of the typical interval signal, obtained under normal resting circumstances.

5.2.1.2. Components of the interval signal

There are three main contributions to the interval signal (Sayers 1971, 1973). Two of these are of vasomotor origin, and the other is respiratory or respiratory-linked; additionally, some random fluctuations, and certain isolated transients due to postural changes, and others of unknown genesis, also exist. The various underlying factors influence the tonic and phasic activity flowing to the sino-atrial node and so generate variations in heart rate generally known as sinus arrhythmia. However, it is often possible to identify the individual contributions, or at least to confirm their existence, and reference to the general effect of sinus arrhythmia is not useful here.

The two vasomotor contributions appear primarily in records of intra-arterial blood pressure, or of blood flow, but appear also in the interval signal. Both originate in underlying feedback control mechanisms that generate incidental spontaneous activity because of their particular structure, and it is this activity that can be identified in the interval signal thus indicating a contribution due to the underlying control system. Both kinds of spontaneous activity alter in various ways due to various physiological changes, and at least some relevant changes are linked to the situation of interest here.

The slower of the two vasomotor components in the interval signal is believed to originate in the system responsible for regulating body temperature. This system certainly operates at two levels of response but in the first instance the response to small thermal unbalance causes a re-adjustment of superficial blood flow to alter the rate of heat loss without invoking the more elaborate machanisms of shivering or sweating. The change of superficial blood flow is reflected in blood pressure and this influences the carotid-sinus and aortic arch baro-receptors and hence heart rate, as discussed below. The control system responsible for first-level response to slight thermal unbalance is believed to operate broadly in the following way: the primary sensors are skin temperature-gradient receptors, the outflow from which initiates hypothalamic activity that effects any necessary adjustments of superficial blood-flow. The system, and models of it based on detailed physiological information, show a spontaneous oscillation which is manifested in periodic fluctuations of blood flow, with a period of about 25 sec in man. This fluctuation is normally present in both blood flow and interval-signals but is subject to considerable frequency change, perhaps because of small fluctuations of blood temperature and possibly for other reasons also (Kitney 1974). From evidence that frequency-selective entrainment of the spontaneous oscillations can be achieved when a repeated thermal stimulus of sufficient frequency is applied, it is known that the control system is essentially non-linear. This is significant in that such non-linear systems may oscillate without in any way affecting their efficiency of control; the same structure that allows the system incidentally to oscillate, also allows fast and precise response to demands of any small thermal unbalance (Kitney 1972).

Hence fluctuations with periods in the vicinity of 25 sec or so (say 20–50 sec) in the interval signal may be attributed to the thermal control system; in fact an entrainment experiment (using a periodic thermal stimulus) establishes that these so-called thermal fluctuations do disappear when the corresponding blood flow oscillations are entrained, and that in the resting adult the fluctuations of thermal origin usually account for perhaps 70–80 per cent of the signal power due to low frequency signal components.

The faster of the two fluctuations of vasomotor origin is much more stable in period, and subject to much slower alterations. However this oscillation, which has a typical period of 10 sec in man, is subject to a switch-on/switch-off kind of effect; the oscillation may cease abruptly and restart later, under the influence of several factors. The oscillation originates in the mechanism regulating short-term mean arterial blood pressure against postural and other distributions (Hyndman, Kitney and Sayers 1971). It is posture-dependent and not readily seen in the recumbent subject. It is also subject to frequency-selective entrainment by broadly-periodic respiratory movements of sufficient rate and depth.

This oscillation can be seen in blood pressure, blood flow, and interval signals, and the same component is certainly involved in all the signals since coherence coefficients in the order of 0·9 have been found for the relevant frequency components. There is no significant difference between the blood flow signals recorded simultaneously at different peripheral sites in the body as far as the 10-sec vasomotor oscillation is concerned, either in frequency or relative phase. However, there is a time-delay (in the order of 1 sec or so) between the fluctuations at the spontaneous frequency as seen in the interval signal and as seen simultaneously in the blood flow or pressure signal and this time-delay is believed to originate in the brain-stem. As the frequency of oscillation alters, so does the time-delay. As the time-delay diminishes, the system is able to oscillate only at progressively higher frequencies. Hence the spontaneous frequency rises. But when the time-delay diminishes sufficiently, oscillation cannot be sustained at all, and abruptly ceases.

Hence there are two mechanisms by which the oscillation in spontaneous blood-pressure vasomotor activity can be suppressed—by a change in respiratory pattern, and by a change in transmission time-delay for relevant signal transmissions through the brain stem (perhaps effected by hypothalamic control). Both are relevant to the present problem.

The third major contribution to the interval signal originates with respiration and respiratory-linked movements. Respiration alters intra-pleural pressure because the diaphragm operates to some extent as a piston compressing or expanding the volume contained within the thoracic cage. The baro-receptors in the aortic wall are actually stretch-receptors, sensitive to transmural pressure and so to intra-pleural pressure; lung stretch receptors also respond to thoracic movements, and through both pathways respiratory and related movements influence the interval signal. The effect is not proportional and while the presence of a respiratory-linked fluctuation in cardiac interval is clear, the detailed waveform of respiratory movement cannot be recovered from the interval signal.

Respiratory sinus arrhythmia is well-known and readily detected; respiratory rates are usually rapid compared to blood pressure or temperature vasomotor oscillatory periods and so the direct effect on the interval signal is easily observed. However, if measurements are to be carried out in a realistic industrial situation, speech activity of the subject may be unavoidable, and it must be noted that speech utterance can substantially influence blood pressure or flow signals, and the interval-signal. The process of speech production involves controlled release of breath, and in many subjects is also linked to small postural changes that additionally influence heart rate. The effects are often considerable, as illustrated in Figure 5.3 and may quite dominate when present.

5.2.1.3. Analysis of the interval signal

Given that there are three individual kinds of consistent contribution to the interval signal, it is possible to devise a method that will separate any interval signal record into contributing components, at least to some extent. The most readily isolated component is that due to the vasomotor oscillation in the blood pressure system; the oscillation is either clearly present or clearly absent in most signal lengths and when present tends to persist on average only for about four complete periods. The frequency of oscillation usually remains close to about 0·10 Hz (period 10 sec) compared to extreme values of 0·08 and 0·12 Hz, and alters relatively little within each burst of oscillation. On the other hand, respiratory rates, depth, and detailed pattern do alter very considerably and it is not often possible to identify any simply periodic effect due to respiration in the interval signal. However, under resting conditions, respiratory rates in the normal adult are of higher frequency than either of

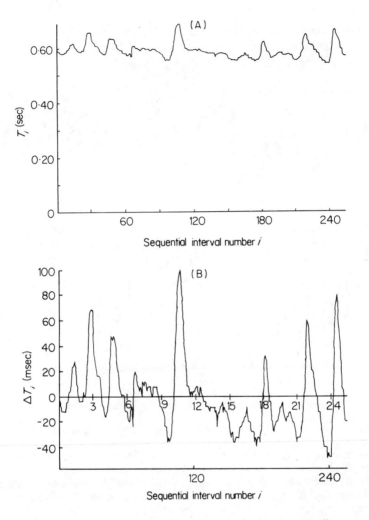

FIGURE 5.3. (A) A cardiac interval sequence showing the effect of speech utterances (6 major transient periods occurred during this record). (B) An amplified version of the interval variations about the mean

the vasomotor fluctuations (e.g., 0·3 Hz compared with 0·1 Hz for pressure system oscillation and perhaps 0·022–0·05 Hz for the thermal system activity) so it is then possible to separate components on the basis of frequency bands.

A digital filter or a frequency-domain filter will serve to select the individual bands. On the basis of a mean interval duration of say, 0·6 sec, a length of 256 intervals = 154 sec giving a fundamental frequency of 1 cycle per 154 sec. The upper limit of the thermal band is then the 8th harmonic of the fundamental, the pressure–vasomotor band is selected by the range 14–25 harmonics and the resting respiratory activity oscillation is selected by the band above harmonic

25. It is important to utilize the widest possible band in each case, to allow the onset and cessation, or the frequency shifts, or other features of this relevant waveform, to be reproduced with reasonable validity.

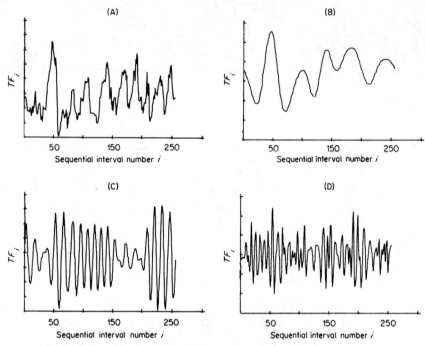

FIGURE 5.4. An interval T_i sequence (A), and three differently-band-filtered versions TF of the original, emphasizing respectively the slow fluctuations largely originating in the thermal control system (B), the quasi-oscillatory components originating in the blood pressure control system (C), and the respiratorily-contributed components (D). Each record is independently scaled for display purposes. It will be noted in record (C) that two bursts of oscillation occur, with oscillatory period equal to about 10 sec

Figure 5.4 shows a typical signal processed in this way; the original sequence of intervals can be compared with the three selectively band-filtered signals (due mainly to the components identified above). Figure 5.5 shows two typical interval spectra, indicating the amplitude of Fourier components of the interval signal, referred to a fundamental frequency of 1 cycle/256 intervals.

5.2.1.4. Spontaneous variability of contributing components

As a basis for considering any alterations that may be imposed by informational-loading of the subject, the spontaneous variability of each of the components must be investigated; this can be based conveniently on the coefficient of variation (CV) of the power in the band-limited signal. The power in each band (thermal, pressure, respiration), evaluated for successive signal lengths,

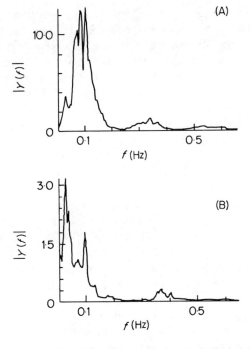

FIGURE 5.5. Two cardiac interval spectra (expressed in Hz) from the same individual (A) before and (B) during a period of demanding, decision-making mental work in an industrial environment. The magnitude of the thermal component is similar in both records (note scaling differences) but the 0–1 Hz band component is suppressed to insignificant levels in record (B); the regular respiratory component at about 0·35 Hz (a period of 3 sec or so) is shifted to a slightly higher frequency in (B)

leads to the mean power and standard deviation of the power in each band, and so to their ratio, CV. The following values can be taken as broadly representative of figures for the normal seated, resting adult:

	CV of Power	95 per cent confidence limits of Power
Band:		
Thermal	0·40	0·4 P; 3·75 P
Pressure	0·30	[0·5 P; 3·05 P]
Respiratory	0·35	0·6 P; 2·2 P

The confidence limits have been estimated on the basis, as found, that the distribution of power is approximately x^2 with an appropriate number of degrees of freedom; P is the power in the given band in the given single length of record. This can be used to test for significant alterations in the original signal, but since the 10-sec (pressure) component may be present or absent, the confidence limits for the corresponding band are not as realistic as those for the other bands. In fact, the important issue about the 10-sec component is the fraction of time for which it occurs. The component obviously cannot be identified by less than two complete cycles of its waveform (say 20 sec in duration), so the individual signal length of say, 256 intervals (mean duration T_0 sec) can be divided into 20-sec segments (256 $T_0/20$ in all) and, because interest is focused only on the presence or absence of the oscillation, the successful identification of the component in each segment can be treated as a binary variable. If successive occurrences were independent then the number of occurrences would be distributed binomially and the mean and standard deviation of the number of segments per 256 interval in which the oscillation appears could be determined, leading to a confidence-limit estimation. If the power in the oscillation is constant each time it occurs, then the confidence limits for the power in the band could then be calculated directly. However the mean duration for which the 10 second oscillation continues is probably at least 30 sec, so occurrences in successive 20-sec segments are not totally independent; also as far as the interval signal is concerned, the oscillatory power is by no means constant at successive occurrences, although this is probably not the case when the oscillations are viewed in the blood pressure or flow signal.

Finally, the vasomotor oscillation in blood pressure, as seen in the interval signal, is somewhat age-dependent (as in the respiratory effect) and older groups of subjects show reduced power, somewhat more variable, 10-sec oscillations. For all these reasons, the key parameter in respect of this component is best taken as the presence or absence of the oscillation as assessed by the relative duration of the oscillatory burst in the interval sequence. Nevertheless some idea of the variation of this and other components can be obtained by evaluating the power in the three bands for each of a number of sequential sections of interval signal, as in Figure 5.6 for which 25 sections of signal were employed.

5.2.2. Peripheral blood flow

The most directly relevant single circulatory variable would be intra-arterial blood pressure, but it is not feasible in practice to measure this variable. Hence the non-invasive measurement of blood flow is used instead to achieve an indication of the waveform changes of the blood pressure signal. The relationship is not fully proportional since, for the low frequency fluctuations of concern here, the vascular hydraulic impedance is not completely resistive. Also, of course, superficial blood flow is itself a significant variable entering directly into the thermal control operations and this certainly affects total

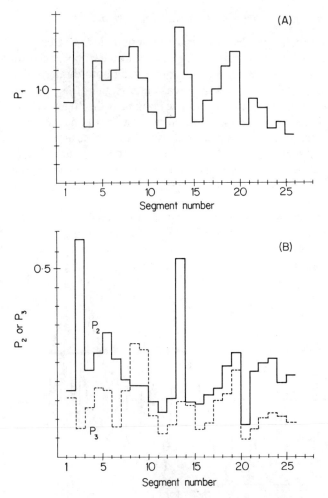

FIGURE 5.6. (A) Signal power (a relative measure) in 25 successive segments, each 256 cardiac intervals, illustrating typical variability. (B) Signal power (on the same scale and for the same period as A) in the blood-pressure vasomotor band (P_2) and simultaneously in the respiratory band (P_3) throughout the set of 25 successive segments. The variability in P_2 is typical of circumstances in which the pressure vasomotor component is active during most of some segments but inhibited during much of others

required blood flow. On the other hand, vasomotor pressure oscillations should be similar (apart from magnitude) in different vascular regions. Also, the peripheral blood flow signal is most attractive because of the ease with which it can be recorded; furthermore, it is a continuous signal in real time and not subject to the slight ambiguities inevitable with a signal having interval-number rather than time, as the independent parameter.

5.2.2.1. Acquisition of the peripheral blood flow signal

The photoelectric plethysmograph is a simple device relying on the visible alteration of the opacity of say, a finger-tip or an ear lobe, according to blood flow in the tissue concerned. A source of light, a photo-diode, and an electronic amplifier are sufficient to produce a reasonable signal; the only slight difficulty is that a light source like a small electric lamp near the finger will heat the tissue and cause a slow alteration in local blood flow that appears in the transducer output, and may be inconvenient, but use of a more distant light source and a light guide eliminate the difficulty. The appropriate sampling rate for this signal is fixed by the fastest feature of the cyclic pressure component harmonic with heart rate and it is rare for a sampling rate above 20 per sec to be needed.

No very substantial relevant differences occur from site to site but the ear lobe or any of the fingers allow satisfactory recordings; however signals obtained from the lower extremities do not usually produce a very satisfactory 0·1-Hz waveform at any time. Figure 5.7 shows a typical finger-blood-flow recording.

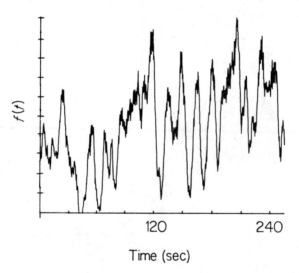

FIGURE 5.7. Digit photo-plethysmogram recorded in a resting individual, showing typical fluctuations in blood-flow

5.2.2.2. Analysis of the blood flow signal

The use of zero phase-shift digital filters will allow the two slower major components to be extracted from this signal without risk of time-shift; the respiratory fluctuations do not always appear strongly in recordings from the extremities. However vasomotor components thought to originate in blood pressure and thermal control operations are readily seen.

There is a time delay between the 10-sec oscillations in blood flow (or pressure)

and the same component in heart rate; as explained previously, this appears to be related to oscillatory frequency and to the fact that the oscillation may cease from time to time. It should be recognized, however, that there is probably no significant change in the effectiveness of the underlying control operation whether or not the system is in spontaneous oscillation.

The entrainment effects reported for thermal and pressure oscillations in the interval signal are duplicated directly in the blood flow signal and indeed there is a high correlation for most of the spectral components in the pressure-vasomotor band, or somewhat less in the thermal band, as between the blood flow and interval signals. (Low frequency effects due to slow changes of mean flow to individual peripheral segments of the circulation are not duplicated in the interval signal.)

5.2.3. Respiration

The most directly derived features of respiration are rate and depth; however, the pattern of respiratory waveforms is subject to appreciable change and this fact is relevant to the present matter. Additionally, a respiratory-linked activity like speech also contributes because it alters the pattern of thoracic movement due to the fact that speech requires the controlled release of breath. The special relevance of respiratory activity is first, that the pattern of breathing frequency alters characteristically when the subject undertakes a mental task (and this may be the most readily observed initial response), and second, that because respiratory activity is linked into the blood pressure and heart rate systems, it not only contributes to these other variables but (because the pressure-control system is non-linear) may produce entrainment of spontaneous oscillation in this system. Also, again because of the non-linearity of the pressure–vasomotor system, the respiratory waveform may produce a wave-form interaction with the spontaneous oscillations of blood pressure as well as a summation, and this can be seen in the blood pressure, blood flow, or cardiac interval signal. It appears as an amplitude modulation of the higher frequency signal (respiration) by the lower frequency signal (vasomotor oscillation); the effect disappears, of course, when the vasomotor oscillation ceases (as a result of entrainment or by another mechanism, for example, a reduction of control-loop time delay). It should also be noted that respiration itself is subject to considerable alteration due to the requirements of speech production.

Respiration is a complex variable, subject to modifying inputs from voluntary and involunatary nervous pathways as well as serving several functions in body metabolism and homeostasis. It seems (Priban and Fincham 1966) that respiratory patterns alter with blood chemistry, as part of the mechanism designed to regulate the state of the blood (in respect of pH, pCO_2, pO_2); hence on this basis, metabolic and other alterations that influence the chemical state of the blood will cause an alteration in respiratory patterns. For these various reasons, the investigation of any respiratory changes that might occur as a result of external disturbances, or mental tasks, or sensory loading, requires some investigation of the details of respiratory activity and cannot be adequately considered simply by study of respiratory rate and depth.

5.2.3.1. Acquisition of the respiratory signal

Most of the linkage between respiration or respiratory-linked movements and the blood pressure or heart rate systems, takes place as a result of intra-thoracic pressure fluctuations. Consequently, breath-flow is not a primary variable here; instead it is desirable to assess intrathoracic pressure, which can be achieved in a somewhat indirect way by monitoring upper abdominal movement, on the grounds that the primary forces producing respiration originate in the diaphragm. Even simple devices are suitable; for example, a displacement transducer to measure circumference of the upper abdomen, in which stretch of a belt changes the pressure on a graphite loaded sponge, for example, the resistance of which is measured electrically, operates satisfactorily with minimal discomfort to the subject. Circumferential rubber tubes filled with conducting material, that reduce radius with stretch, and so increase resistance to current-flow, are also simple and effective, with adequate speed of response. An account of various methods of measurement will be found in Yanov (1972). Figure 5.8 shows a typical signal.

The problem of respiratory signal variability is considerable since rate, depth, and pattern alter greatly and rapidly; artefacts due to coughing and postural change are also present.

Spectral descriptions of the complete signal are of little value in this situation; some rational simplification is required, and the use of individual breath parameters is convenient. In addition to rate and depth measurements, such measurements as expiratory–inspiratory movement, time to peak inspiration (referred to the start of the breath), time to maximum inspiratory rate (and its magnitude), offer a somewhat more detailed picture of respiratory pattern. For some physiological purposes, these measures of breath pattern are useful, especially when treated as a multi-dimensional description, and the same is true here.

5.2.3.2. Analysis of the respiratory signal

Utilizing a semi-automatic editing scheme similar to that mentioned above (5.2.1.1) for acquisition of individual breath parameters, a single or multi-dimensional analysis can be carried out. The signal maxima of peak inspiration, and peak expiration can be detected automatically, subjected to visual checking and correction as described before and from these points the required intervals, magnitudes and ratio of change (for example) can be computed for each breath. In view of the usually large breath-by-breath variability, it is necessary to collect data for a series of sequential breaths (called an ensemble) in order to characterize respiratory activity. With an adequate ensemble of N observations (i.e. one measurement from each of N breaths), the usual statistical measures

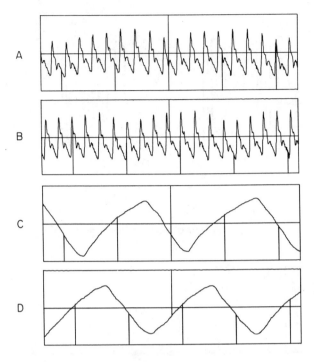

FIGURE 5.8. Respiratory (A, B) and simultaneous intra-arterial blood pressure (B.P.) waveforms (C, D) in the resting individual, in this case with a forced respiration to emphasize the resulting arrhythmia. Each record is 15 sec in duration and the B.P. signal shows both the characteristic respiratory-rate modulation and an amplitude modulation due to the breathing movements. The respiratory activity is assessed in this case by measuring thoracic movements. A and B are continuous, as are C and D

can be calculated, but another approach has been found more useful.

The N observations of the specific parameter chosen for study (say, for example, peak inspiratory magnitude) are re-ordered in a ranked amplitude sequence (RAS). This sequence, as illustrated in Figure 5.9, has a characteristic shape, and a single mathematical curve (say, a third-order polynomial) can be fitted to the sequence to achieve a quantitative description of the parameter. (It will be recognized that this procedure is related to the analysis of a histogram of magnitudes, but simpler). For the present purposes, the average slope of the main part of the RAS, and its intercept at the start of the sequence, are sufficient to represent the group of breaths concerned.

The result of this kind of analysis suggests that the pattern of individual breaths observed is drawn from a repertoire of available breath patterns; the increments in size of the variable and the range of values being utilized alter consistently as time passes. A change in step size of the variable from any

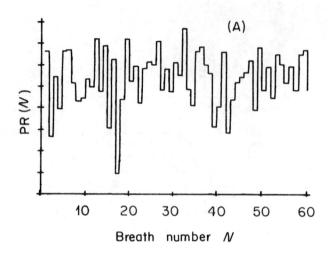

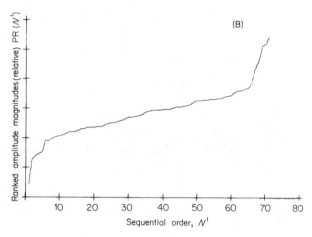

FIGURE 5.9. (A) Part of a sequence of 60 successive peak-inspiratory magnitudes PR (N) extracted from the original respiratory signal. (B) Ranked amplitude sequence of 70 peak-inspirations PR (N') from the same succession of breaths as in A. The signal is re-ordered according to sample magnitude and the resulting curve can be quantified by curve-fitting procedures (using for example a third-order polynomial)

magnitude to the next larger, if common throughout the range of values, will produce a change in slope of the main, approximately linear, part of the RAS, whereas if a net change in the variable is achieved by adding some larger values, the linear part will be extended and the overall slope of the curve altered. Both kinds of change are observed, and when this kind of analysis is carried out with different descriptive variables (e.g., time to peak inspiration, magnitude of peak inspiratory rate of change), a detailed and useful representation of the breath pattern can be achieved.

5.3. RESPONSES TO AN INFORMATION-HANDLING TASK

When decision-making tasks are undertaken, various physiological changes occur. For purposes of practical investigation, only readily measurable variables observed by non-invasive measurements can be employed; for this reason, attention is focused here on the cardio-respiratory variables that have been discussed: the cardiac interbeat signal (or the heart rate signal), peripheral blood flow, and respiratory and respiratory-linked movements.

The range of effects noted, both in laboratory investigations and industrial studies, can be outlined briefly. When a subject is presented with a difficult information-handling task, there may be a change in the pattern of heart rate or of respiratory rate; sometimes the power (variance) of the cardiac interbeat interval signal diminishes, but this cannot always be relied upon. A similar situation exists with other variables such as blood flow. However, certain detailed physiological changes can now usually be identified and their separate changes, and interactions, are often very instructive. In particular, the pattern, rather than simply the depth, of respiration alters in a way that can be measured and quantified; also, the relative fraction of time for which the pressure–vasomotor oscillation can be identified, is likely to decrease sharply with increased demands of the task. Furthermore, alterations in the interaction between respiratory and slower (pressure or thermal) fluctuations can occur.

The respiratory-pattern changes appear to be basic in the sense that changes in at least some other variables (e.g. in heart rate or in pressure vasomotor oscillations) seem usually to flow from, rather than cause respiratory effects. The inhibition, to some extent, of pressure vasomotor oscillations originates in either of two possible causes. First, the alteration in respiratory rate, depth, or pattern, may be sufficient to entrain the pressure–vasomotor oscillation; second, the operation of a mechanism that alters transmission time-delay for pressure signals traversing the brain-stem can also be inferred, and in an informational-load situation, may inhibit the spontaneous oscillation for long periods of time. The apparently altered interaction between vasomotor oscillations and respiratory fluctuations occurs when the patterns of respiratory activity become too irregular to be clearly characterized, and possibly also when alterations occur in the effects presumed to arise in the brain-stem.

Thus in the cardiac interval signal, the pressure vasomotor ($0 \cdot 1$ Hz) component may occur less often and the effect is frequently if not always progressive with load; respiratory patterns may alter in rate and detailed waveshape, and as a result, may produce a very considerably altered contribution to the interval signal. The loss of the $0 \cdot 1$ Hz component will diminish the total signal power, and the spectral profile of the signal will lose the characteristic and substantial contribution due to the $0 \cdot 1$ Hz component and will become noticeably biased towards lower frequency components. Because of this, the auto-correlation function of intervals will then exhibit a substantial broadening in shape, as sometimes reported (Parin and Baevsky 1967), and this follows follows directly and totally from the change in signal spectrum.

On the other hand, it must be remembered that the structure of the relevant control system certainly involves a non-linear element; so if a change in respiratory rate or pattern, or both, occurs, it is possible for signal power to increase again for this reason. As a result, despite the loss of the 0·1 Hz component, the total signal power may experience a net increase. Consequently, the total signal power (i.e., variance) should not be expected to produce invariably consistent indications of informational loading. In short, the most evident usual change in the signal when an informational-loading task is undertaken, can be identified as a progressive inhibition of the bursts of spontaneous pressure vasomotor oscillation that normally occur; however, the effect of any simultaneous respiratory change may be to counterbalance the resulting loss of power. Hence a more detailed analysis of effects is justified than is provided by a simple power (variance) measure applied to the cardiac interval signal.

5.3.1. Respiratory effects

Changes occur in respiratory pattern in response to an information-handling task. First, a decrease of respiratory rate sometimes occurs; the spectral effect, the still broadly-regular respiratory contribution to the interval (or blood flow) signal, will then spread downwards towards the band usually associated with the pressure–vasomotor activity. If the respiratory depth increases, at whatever rate, entrainment of the 0·1 Hz pressure vasomotor component can occur and might be followed by the appearance of respiratory components in the 0·1-Hz region.

Second, quite distinct from this, substantial changes not only in respiratory regularity but also in the range of breath patterns, may be observed (the latter sometimes without change in rate or depth). This has a significant effect on the interval or blood flow signal; in particular, the bursts (typically 30 sec or so) of 0·1-Hz activity become less frequent, and the signal power in that band of the spectrum is generally reduced. The effects of an informational-loading task on respiratory pattern are illustrated in Figure 5.10; the ranked amplitude sequence method has been applied to the thoracic movement signal acquired as previously described, and represented by a single index per breath.

Virtually any parameter that refers to a specific breath feature exhibits changes, but perhaps the most noticeable feature is the progressive change in breath-by-breath pattern variability assessed over say, 20 breaths or more (even excluding extreme values and even when breath rate is constant) as the task becomes more difficult. Also, it must be noted that while variability of, say, inspiratory amplitude, usually increases (on average by up to a factor of 3), some individuals (about 20 per cent) invariably demonstrate a decreased variability with load. However, on the basis of experience in this Laboratory of studying 50 individuals in 6 various different age and occupation categories,

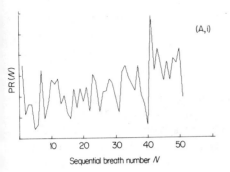

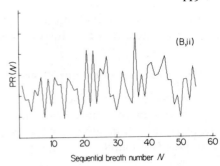

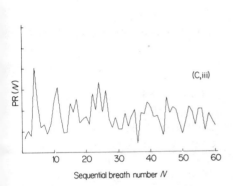

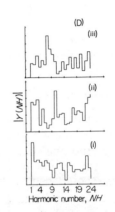

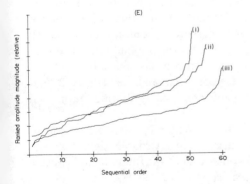

FIGURE 5.10. (A), (B) and (C) illustrate sequences of respiratory peak-inspiratory magnitudes in an individual conducting a decision-making task; 50–60 breaths are shown in each of three work-load situations. These results are typical, qualitatively and quantitatively, of the order-independent responses observed in most individuals when work-load situations are imposed but the original respiratory signal itself is often almost wholly insensitive to any such changes of loading. The three states [light (i), medium (ii) and considerable difficulty (iii)] of the task produce patterns as shown in (A), (B) and (C) respectively. (D) The spectra of the peak-inspiratory magnitudes [corresponding to (A), (B) and (C)] exhibit mainly the low-frequency bias due to within-record trend, and also the presence of other slow fluctuations. No significant differences according to loading can be confirmed in such spectral descriptions, suggesting that serial correlations are not important. (E) The re-ordering procedure produces a marked difference in the distribution of peak inspiratory magnitudes at the high work-load level (iii); records (i) and (ii) are not distinguishable from the fully-resting records. This effect can be qualified by curve fitting

an individual is found to produce similar variability of respiratory responses, always increasing with load, or always decreasing.

5.3.2. Pressure–vasomotor effects

When a subject undertakes an information-handling task, the frequency of bursts of spontaneous vasomotor oscillations diminishes. This has been observed both in subjects who respond to the task with increased variability of breath amplitude fluctuations and in those generating decreased variability. Thus it follows that the progressive inhibition of pressure–vasomotor oscillations is not necessarily a respiratory-linked entrainment effect although without doubt entrainment is relevant in some circumstances. In laboratory tasks, as well as in industrial situations, the effect of greatly increased difficulty of a task is often to terminate the pressure–vasomotor oscillation altogether.

5.3.3. Interactions

As stated above, both the pressure-vasomotor and thermal-vasomotor systems are non-linear, in the sense that the effect of a combined signal in passing a thorough non-linear pathway is different from the sum of independent effects. Interaction between simultaneous on-going components that share common non-linear pathways is possible, and the most common effect is that any higher frequency component (if sufficiently regular) such as due to respiration, is modulated in amplitude by a lower frequency component, like the vasomotor contributions due to thermal and pressure effects. In the resting individual such interactions can commonly be seen, when the respiratory rate is stable enough, in the cardiac interval signal; the effect shows up as a modulation of the respiratory fluctuation usually by the thermal vasomotor component (or much less often by the pressure–vasomotor component). The effect is shown in Figure 5.11 which illustrates the original interval signal, the thermal components obtained by filtering with a pass band from DC to 12 harmonics of the fundamental (1 cycle/256 intervals), i.e. H0-H12, and also the respiratory and other fast components obtained by filtering the original signal from H25-H64.

If the mean interval is say 0·6 sec the H25-H64 filter (chosen widespread to avoid risk of overlooking important parts of this variable signal) selects components with frequencies of 25 to 64 times that of the fundamental (1 cycle per 256 intervals = 1 cycle per $256 \times 0·6$ seconds = 1/154 Hz, with a period of 154 sec) so the components selected have periods of $154/25 = 6·1$ sec to $154/64 = 2·4$ sec which would correspond to regular breathing rates of 10–25 breaths per min. This vasomotor waveform correlates negatively with the envelope fluctuations of the high frequency waveform over parts of the record (when the low frequency signal goes negative from its mean level, the high-frequency signal shows its maximum level and this can be seen most effectively by extracting the 'envelope' of the fast signal, as also shown. These interactions

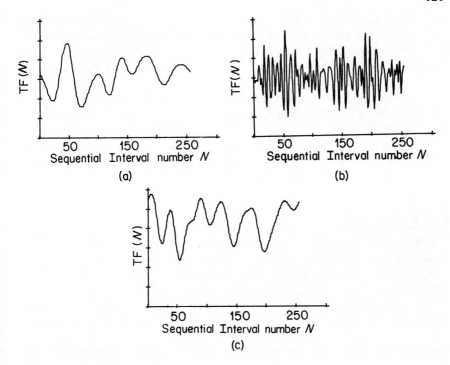

FIGURE 5.11. Interactions between components exhibited by the cardiac interval signal recorded in the resting individual; the signal is the same as in Figure 4. The low-pass filtered version of the signal is shown in (A) (harmonics 1–15), and in (B) the signal is band-filered to select effects of essentially respiratory origin. As in most interval signals recorded in the resting individual, a correlation can be seen over part of the record between the pattern of magnitudes of the band-filtered signal and that of the simultaneous low frequency component of the original signal. Curve (C) shows the envelope signal obtained from (B) and can be compared directly with (A). Note that maximum correlation occurs with a delay of some 15 intervals between the two records and that the effect is most evident in respect of timing rather than in the detailed amplitude of the common fluctuations

are quite significant in scale and contribute appreciably to the power; for example, estimated in 25 subjects, the fraction of signal power in the high frequency region involved in and attributable to the modulation effects is about 0·7 and the fraction of time for which the modulation linkage can be be seen is about 0·4.

It is important to recognise that certain conditions are required for this effect to be seen. First, adequate respiratory depth is needed since otherwise there will be insufficient signal for any modulation; also the respiration must be reasonably stable in frequency or it will be impossible to filter any realistic version of the respiratory signal from other contributions. Since these two conditions are met only some of the time even in resting conditions, the modulation effect will occur overtly and clearly only during part of any record. Also, postural changes will certainly contribute to the fast components of the interval signal without necessarily entering the interaction. Furthermore, it must be recognized that the operating state of the control system can vary (perhaps slowly) for reasons not wholly understood, and may operate for some periods like a linear system; no modulation effects can occur in these circumstances. Finally, the presence of large but slower respiratory-linked variations due to speech will certainly dominate the behaviour of the system and inhibit any modulation effects.

The interactive relation within the interval signal between low-frequency components and respiratory effects alters when the subject undertakes a difficult information-handling task. Several factors may be involved. First, if the pressure–vasomotor component is involved (a relatively infrequent occurrence), the interaction can, of course, no longer be found when this component is inhibited by entrainment or otherwise. Second, if the respiration becomes highly irregular (short interbreath intervals alternating with longer intervals, for example) the interval signal spectral contribution due to respiration will be widely spread and no clear separation from other components can be achieved. Third, the system operating point may be altered, for example by a similar mechanism to that which affects signal transmission time-delay through the brain-stem. Of these three, the latter two are apparently most common and careful separation of records in which a fairly steady respiratory rate is maintained, with or without substantial pattern changes, shows that the third mechanism is apparently operative when the task in hand becomes very difficult for the subject, about the stage when the error rate in the task becomes large.

5.3.4. A summary of effects

The most useful practical physiological indicator of effects that can occur when a listener is presented with a difficult information-handling task is the cardiac intervals (heart rate) signal. In our experience, mean heart rate is not often a useful indicator, and total variability of the signal, as assessed by signal power (variance) also cannot be relied upon for reproducible indications in most subjects. On the other hand, an analysis of the signal power into various contributing components is both illuminating and potentially useful. Rather than to review the already extensive literature on minutae of revelant psychophysiological effects, the aim of this chapter has been to present a selective account of the components that contribute to the cardiac signal and their involvement in the main psychophysiological effects judged to be important, together with an outline of the mechanisms currently believed to be responsible. The detailed justifications are presented elsewhere.

All physiological signals are subject to spontaneous variation for two reasons; the operation of statistical sampling effects, and the influence of altering biological processes that affect the signal. Against the background of spontaneous variability of the cardiac interval signal and its contributing components, the main effects that commonly occur when a subject undertakes a difficult informational-handling task as follows. First, the signal power (variance) often decreases, but not invariably. (Improved sensitivity in this measure can be obtained by excluding very slow fluctuations having periods above 25 sec). Certainly however, there is a redistribution of signal power amongst available spectral components; this is reflected in changes of the cardiac interval auto-correlation sequence, but this particular measure is inconvenient to compute and interpret and is also subject to unattractive statistical sampling variations. Close scrutiny of the amplitude spectra instead, and of spectral variations, indicates several reasons for the changes that occur: respiratory rate, depth or pattern variations, alterations in the recurrence periods of the bursts of roughly 0·1-Hz oscillations that are believed to originate in the blood-pressure vasomotor system and reductions in the interactions between vasomotor fluctuations believed to be of thermo-regulatory origin fluctuations of respiratory origin. When the task is too difficult to be carried out without a significant increase in error rate, it is also observed that pressure–vasomotor oscillations cease altogether, and the interactions that indicate an (incidental) influence due to thermo-regulatory fluctuations on the way respiration appears to affect cardiac intervals can no longer be identified. No effects on the components believed to originate in the thermo-regulatory process have been seen in any subject and there may be advantages, for this reason, in eliminating this component altogether from the signal.

5.4. ACKNOWLEDGMENT

The material presented in this chapter includes work carried out in this Laboratory and supported by the U.K. Medical Research Council.

5.5. REFERENCES

Bendat, J. S. & Piersol, A. G. *Random data: Analysis and measurement procedures.* New York: Wiley-Interscience, 1971.

Ergonomics Research Society (J. M. Rolfe, Ed.), Symposium on Heart Rate Variability, *Ergonomics*, 1973, **16,** 1–12.

Hyndman, B. W., Kitney, R. I. & Sayers, B. McA. Spontaneous oscillations in physiological control systems. *Nature*, 1971, **233,** 339–341.

Kitney, R. I. The use of entrainment in analysis of the human thermo-regulatory system. *Journal of Physiology*, 1972, **229,** 40–41.

Kitney, R. I. Analysis and simulation of the human thermoregulatory control system. *Medical and Biological Engineering*, 1974, **12,** 57–64.

Lynn, P. A. *An introduction to the analysis and processing of signals.* London: MacMillan, 1973.

Monro, D. M. Chirp-z and fourier algorithm. Engineering in Medicine Laboratory, 1973, Report No. 5, Imperial College, p. 19.

Parin, V. V. & Baevsky, R. M. Mathematical models of the heart rhythm and their diagnostic significance. *7th International Conference on Medical and Biological Engineering*, Stockholm, August 14–19, 1967, Digest p. 283.

Priban, I. P. & Fincham, W. P. Self-adaptive control and the respiratory system. *Nature*, 1965, **208,** 339–343.

Rabiner, L. R., Schafer, R. W. & Rader, C. M. The chirp-z transform algorithm and its application. *Bell System Technical Journal*, 1969, **48,** 1249–1292.

Sayers, B. McA. Inferring significance from biological signals. In Clynes, M. & Milsum, J. H. (Eds), *Biomedical Engineering Systems*. New York: McGraw-Hill, 1970.

Sayers, B. McA. The analysis of cardiac interbeat interval sequences and the effects of mental work-load. *Proceedings of the Royal Society of Medicine*, 1971, **64,** 707–710.

Sayers, B. McA. Quantitative methods in cardiology. In, Snellen, H. A., Hugenholtz, P. G. & Van Bemmel, J. H. (Eds), *Quantitation in cardiology*. University of Leiden Press, 1972, pp. 5–23.

Sayers, B. McA. Analysis of heart rate variability. *Ergonomics*, 1973, **16,** 17–32.

Vahl, S. P., Vickery, J. C., Monro, D. M. & Tinker, J. An interactive computer-based editing system for physiological data. *Computers in Medicine and Biology*, 1971, **1,** 317–322.

Yanov, H. M. *Biomedical electronics*. (2nd ed.) Philadelphia: F. A. Davis & Co., 1972.

Chapter 6

Sleep

LAVERNE C. JOHNSON

*Navy Medical Neuropsychiatric Research Unit
San Diego, California*

6.1. SLEEP AS AN EXPERIMENTAL VARIABLE

The richness and complexity of the activity we call 'sleep' has been brought to our awareness through the variety of recordings of physiological measures. There is now no doubt that sleep is an active process with a great deal of sensory processing and decision-making, though we are generally unaware of such mentation. In recognition of this active internal state and its interaction with the external environment, sleep researchers named their society the Association for the Psychophysiological Study of Sleep (APSS). While the name alone would qualify the research done by this Society's members for inclusion in this volume, the richness of the information contributed from sleep laboratories makes its inclusion mandatory and the task of summarizing the critical findings in a single chapter a formidable one. Fortunately, an extensive review of the psychophysiology of sleep has been published by Snyder & Scott (1972). A recent review by Williams, Holloway & Griffiths (1973) surveys other aspects of sleep in addition to psychophysiology.

Sleep as an experimental variable affords many unique advantages even though it is generally not discussed in most experimental psychology textbooks. If sleep is mentioned, it is usually in the context of memory and retention. Sleep was felt to be an excellent condition to investigate the concepts of disuse and retroactive inhibition on memory. In one of the earliest studies of sleep as an experimental variable, Jenkins & Dallenbach (1924) reported that retention was consistently higher after an interpolated period of sleep than waking. The effect of sleep on retention has continued to be an area of interest, with Van Ormaer (1932) essentially replicating the results of Jenkins & Dallenbach. More recently, Ekstrand (1967) asked the question whether a period of sleep facilitated retention by reducing proactive rather than retroactive inhibition. Ekstrand also found that recall was significantly higher when the interval was spent in sleep rather than waking. The positive effect of sleep was not contingent upon interference from prior lists learned in the laboratory.

These studies, thus, presented clear evidence that sleep during the period following acquisition facilitates retention. In these early studies, sleep was viewed as a single state and Jenkins and Dallenbach, and Van Ormer, were probably unaware that sleep stages and sleep cycles existed. With the discovery of sleep stages, there has been a reawakening of interest in the effect of sleep on learning and memory with particular interest in the relative importance of various sleep stages in the consolidation of memory traces (Ekstrand, Sullivan, Parker & West, 1971; Empson & Clarke, 1970; Fowler, Sullivan & Ekstrand, 1973; Grieser, Greenberg & Harrison, 1972; Pearlman, 1971; Portnoff, Baekeland, Goodenough, Karacan & Shapiro, 1966; Yaroush, Sullivan & Ekstrand, 1971). A more detailed discussion of information processing during sleep will be presented later in this chapter.

It is for those interested in the psychophysiology of altered states that sleep is a most useful experimental variable. Sleep offers cyclic and predictable state changes uncomplicated by use of drugs, brain stimulation, or lesions. The ability clearly to delineate the changes in sleep stages from electrophysiological data permits the researcher a unique opportunity to study changes in responses as the subject goes from awake through the various sleep stages. In contrast to the continual shifting and fluctuations in arousal level and attention present in the awake subject, for several minutes and, in some instances for several hours, a sleeping subject remains in a relatively steady state. The constant impinging of external stimuli which often complicates interpretation of results can be reduced to near zero in the sleeping subject. Though mental activity does not cease with sleep onset, there is now information as to the changes in quality and quantity of mental activity as the sleeper changes sleep stages. In addition to those interested in learning and memory, these advantages of sleep have not been overlooked by those concerned with effect of state on the orienting response (OR), changes in basal and spontaneous physiological activity, neuroendocrinology, neurophysiology, neuroanatomy, and neurochemistry. Sleep has truly become a period for study of the total subject, as reflected in the proceedings of the First International Congress on Sleep (Chase, 1972).

For the many psychophysiologists who have, without hesitation, reported that their data were obtained from awake subjects, sleep may have become an unreported source of error variance. One often wonders how frequently their reported awake subjects had, in fact, succumbed to the soporific qualities of the laboratory and drifted into a drowsy or sleep state. In addition to expected changes caused by drowsiness in attention, memory, and behavioural responses, there are other state specific changes of which psychophysiologists might be unaware. Johnson & Lubin (1972) have discussed level of activation (arousal) as an experimental variable and cautioned against neglect of this source of error variance. For example, habituation curves for the cardiovascular measures of heart rate (HR) and finger pulse response (FPR) were not found in drowsy subjects (McDonald, Johnson & Hord, 1963). During stage 2 sleep, there was, in fact, an increase in evoked HR response (Hord, Lubin & Johnson, 1966). In the awake state, a high rate of background spontaneous electrodermal activity (EDA) is associated with large ED responses to stimuli and slow habituation. During all sleep, an ED response to external stimuli is difficult to obtain even though during certain sleep stages there is a high rate of background spontaneous activity (Johnson & Lubin, 1966).

Evoked EEG responses also change considerably in waveform and amplitude with changes in arousal level. Williams, Tepas, and Morlock (1962), in a detailed study of EEG evoked response to clicks during awake and various stages of sleep, found with sleep onset an increased first positive component (P_1) but a decreased first negative (N_1) and second positive (P_2) component. Only subject state was varied in their study.

In contrast, the contingent negative variation (CNV) or expectancy wave decreases in amplitude with drowsiness and disappears with sleep. In Figure 6.1 is an example of the increase in CNV as the subject is encouraged to 'try harder' and its decrease after the subject is told to 'go to sleep' and sleep ensues. This finding was not unexpected since no build-up in expectancy was anticipated during sleep, but unpredicted was the similar decrease in CNV in the awake subject following sleep deprivation reported by Naitoh, Johnson & Lubin (1971). Sleep loss will be discussed in another chapter of this volume (Naitoh).

Other examples could obviously be given to illustrate changes in response with changes in state, but perhaps these will suffice to sensitize the reader to the possible systematic biases induced by the subject's change from an alert awake state to a drowsy or sleep state. Of course these 'error variances' are intriguing results for those concerned with the psychophysiology of sleep.

Detection of changes in background EEG, detailed below, is the usual procedure for partialing out changes in arousal level. But if EEG recording is not possible and if your study requires a constant awake state, are there techniques to ensure that the subject remains awake? We know of no completely foolproof technique. We have had some success with asking the subject to count repeatedly from 1 to 9 by pressing one of nine buttons. This task was not completely successful in keeping the subject awake but, in the absence of EEG data, lapses in counting rate usually indicated lapses in arousal level. Peter Venables asks his subjects to exert a constant pressure on a handgrip, and auditory feedback is used to arouse the subject if pressure slackens (personal communication). As the contributions made by changes in arousal levels to the error variance become more widely known, we are certain more effec-

128

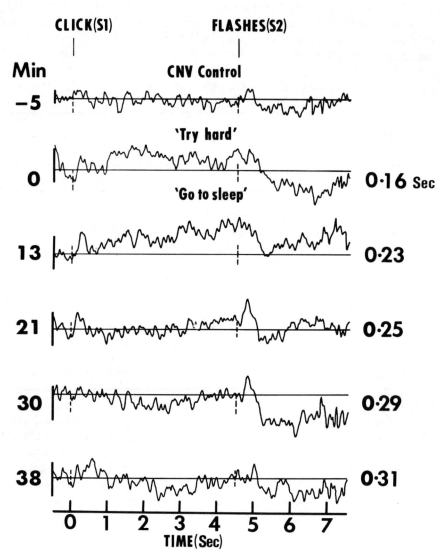

FIGURE 6.1. Changes in CNV with changes in arousal. With onset of drowsiness (21 min), the CNV amplitude is decreased and disappears with sleep onset (30 min)

tive techniques for maintaining a minimum level of arousal will be found.

In this chapter, we will first describe the electrophysiological and autonomic activity that justify the classification of sleep as a unique state and the division of sleep into stages. Then information processing during sleep, with particular attention to the OR during sleep, is discussed to illustrate the knowledge that can be obtained from sleep studies and the problems involved in studying a well-defined awake measure, such as the OR, during sleep.

6.2. SLEEP AS A UNIQUE STATE

6.2.1. Electrographic correlates

No one denies that the awake state differs from sleep, but the extent of this difference varies depending upon the area or behaviour being compared. The stages of sleep have been defined by the APSS Manual (Rechtschaffen & Kales, 1968) in terms of electrophysiological criteria. In Figure 6.2 are 20-sec samples of the electroencephalographic (EEG) and electrooculographic (EOG) activity during awake and each sleep stage.

In sleep laboratories, brain waves and eye movements, recorded on a polygraph, have replaced the traditional behavioural criteria (closed eyes,

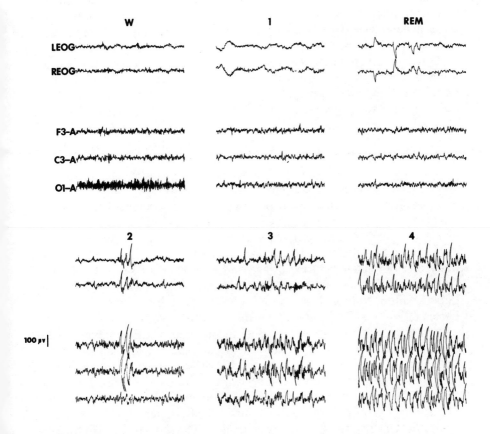

FIGURE 6.2. EEG stages of sleep following revised scoring criteria of Rechtschaffen & Kales (1968). The bursts of alpha are clearly seen in the 0_1–A lead during REM sleep. Abbreviations: W = awake; REM = rapid eye movement sleep; LEOG, REOG = left and right electrooculogram; F_3–A, C_3–A, O_1–A = frontal, central, and occipital electrode placements referenced to mastoid according to the International 10–20 system for EEG electrode placement. (From Hilbert, R. & Naitoh, P. *Psychophysiology*, 1972, **9**, 533–538, with permission.)

absence of speech, recumbent posture, etc.) for defining sleep. As currently defined in the APSS Manual, stage 1 consists of low-amplitude mixed-frequency EEG activity without sleep spindles, K-complexes, or rapid eye movements (REMs). In stage 2, there is low-amplitude mixed-frequency activity with K-complexes and 12–14 Hz sigma rhythms (sleep spindles). K-complexes are waveforms, lasting 1–2 sec, with a well-defined negative sharp wave and slow-wave component often followed by sigma spindles. Usually sleep spindles occur in bursts of 0·5–1·0 sec duration. Both K-complexes and bursts of sleep spindles are seen in stage 2 sleep, in Figure 6.2. Sleep spindles are also present in stages 3 and 4, but detection of K-complexes in stages 3 and 4 is difficult because of the high-voltage, slow-wave activity characteristic of these two stages. In stage 3, at least 20% of the EEG consists of high-amplitude slow delta waves (2 Hz or slower and at least 75 μV peak-to-peak). In stage 4, at least half the record is dominated by these high-amplitude slow waves. During REM sleep, there is low-amplitude mixed-frequency (stage-1-like) EEG activity with bursts of REMs and, in many instances, a markedly decreased tonus of certain head and neck muscles. In contrast, when stage 1 EEG is present at sleep onset, slow eye movements of about 1 per sec are seen, REMs do not occur, and the muscle tonus of head and neck muscles is higher than the levels seen during the stage 1 EEG of the REM sleep periods. Stages 2, 3, 4, and stage 1 without REMs, are collectively referred to as non-rapid-eye movement (NREM) sleep. The format of Figure 6.2 places the stages into the two groups which, for us, appear by several indices to be similar; i.e. stages awake, stage 1, and REM *vs* sleep stages, 2, 3, and 4.

While sleep clearly has behavioural characteristics different from waking, the questions 'Are there unique electrophysiological differences between the two states?' and 'Are there brain wave patterns unique to each sleep stage?' were not easily answered. Utilization of computers has enabled a detailed study of EEG activity during awake and each stage of sleep (Caille, 1967; Dumermuth, Walz, Scollo-Lavizzari & Kleiner, 1972; Johnson, 1972; Johnson, Lubin, Naitoh, Nute & Austin, 1969; Johnson, Naitoh, Lubin & Moses, 1972; Larsen & Walter, 1970; Lubin, Johnson & Austin, 1969).

We use spectral analysis to compute the amount of EEG activity for each frequency, and cross-spectral analysis to compute the amount of coherent EEG activity common to any two sites on the scalp at each frequency. Other computer methodologies have also been applied to the sleep EEG; for a more detailed discussion of computer use in sleep research, see Johnson (1972). The spectral profile, based upon Fourier analysis, represents the intensity of electrical energy as a function of frequency. The ordinate at each frequency reflects both the amplitude of the waveform and the prevalence of that frequency during the specific time period being analysed. For high alpha subjects, the awake EEG has a spectral peak near 10 Hz, as seen in Figure 6.3, awake (W) spectra.

Pairwise coherence (e.g., activity recorded from the F_3 and C_3 sites, see Figures 6.3 & 6.4) expresses the strength of the linear relation between activity

at one scalp site and EEG activity at another site. These coherences are calculated for each EEG frequency of interest. Coherence values lie between
0 and 1 and can be interpreted as squared correlations. High coherence between
brain areas at a specific frequency is consistent with the hypothesis of a common
generator or source for that specific frequency. The phase angle associated
with each coherence tells us whether activity at one electrode tends to lead
the other.

In our several computer analyses of awake and asleep EEG, we have consistently found that delta and alpha activity are present during both awake and
asleep. Inspection of the spectral and coherence profiles in Figures 6.3 and

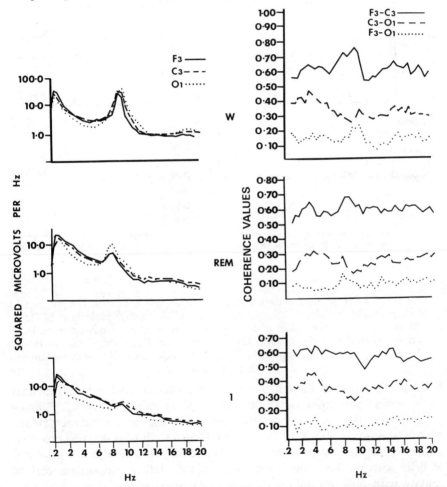

FIGURE 6.3. EEG spectra and coherence profiles for awake (W), stage REM, and
stage 1 ($N = 8$). In this figure, stage REM is placed below awake to highlight the
similarity of spectral and coherence profiles. There are no spectra and coherence
peaks in the 12–14 Hz area. (From Johnson, L. C., in Chase, M. H. (Ed) *The Sleeping
Brain*, 1972, pp. 277–321. Los Angeles: Brain Research Institute, with permission.)

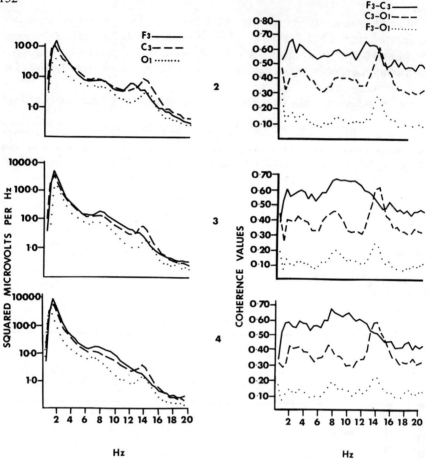

FIGURE 6.4. EEG spectra and coherence profiles for stages 2, 3 and 4. The presence of sleep spindles are clearly reflected in the C_3 and O_1 spectral peaks near 14 Hz and the high coherence values of these spindles are seen in the coherence peaks near 14 Hz in the C_3-O_1 profiles. (From Johnson, L. C., in chase, M. H. (Ed) *The Sleeping Brain*, 1972, pp. 277–321. Los Angeles: Brain Research Institute with permission.)

6.4 indicate that even though there is an increase in delta spectral intensity as the subject goes from awake through the sleep stages of stages 2, 3, and 4 (Figure 6.4), there is no associated increase in the delta coherence values. Naitoh, Johnson, Lubin & Wyborney (1971), in a study of generating processes during waking and sleep, suggested that there may be several possible sources of delta activity. The slow waves of sleep may reflect endogenous cortical activity with little regulation by subcortical pacemakers.

In contrast, the coherence values of alpha, especially in F_3-O_1 leads, change with onset of sleep and vary as the subject goes through the sleep stages. Naitoh *et al.* (1971) reported that there were at least two possible 'generators' or sources of alpha activity.

Sleep spindles, as Loomis, Harvey & Hobart (1935) suggested, appear to be unique to sleep stages 2, 3, and 4. As far as we know, waveforms with the morphological characteristics, distribution, and coherence values that characterize sleep spindles during sleep stages 2, 3, and 4 do not consistently occur in any state other than stages 2, 3, and 4. The high coherence values plus the results by Naitoh et al. (1971) suggest that the spindle waveforms are from a single source or generator. An early suggestion by Grey Walter (1953) that sleep spindles are associated with dreams has not supported.

Our work supports the suggestion made by Snyder & Scott (1972) and by Agnew & Webb (1972) that the appearance of the first sleep spindle can be used as an objective EEG measure of sleep onset. Sleep spindles are present in all human and most animal sleep records. Stage 1, with its fluctuating behavioural and EEG activity, appears to be a transition period between awake and sleep, and is often associated with hypnagogic phenomena. Stage 1 also does not appear to have restorative value; sustained stage 1 EEG patterns in our sleep-deprived subjects do not alleviate their expressed sleep needs or reverse the pattern of performance decrement.

Our spectral and coherence analyses, illustrated in Figure 6.4, clearly separated stages 2, 3, and 4 from REM with respect to EEG activity. EEG activity during REM is similar to awake and stage 1. This difference in EEG and the numerous differences in autonomic, mental, and motor activity between REM and stages 2, 3, and 4, support those sleep researchers who divide sleep into only two types; REM and NREM.

Larsen & Walter (1970) at the University of California, Los Angeles, subjected our EEG sleep data to quadratic function discriminating analysis and came to a similar conclusion. Stages 2, 3, and 4 formed one grouping; awake, REM, and stage 1 a second grouping.

The question is often asked whether hypnosis produces a state of sleep. In a quantitative analysis of the EEG during hypnosis, Ulett, Akpinar & Itil (1972) used digital period analysis and analogue filters to test the significance of EEG changes during both hypnotic induction and hypnotic trance. They found that the hypnotic-induced EEG changes were far from the drowsiness or sleep EEG patterns. In the good hypnotic subjects, hypnotic induction and trance were associated with a significant decrease of slow activity and an increase of alpha and beta waves.

6.2.2. Physiological correlates

The physiological correlates of sleep, like the EEG activity, clearly cluster into REM and NREM patterns. The rapid eye movements and other physiological correlates of REM sleep have received most attention (see Snyder & Scott, 1972). Early association of REM sleep with reports of dreaming led to the reasonable hypothesis that the eye movements and the large fluctuations in heart rate, blood pressure, and respiration seen during this sleep period were directly associated with dream content; in particular, that the rapid

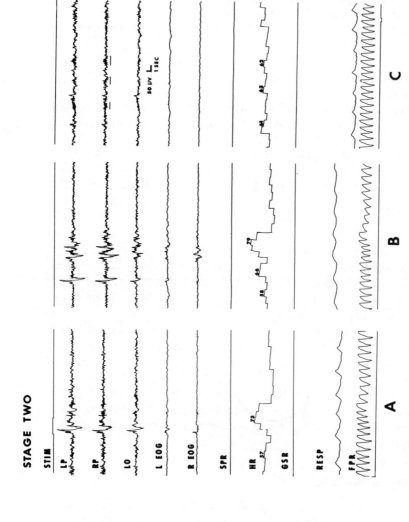

FIGURE 6.5. Autonomic responses to stimulus evoked K-complex (A), to a spontaneously produced K-complex (B), and absence of autonomic response during bursts of sleep spindles (C). Abbreviations: Stim = stimulus; LP and RP = left parietal and right parietal; LO = left occipital EEG; SPR = skin potential response; HR = heart rate; GSR = galvanic skin response; RESP = respiration; FPR = finger pulse responses. Other abbreviations are as used in previous figures. (From Johnson, L. C. & Karpas, W. E. *Psychophysiology*, 1968, **4**, 444–452, with permission.)

eye movements were tracking the visual content of dreams (Dement & Wolpert, 1958; Roffwarg, Dement, Muzio & Fisher, 1962). Several findings have cast doubt upon this attractive hypothesis, however. First, though less vivid and complex than stage REM reports, dream reports have been obtained upon awakenings from NREM stages of sleep. Second, there is no invariant relation of eye movements to the visual activity reported in dreams. Third, REMs have been reported in congenitally blind subjects. Fourth, newborn humans and animals, raised without any visual stimulation, have rapid eye movements during sleep. Fifth, the rate and distribution of REM bursts have been found to be consistent within subjects from REM period to REM period and from night to night; there is a consistent individual subject bias in eye movement direction; and there is a consistent relation between REM bursts and autonomic changes (Spreng, Johnson & Lubin, 1968). These latter results by Spreng *et al.* support the hypothesis proposed by Aserinsky (1965) that a neurophysiological mechanism, rather than the visual imagery of dreams, might be associated with the REM bursts and accompanying autonomic changes. Koulack (1972), after reviewing the studies concerning eye movements and imagery, concluded that 'the initial hypothesis of a constant isomorphic relationship between REMs and visual imagery seems to be untenable'.

Though it has received less attention, NREM sleep also has unique phasic events which are similar, in many ways, to the phasic eye movements of stage REM. Sleep spindles have already been mentioned as unique to stages 2, 3, and 4, but the K-complex is also a phasic event unique to NREM sleep. It was initially thought that K-complexes were always arousal responses evoked by external or internal stimuli. Careful monitoring has indicated that, like other phasic events during sleep, the K-complex also occurs spontaneously, i.e. without a known cause (Johnson & Karpan, 1968). Like REMs, spontaneous K-complexes occur with considerable regularity with a range over subjects of 0·75 to 2·00 per min. Each person's rate appears to be consistent over several nights of sleep. Both the spontaneous and evoked K-complexes were significantly associated with brief increases in heart rate (HRRs), finger vasoconstrictions (FPRs), and, in rare instances, with a brief decrease in skin resistance (SR) (see Figure 6.5). (In our earlier studies, as reflected on some figures, we used 'GSR' as our abbreviation for skin resistance response. We now use the more accepted 'SR' for skin resistance and 'SRR' for skin resistance response.) No autonomic changes have been associated with sleep spindles.

While K-complexes have many similarities to REMs with respect to autonomic correlates, there have been no serious suggestions that they are associated with dream content. The preferred hypothesis is still that K-complexes are related to brief increases in arousal. In support of the arousal hypothesis are the findings that body movements are almost always preceded by K-complexes (Sassin & Johnson, 1968) and that the evoked autonomic response to an external stimulus is significantly larger if the stimulus evoked a K-complex than when no K-complex is seen (Johnson & Lubin, 1967).

If there is a quiet period of sleep, slow-wave sleep (SWS), stages 3 and 4,

Stage 4

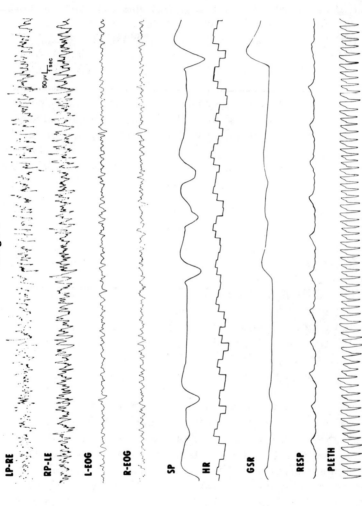

FIGURE 6.6. Example of spontaneous electrodermal activity (SP and GSR) during stage 4 sleep. No spontaneous fluctuations are evident in the other variables reflecting the dissociation among autonomic variables that occur during sleep. Abbreviations: LP–RE = left parietal to right ear; RP–LE = right parietal to left ear; SP = skin potential; PLETH = plethysmograph (a measure of finger pulse amplitude recorded from finger). Other abbreviations previously used. (From Johnson, L. C. & Lubin, A. *Psychophysiology*, 1966, **3**, 8–17, with permission.)

is generally thought of as that state. Body motility is lowest during this period and, when awakened, it takes longer for the person to respond effectively than if awakened from REM sleep or stage 2. But SWS has its own pattern of heightened activity; an increase in spontaneous SRRs and skin potential responses (SPRs). Though these spontaneous responses usually begin in stage 2, their rate of occurrence increases as the person enters stages 3 and 4. An example of this spontaneous EDA is seen in Figure 6.6. Figure 6.6 also clearly reflects the dissociation among autonomic variables during sleep. The spontaneous EDA, larger than that usually seen during waking, is not associated with increases in heart rate, respiration, or the finger pulse amplitude (FPR). The significance of the spontaneous EDA is unknown. Lester, Burch & Dossett (1967) have reported that sleep EDA increased as daytime stress increased, being especially great on nights preceding important school examinations, in 53 healthy students. In our studies, spontaneous EDA has shown no clear relation to activities of the previous day, the psychological state, or to awake levels of EDA. Johnson & Lubin (1966) have suggested that, as with EEG phasic activity and REMs, these spontaneous electrodermal discharges are related to the release of inhibitory mechanisms during NREM sleep.

The heightened and varying physiological activity associated with REM and NREM sleep removed any lingering beliefs in sleep as a steady state or a passive quiet state. Troublesome to the traditional psychophysiologist was the appearance of autonomic activity (e.g. evoked HRR, spontaneous EDA) similar to or greater than that seen in the awake state, but obviously without the same significance. This apparent paradox was discussed by Johnson (1970) when he raised the question, "If the same physiological responses or visceral changes occur in more than one state of consciousness, can we infer that they have the same behavioural meaning (e.g., high or low arousal) and the same physiological significance in each state? [p. 502].' The occurrence of alpha activity during REM sleep (see Figure 6.7) and the spontaneous EDA during NREM sleep were chosen as striking examples (Figure 6.6). The evoked alpha response during awake and the evoked alpha response during REM were clearly different (see Figure 6.8). In the awake state, high rates of spontaneous EDA are associated with large ORs. During NREM sleep, it is extremely difficult to obtain an evoked electrodermal response (EDR). (The OR during sleep will be discussed in more detail later.) In his review, Johnson concluded that 'indeed similar physiological activity can occur in dissimilar states ... instead of using autonomic and EEG measures to define state, it may be necessary to first determine the state before interpreting the physiological activity [p. 515]' (Johnson, 1970).

6.3. INFORMATION PROCESSING DURING SLEEP

6.3.1. Response alternatives

Sleep has often been viewed as an unconscious state, devoid of complex

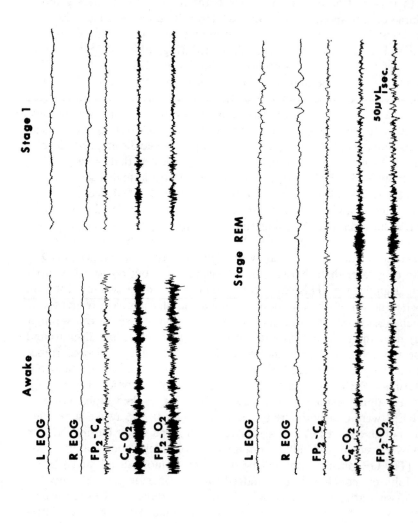

FIGURE 6.7. Alpha activity during awake, stage 1, and stage REM sleep. International 10–20 system used for electrode placement. (From Johnson, L. C. *Psychophysiology*, 1970, **6**, 501–516, with permission.)

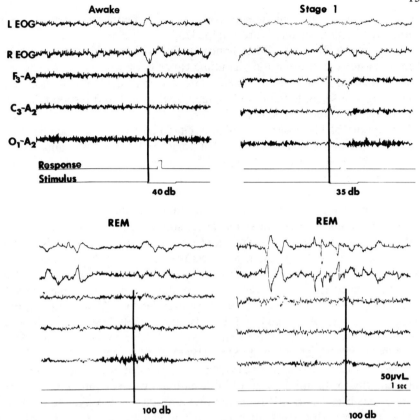

FIGURE 6.8. Illustration of alpha blocking to a stimulus during awake, alpha enhancement during stage 1, and absence of alpha response to a stimulus during REM sleep. International 10–20 system used for electrode placement. (From Johnson, L. C. *Psychophysiology*, 1970, **6**, 501–516, with permission.)

mental functions and behaviours. While psychophysiologists might be interested in the background and phasic physiological activity during the stages of sleep, it is the relation of mental functions and behaviour to physiological activity that is of major concern to psychophysiologists. Snyder & Scott (1972) were also concerned about the subject's capacity to respond during sleep and felt that two important aspects of sleep constitute the basis for research concerned with the psychophysiology of sleep. 'First, the absence of capacity for waking behaviours is only relative—as Lucretius expressed it, some part of the soul remains behind, ready to respond to appropriate external stimulation by awakening . . . Second, sleep involves dreaming, that mode (or modes) of mental functioning intrinsic to sleep and more or less peculiar to it [p. 645].' But what are the response alternatives of the sleeping subject? Are the mechanisms of information processing available to the waking subject intact during sleep? Dement (1972) has stated that '. . . with neither perceptual processes nor memory processes operating, the organism has no will, no motivation, and in fact, about the only meaningful response to either external or internal stimuli left in its repertoire is arousal [p. 323]'.

Williams (1972) on the other hand concludes that neither psychophysical threshold nor the information—handling capacity of sensory systems is necessarily impaired during sleep. 'There is now a great deal of evidence that in some stages of sleep, humans and animals *can* analyse and respond differentially to complex auditory stimuli.'

In support of his position, Williams cites the finding of Buendia, Sierra, Goode & Segundo (1964), Granda & Hammack (1961), and Williams, Morlock & Morlock (1966) that differentiated responses acquired during waking persist during sleep. Oswald, Taylor & Treisman (1960) reported that a subject's own name was more likely to produce an EEG and behavioural response than another name with no personal significance. In addition to discriminating stimuli, in terms of personal significance, stimuli with differing motivational value are also effectively discriminated during sleep. Zung & Wilson (1961) found that motivation by monetary incentives enhanced the responses to any sounds in all stages. Similar results were obtained by Williams *et al.* (1966) who threatened to sound a very loud fire alarm bell if the subject failed to respond. Generally, the frequency of responses decreases from stage 1 through stage 4 (Frazier, McDonald & Edwards, 1968; Williams *et al.*, 1966). The more complex responses are usually seen only during REM sleep (Evans, Gustafson, O'Connell, Orne & Shor, 1966).

There is, therefore, impressive evidence that the sleeping subject can respond differentially to stimuli in terms of informational value acquired in the waking state. It has been frequently observed that a mother will awaken to her baby's cry and sleep undisturbed through much louder noises. The arousal value of a stimulus, therefore, depends on its quality as well as its strength. The sleeping subject can discriminate among various stimuli and awaken or remain asleep depending upon the information transmitted by the stimuli. Does he have an alternative response to arousal? The data on this question are not consistent. Keefe, Johnson & Hunter (1971) found that in all stages of sleep a motor response signalling detection of an auditory stimulus never occurred without associated EEG signs of arousal. Buendia *et al.* (1964), in their study of discriminated motor responses during sleep in cats, also found that motor responses were invariably preceded and accompanied by EEG desynchrony. Williams *et al.* (1966), on the other hand, have reported that in their sleeping human subjects many motor responses to designated auditory signals occurred without prior signs of awakening. These responses were most often seen during stage REM and stage 2 sleep. Evans *et al.* (1966), as well as Salamy (1971), have found that it is easier to obtain instrumental motor responses (without prior awakening) during REM sleep than during NREM sleep. Instrumental motor responses are seldom reported during SWS.

Based upon the results of differential responses during sleep, Williams (1972) stated, '... brain mechanisms must be available during sleep for transduction and transmission of acoustic information, interrogation of LTM [long-term memory], feature testing and classification. These encoding and categorizing operations take time, and therefore require a viable mechanism for short-term storage.'

A complete discussion of learning during sleep is beyond the scope of this chapter, but a brief mention is in order because the subject continues to surface in publications (Rubin, 1968) and through sale of sleep-learning equipment. The support for sleep learning is stronger in Europe, and particularly in Russia, than in the United States. Snyder & Scott (1972) noted that no studies had refuted the conclusions by Simon & Emmons (1955) that there was no evidence of learning complex verbal material as long as the EEG pattern clearly indicated the subject was asleep. Cooper & Hoskovec (1972) hypnotized subjects before sleep and told them while under hypnosis they would be given some words during sleep that they were to remember. They found some evidence of learning of Russian words presented during REM sleep in hypnotically susceptible subjects, but they concluded that learning during sleep was not practical. Much of the sleep learning reported in the Russian studies appears to have occurred during the stage 1 drowsy period. The general conclusion at this time is that while information may be processed, stored, and even recalled during sleep, particularly during stage REM sleep (Evans et al., 1966), there is little evidence to indicate that the information first presented and processed during sleep is available to the subject when awake. The processing and availability of the information only while the subject is in REM sleep is similar to the state-dependent learning produced by alcohol (Goodwin, Powell, Bremer, Hoine & Stern, 1969; Overton, 1972; Weingartner & Faillace, 1971) and in some states of hypnosis. The possibility of state dependent learning during stages of sleep opens the possibility for intriguing research into memory storage and retrieval.

6.3.2. The orienting response (OR)

The above data and the conclusion by Williams indicate that, with respect to sensory threshold and information processing capabilities during sleep, sleep is an entirely appropriate state for psychophysiological research and the OR has been one area of such study.

6.3.2.1. Defining the OR

The OR is an important psychophysiological phenomenon whose characteristics have been well-defined for the awake state. Attempts to identify similar characteristics of the OR during sleep, or to even state with certainty that there is an OR during sleep, clearly illustrate the problem of generalizing the findings from one state to another.

Sokolov (1963) imposed three conditions for the OR or 'what is it' response:

(i) It must be nonspecific with regard to the quality of the stimulus.
(ii) It must be nonspecific with regard to the intensity of the stimulus.

(iii)   It must decrease in amplitude with repeated stimulation.

To these three, Stern (1972) has added a fourth criterion that the response is time locked to either the onset of the stimulus or the offset.

One of the first problems in defining the OR during sleep is that of detecting the stimulus-evoked response from the background spontaneous fluctuations. In all stages of sleep, one or more of the autonomic variables demonstrate high rates of background activity. During REM, there are large fluctuations in HR, respiration, FPR, and blood pressure. During NREM, the high rate of spontaneous EDA has been noted earlier. How can the evoked response be detected among the numerous spontaneous changes? Figure 6.9 illustrates the problem for evoked EDA. Stern's requirement that the response be time locked to the stimulus would not suffice as some spontaneous responses will fall within the time criteria for an evoked response. This problem has been discussed at length by Johnson & Lubin (1967, 1972) and a pseudostimulus approach is recommended. The response to a carefully placed pseudostimulus is determined and this is subtracted from the response obtained following the real stimulus. In the Johnson & Lubin (1967) study of evoked EDA during sleep, the difference between the rate for the pseudostimuli and real stimuli was insignificant during stages 2, 3, and 4 indicating that, in this instance, references to a stimulus-evoked ED OR would have been in error.

As indicated earlier, during sleep spontaneous EDA is dissociated from spontaneous cardiovascular activity. Similarly, the evoked HRR is maximal at a time (stage 2) when it is difficult to prove there is any evoked SRR. In addition, a clear difference in auditory response thresholds exists among autonomic and EEG measures during sleep that is not present when awake. These threshold differences were detailed by Keefe et al. (1971) in a study concerned with the response hierarchy of EEG and autonomic variables to tones of increasing intensity during awake and sleep stages 2, REM, and SWS. In the awake state, statistically significant responses were found for EEG, finger pulse, early heart rate deceleration, skin potential, and skin resistance to the tone at awake auditory threshold, but not to tones at lesser dB levels which subject reported he could not hear. During sleep, significant EEG responses were present to tones 30–25 dB below arousal threshold, finger pulse 20–15 dB below, and heart rate acceleration 20–25 dB below. The subject reported hearing none of these tones and there were no changes in EEG indices of sleep stage. Significant skin potential, skin resistance, and motor responses were seen only at arousal threshold, i.e. there were EEG signs of awakening and the subject reported he had heard the tones (see Figure 6.10). Thus, in sleep, there were clear responses to stimuli below the arousal threshold, and there was definite ordering of the appearance of the various responses: EEG preceded the cardiovascular, with electrodermal and motor occurring only at arousal. This order was constant over sleep stages (see Figure 6.11).

The shape of the HR also differs from that seen during waking. Graham & Clifton (1966) have identified the HR OR as a deceleratory response and an increase in HR as a defensive response. During sleep, the response to stimuli

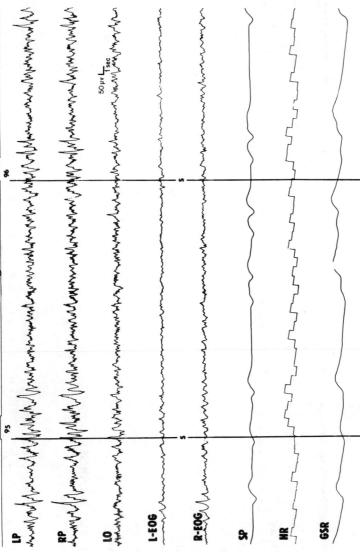

FIGURE 6.9. Example of problem of detecting evoked GSRs and SPRs from spontaneous changes. The beat-to-beat HR variability is also clearly illustrated. Abbreviations: 95 and 96 = the 95th and 96th stimuli. Other abbreviations are as previously used (From Johnson, L. C. & Lubin, A. *Electroencephalography and Clinical Neurophysiology*, 1967, **22**, 11–21, with permission.)

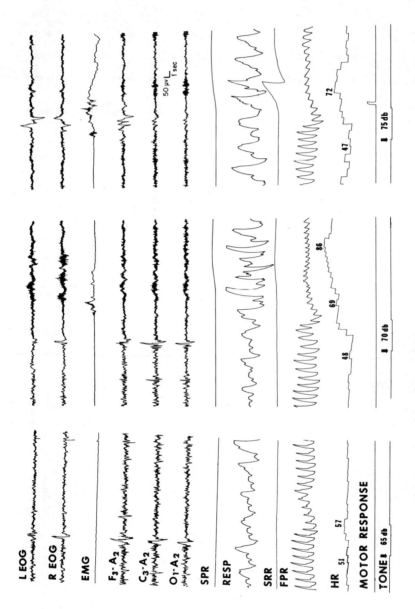

FIGURE 6.10. Illustration of differential response threshold to 65-dB tone. Skin potential (SPR) and skin resistance responses (SPR) are not present until signs of EEG arousal occur at end of 70-dB tone. Responses in all variables are seen to 75-dB tone when subject is awake. Abbreviations: EMG = electromyogram. Other abbreviations are as previously used. (From Johnson, L. C. *Psychophysiology*, 1970, **6**, 501–516, with permission.)

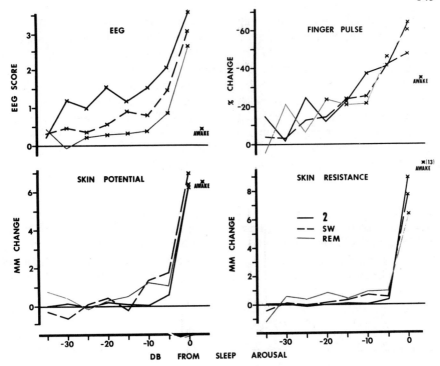

FIGURE 6.11. Relative threshold levels during awake and sleep stages 2, REM, and SWS. 0 indicates arousal threshold from sleep. Asterisk (*) indicates dB level at which response was significant as compared to pseudostimulus, e.g. significant EEG responses were present beginning at 30-dB below arousal (2 and SW), beginning at 25-dB below arousal (REM), and at awake. Skin potential and skin resistance responses (in mm pen-deflection) were significant only when subjects were awake or showed clear signs of arousal from sleep. (From Keefe, F. B., Johnson, L. C. & Hunter, E. J. *Psychophysiology*, 1971, **8**, 198–212

well below the awake threshold is always an increase in HR followed by a decrease (Hord, Lubin & Johnson, 1966). Thus, is it correct to classify a response during sleep as a 'what is it' OR response or should it be labelled a defensive response? With stimuli below arousal threshold, there are no stage changes and, in most instances, no increase in muscular activity that would reflect any type of motor response. When awakened, the subjects are unaware that external stimuli, usually auditory, have been presented.

One of the earliest observations on the OR and sleep was the report by Jung (1954) that stimuli which had become ineffective in the waking state evoked an FPR during sleep. In a 1960 study, Sokolov reported similar findings. Johnson & Lubin (1967), in a study of several autonomic variables as well as EEG activity, and recently Townsend & House (1973), in a study of the auditory evoked EEG response, have reported that previously habituated responses returned with sleep onset. Johnson & Lubin (1967) found that the magnitude of the returned response during sleep was not consistent over variables and varied from one sleep stage to another (see Figure 6.12). Compared to waking, the evoked heart rate and finger pulse responses are clearly larger during sleep than are the electrodermal responses. Hord *et al.* (1966) as well as McDonald & Carpenter (1966) also found that the evoked HR response during sleep was larger than that to the same stimulus presented when awake. Ackner & Pampiglione (1955) and Oswald (1962) found that during light sleep a stimulus no longer evoked SRRs although, according to Oswald, these would return as sleep progressed. Broughton, Poire & Tassinari (1965) reported no marked inhibition of the SPR with sleep onset and a lower SPR threshold during stages 2, 3, and 4 when compared to waking. Tizard (1966) found a decrease in SPRs from the waking state to sleep stage 2, and McDonald and Carpenter (1966) reported a decrease in evoked SPRs with sleep onset and a complete absence of SRRs. Johnson & Lubin (1967) have also noted that of the two ED measures, SRR and SPR, both the spontaneous and evoked SPRs are more likely to be present during sleep. It is difficult to evaluate the SRR findings in those studies that did not take into account the rate of spontaneous SRRs during sleep.

During sleep, *per se*, Johnson & Lubin (1967) found that the evoked HR response was larger during REM and stage 2, smaller during SWS. For FPR and SRR, the lowest percent of evoked responses occurred during REM

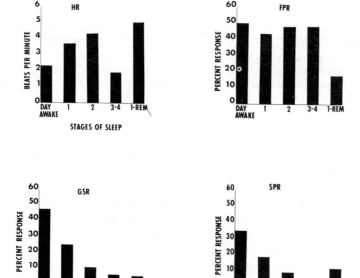

FIGURE 6.12. Mean response patterns for day awake and stages of sleep. (From Johnson, L. C. & Lubin, A. *Electroencephalography and Clinical Neurophysiology*, 1967, **22**, 11–21, with permission.)

sleep. Like Williams, Morlock, Morlock & Lubin (1964), Townsend & House (1973) found that the average peak-to-peak amplitude of the EEG evoked response was smaller in stage REM than in any other sleep stage.

Whether due to a release of cortical inhibition or inhibition of Sokolov's neuronal analyser, an OR habituated during awake does dishabituate with sleep onset, though its magnitude varies from variable to variable and changes as the sleep progresses from one sleep stage to another.

6.3.2.2. OR habituation during sleep

If Sokolov had been a sleep researcher, he probably would not have listed habituation as one of his criteria for the OR or would have made his definition state specific. Nearly two decades of active research on sleep and the responses during sleep have failed to resolve the question of whether autonomic and EEG response habituation occurs to stimuli presented when one is asleep.

Sokolov & Paramonova (1961) early noted the difficulty in habituating a vasomotor response, but in spite of its greater persistence they reported such a response could be regularly extinguished. Williams, Hammack, Daly, Dement & Lubin (1964), on the other hand, found no extinction of a finger pulse vasoconstriction response to an auditory stimulus repeated throughout all-night sleep. Williams et al. (1964) also found the vasoconstriction response was of constant duration throughout all stages of sleep, but Ackner & Pampiglione (1957) found that as sleep progressively deepened, the evoked FPR ceased to occur. McDonald & Carpenter (1966) found habituation of both HR responses and FPR during all stages of sleep in 46 subjects. The response in both variables was never completely extinguished, however, and the 'habituated' response during sleep for HR was still larger than the awake OR to the initial stimulus. Johnson & Lubin (1967) reported that the 'dishabituated' HRR and FPR continued at the same magnitude throughout the entire night which involved exposure to 10,544 tone presentations. In a more recent study of the response to auditory stimuli during sleep, tones of 80–85 dB, approximately 1 sec in duration and with an interstimulus interval (ISI) of 45 sec were presented 24 hours a day for 15 days. The data reported by Johnson & Lubin in 1967 were reconfirmed. There was a return of the waking habituated EEG response, the HRR, and the FPR with sleep onset on each of the 15 nights. The percent response and magnitude of response on the 15th night was not significantly different from that on the first night. To see if there was a response decrement which occurred to the first tones after sleep onset, additional analysis of the first 10 tones after sleep onset was done. No significant response decrement was seen in these 10 tones. In our laboratory, over several studies, we have found that EEG, respiratory and cardiovascular responses habituated during awake, return with sleep onset and do not exhibit a clear habituation curve during sleep.

The habituation data for the ED responses are even more confusing because of the difficulty in obtaining consistent evoked ED responses during sleep and the problem of separating the evoked responses from the spontaneous activity during NREM sleep. Sokolov & Paramonova (1961) reported that the SRR could be habituated during sleep, but Oswald (1962) reported no habituation. Johnson & Lubin (1967) found no habituation of the few responses seen, and McDonald & Carpenter (1966) felt their results were inconclusive for SPR habituation since most of the variance was contributed by a few subjects. McDonald & Carpenter reported a complete absence of the SRR during sleep.

Firth (1973), in an attempt to partial out some of the variance reported in previous studies, looked at the effect of varying interstimulus intervals from 10–30 sec for a 70 dB, 1000 Hz, tone of 1-sec duration in three subjects. Firth analysed SP, HR and EEG response in a drowsy state and during stages, 2, 4, and REM sleep.

Within-subject analysis indicated there was no significant HR habituation at any ISI during REM sleep or in the daytime recording. There was habituation of HR during stage 2 for all ISI. Firth reported SPR habituation at all ISIs for all conditions, but the EEG response was not seen during the 30-sec ISI in any condition.

In an as yet unpublished study, we presented tones of 75 dBA, 2-sec duration with an ISI which varied between 20–45 sec, with an average ISI of 30 sec, to eight sleeping subjects during stage 2 and to seven subjects during stage REM. The subjects had no prior exposure to these tones and showed no EEG signs of arousal to the tones. Like Firth, we found some HR habituation during stage 2, but no habituation during REM sleep or when the tones were presented after morning awakening. There was a similar pattern of habituation for FPR. Like Firth, for his 30-sec ISI, we also found no hibituation of the K-complex during stage 2. Unlike Firth, however, we found few scorable EEG responses during REM sleep and few scorable SRRs that could be separated from background spontaneous activity during stage 2 or REM. In both instances, the number of responses were too few to measure habituation. Firth reported EEG and SPR habituation in both stage 2 and REM.

Question: Does habituation occur during sleep? Answer: Maybe. A more definitive answer does not appear to be possible at this time. In addition to problems of defining what is significant habituation, there is the question of which variable in what stage of sleep. If the response is a return of a previously habituated response, habituation does not appear to occur; but if the response is to a stimulus first presented during sleep, no simple answer can be given.

Question: Then is there an OR during sleep? Answer: Depends upon your definition. The answer must be 'no' if you apply the waking criterion of habituation to the response pattern during sleep. But that is the problem. Is there a psychophysiology for all states or must the state be specified before the response can be interpreted?

6.4. ACKNOWLEDGMENTS

This research was supported in part by National Science Foundation grants to the San Diego State University Foundation, and by Department of the Navy, Bureau of Medicine and Surgery.

The opinions and assertions contained herein are the private ones of the author and are not to be construed as official or as reflecting the views of the Navy Department.

The author wishes to thank Ardie Lubin, Paul Naitoh, Walter Wilkins, John House, and Richard Townsend for their contributions to this manuscript.

6.5. REFERENCES

Ackner, B. & Pampiglione, G. Combined EEG, plethysmographic, respiratory and skin resistance studies during sleep. *Electroencephalography and Clinical Neurophysiology*, 1955, **7**, 153.

Ackner, B. & Pampiglione, G. Some relationships between peripheral vasomotor and EEG changes. *Journal of Neurology, Neurosurgery and Psychiatry*, 1957, **20**, 58–64.

Agnew, H. W., Jr. & Webb, W. B. Measurement of sleep onset by EEG criteria. *American Journal of EEG Technology*, 1972, **12**, 127–134.

Aserinsky, E. Periodic respiratory pattern occurring in conjunction with eye movements during sleep. *Science*, 1965, **150**, 763–766.

Broughton, R. J., Porie, R. & Tassinari, C. A. The electrodermogram (Tarchanoff effect) during sleep. *Electroencephalography and Clinical Neurophysiology*, 1965, **18**, 691–708.

Buendia, N., Sierra, G., Goode, M. & Segundo, J. P. Conditioned and discriminatory responses in wakeful and sleeping cats. *Electroencephalography and Clinical Neurophysiology*, 1964, Suppl. 24, 199.

Caille, E. J. Apport de l'analyse spectrale de l'E.E.G. dans l'etude des relations entre sommeil lent et sommeil onirique. Centre d'Etudes et de Recherches, Toulon-Naval, France, Etude No. 12/67, 1967.

Chase, M. H. (Ed.) *The sleeping brain.* Los Angeles: Brain Research Institute Publications Office, University of California, Los Angeles, 1972.

Cooper, L. M. & Hoskovec, J. Hypnotic suggestions for learning during stage 1 REM sleep. *American Journal of Clinical Hypnosis*, 1972, **15**, 102–111.

Dement, W. C. Sleep deprivation and the organization of the behavioral states. In C. D. Clemente, D. P. Purpura & F. E. Mayer (Eds), *Sleep and the maturing nervous system.* New York: Academic Press, 1972, pp. 319–361.

Dement, W. & Wolpert, E. The relation of eye movements, body motility, and external stimuli to dream content. *Journal of Experimental Psychology*, 1958, **55**, 543–553.

Dumermuth, G., Walz, W., Scollo-Lavizzari, G. & Kleiner, B. Spectral analysis of EEG activity in different sleep stages in normal adults. *European Neurology*, 1972, **7**, 265–296.

Ekstrand, B. R. Effect of sleep on memory. *Journal of Experimental Psychology*, 1967, **75**, 64–72.

Ekstrand, B. R., Sullivan, M. J., Parker, D. F. & West, J. N. Spontaneous recovery and sleep. *Journal of Experimental Psychology*, 1971, **88**, 142–144.

Empson, J. A. C. & Clarke, P. R. F. Rapid eye movements and remembering. *Nature*, 1970, **227**, 287–288.

Evans, F. J., Gustafson, L. A., O'Connell, D. N., Orne, M. T. & Shor, R. E. Response during sleep with intervening waking amnesia. *Science*, 1966, **152**, 666–667.

Firth, H. Habituation during sleep. *Psychophysiology*, 1973, **10**, 43–51.

Fowler, M. J., Sullivan, M. J. & Ekstrand, B. R. Sleep and memory. *Science*, 1973, **179**, 302–304.

Frazier, R., McDonald, D. G., & Edwards, D. Discrimination between signal and non-signal stimuli during sleep. *Psychophysiology*, 1968, **4**, 369. (Abstract)

Goodwin, D. W., Powell, B., Bremer, D., Hoine, H. & Stern, J. Alcohol and recall: State-dependent effects in man. *Science*, 1969, **163**, 1358–1360.

Graham, F. K. & Clifton, R. K. Heart-rate change as a component of the orienting response. *Psychological Bulletin*, 1966, **65**, 305–320.

Granda, A. M. & Hammack, J. T. Operant behavior during sleep. *Science*, 1961, **133**, 1485–1486.

Grieser, C., Greenberg, R. & Harrison, R. H. The adaptive function of sleep: The differential effects of sleep and dreaming on recall. *Journal of Abnormal Psychology*, 1972, **80**, 280–286.

Hilbert, R. & Naitoh, P. EOG and delta rhythmicity in human sleep EEG. *Psychophysiology*, 1972, **9**, 533–538.

Hord, D. J., Lubin, A. & Johnson, L. C. The evoked heart rate response during sleep. *Psychophysiology*, 1966, **3**, 46–54.

Jenkins, J. G. & Dallenbach, K. M. Obliviscense during sleep and waking. *American Journal of Psychology*, 1924, **35**, 605–612.

Johnson, L. C. A psychophysiology for all states. *Psychophysiology*, 1970, **6**, 501–516.

Johnson, L. C. Computers in sleep research. In M. H. Chase (Ed.), *The sleeping brain*. Los Angeles: Brain Research Institute Publications Office, University of California, Los Angeles, 1972, pp. 277–321.

Johnson, L. C. & Karpan, W. E. Autonomic correlates of the spontaneous K-complex. *Psychophysiology*, 1968, **4**, 444–452.

Johnson, L. C. & Lubin, A. Spontaneous electrodermal activity during waking and sleeping. *Psychophysiology*, 1966, **3**, 8–17.

Johnson, L. C. & Lubin, A. The orienting reflex during waking and sleeping. *Electroencephalography and Clinical Neurophysiology*, 1967, **22**, 11–21.

Johnson, L. C. & Lubin, A. On planning psychophysiological experiments: Design, measurement and analysis. In N. S. Greenfield & R. A. Sternbach (Eds), *Handbook of psychophysiology*. New York: Holt, Rinehart & Winston, 1972. pp. 125–158.

Johnson, L., Lubin, A., Naitoh, P., Nute, C. & Austin, M. Spectral analysis of the EEG of dominant and non-dominant alpha subjects during waking and sleeping. *Electroencephalography and Clinical Neurophysiology*, 1969, **26**, 361–370.

Johnson, L., Naitoh, P., Lubin, A. & Moses, J. Sleep stages and performance. In W. P. Colquhoun (Ed), *Aspects of human efficiency*. London: English Universities Press, 1972. pp. 81–100.

Jung, R. Correlation of bioelectrical and autonomic phenomena with alterations of consciousness and arousal in man. In J. F. De la Fresnaye (Ed), *Brain mechanisms and consciousness*. Oxford: Blackwell Scientific Publications, 1954. pp. 310–344.

Keefe, F. B., Johson, L. C. & Hunter, E. J. EEG and autonomic response pattern during waking and sleep stages. *Psychophysiology*, 1971, **8**, 198–212.

Koulack, D. Rapid eye movements and visual imagery during sleep. *Psychological Bulletin*, 1972, **78**, 155–158.

Larsen, L. E. & Walter, D. O. On automatic methods of sleep staging by EEG spectra. *Electroencephalography and Clinical Neurophysiology*, 1970, **28**, 459–467.

Lester, B. K., Burch, N. R. & Dossett, R. C. Nocturnal EEG-GSR profiles: The influence of presleep states. *Psychophysiology*, 1967, **3**, 238–248.

Loomis, A. L., Harvey, E. N. & Hobart, G. Potential rhythms of the cerebral cortex during sleep. *Science*, 1935, **81**, 597–598.

Lubin, A., Johnson, L. C. & Austin, M. T. Discrimination among states of consciousness using EEG spectra. *Psychophysiology*, 1969, **6**, 122–132.

McDonald, D. G. & Carpenter, F. A. Habituation of the orienting response in sleep. Paper presented at the meeting of the Society for Psychophysiological Research, Denver, Colorado, October 1966.

McDonald, D. G., Johnson, L. C. & Hord, D. J. Habituation of the orienting response in alert and drowsy subjects. *Psychophysiology*, 1964, **1**, 163–173.

Naitoh, P., Johnson, L. C. & Lubin, A. Modification of surface negative slow potential (CNV) in the human brain after total sleep loss. *Electroencephalography and Clinical Neurophysiology*, 1971, **30**, 17–22.

Naitoh, P., Johnson, L. C., Lubin, A. & Wyborney, G. Brain wave 'generating' processes during waking and sleeping. *Electroencephalography and Clinical Neurophysiology*, 1971, **31**, 294. (Abstract)

Oswald, I. *Sleeping and waking, physiology and psychology.* Amsterdam: Elsevier, 1962.

Oswald, I., Taylor, A. M. & Treisman, M. Discriminative responses to stimulation during human sleep. *Brain*, 1960, **83**, 440–453.

Overton, D. A. State-dependent learning produced by alcohol. In B. Kissin & H. Begleiter (Eds), *The biology of alcoholism.* Vol. 2. New York–London: Plenum Press, 1972. pp. 193–217.

Pearlman, C. A., Jr. Latent learning impaired by REM sleep deprivation. *Psychonomic Science*, 1971, **25**, 135–136.

Portnoff, G., Baekeland, F., Goodenough, D. R., Karacan, I. & Shapiro, A. Retention of verbal materials perceived immediately prior to onset of non-REM sleep. *Perceptual and Motor Skills*, 1966, **22**, 751–758.

Rechtschaffen, A. & Kales, A. (Eds) *A manual of standardized terminology, techniques and scoring system for sleep stages of human subjects.* NIH Publication No. 204. Washington, D. C.: U. S. Government Printing Office, 1968.

Roffwarg, H. P., Dement, W. C., Muzio, J. N. & Fisher, C. Dream imagery: Relation to rapid eye movements of sleep. *Archives of General Psychiatry*, 1962, **7**, 235–258.

Rubin, F. (Ed) *Current research in hypnopaedia.* New York: Elsevier, 1968.

Salamy, J. Effects of REM deprivation and awakening on instrumental performance during stage 2 and REM sleep. *Biological Psychiatry*, 1971, **3**, 321–330.

Sassin, J. F. & Johnson, L. C. Body motility during sleep and its relation to the K-complex. *Experimental Neurology*, 1968, **22**, 133–144.

Simon, C. W. & Emmons, W. H. Learning during sleep? *Psychological Bulletin*, 1955, **52**, 328–342.

Snyder, F. & Scott, J. The psychophysiology of sleep. In N. S. Greenfield & R. A. Sternbach (Eds), *Handbook of psychophysiology.* New York: Holt, Rinehart & Winston, 1972, pp. 645–708.

Sokolov, E. N. Neuronal models and the orienting reflex. In M. A. B. Brazier (Ed), *The central nervous system and behavior.* New York: Josiah Macy Jr. Foundation, 1960. pp. 187–276.

Sokolov, E. N. Higher nervous function: The orienting reflex. *Annual Review of Physiology*, 1963, **25**, 545–589.

Sokolov, E. N. & Paramonova, N. P. Progressive changes in the orienting reflex in man during the development of sleep inhibition. *Pavlovian Journal of Higher Nervous Activity*, 1961, **11**, 217–226.

Spreng, L. F., Johnson, L. C. & Lubin, A. Autonomic correlates of eye movement bursts during stage REM sleep. *Psychophysiology*, 1968, **4**, 311–323.

Stern, J. A. Physiological response measures during classical conditioning. In N. S. Greenfield & R. A. Sternbach (Eds), *Handbook of psychophysiology.* New York: Holt, Rinehart & Winston, 1972, pp. 197–227.

Tizard, B. Repetitive auditory stimuli and the development of sleep. *Electroencephalography and Clinical Neurophysiology*, 1966, **20**, 112–121.

Townsend, R. E. & House, J. F. Auditory evoked potentials in stage 2 and rapid eye movement sleep during a 30-day exposure to tone pulse noises. Paper presented at the 29th annual meeting of the Western EEG Society, San Diego, February 1973.

Ulett, G. A., Akpinar, S. & Itil, T. M. Quantitative EEG analysis during hypnosis. *Electroencephalography and Clinical Neurophysiology*, 1972, **33**, 361–368.

Van Ormer, E. G. Retention after intervals of sleep and waking. *Archives of Psychology*, 1932, **21**, No. 137.

Walter, W. G. *The living brain*. New York: W. W. Norton, 1953.

Weingartner, H. & Faillace, L. A. Alcohol state-dependent learning in man. *Journal of Nervous and Mental Disease*, 1971, **153**, 395–406.

Williams, H. L. Information processing during sleep. Paper presented at the 1st European Congress on Sleep Research, Basel, Switzerland, October 1972.

Williams, H. L., Hammack, J. T., Daly, R. L., Dement, W. C. & Lubin, A. Responses to auditory stimulation, sleep loss and the EEG stages of sleep. *Electroencephalography and Clinical Neurophysiology*, 1964, **16**, 269–279.

Williams, H. L., Holloway, F. A. & Griffiths, W. J. Physiological psychology: Sleep. In P. H. Mussen & M. R. Rosenzweig (Eds.), *Annual Review of Psychology*. Palo Alto, Calif.: Annual Reviews, Inc., 1973. pp. 279–316.

Williams, H. L., Morlock, H. C., Jr., Morlock, J. V. & Lubin, A. Auditory evoked responses and the EEG stages of sleep. *Annals of the New York Academy of Science*, 1964, **112**, 172–181.

Williams, H. L., Morlock, H. C., Jr. & Morklock, J. V. Instrumental behavior during sleep. *Psychophysiology*, 1966, **2**, 208–216.

Williams, H. L., Tepas, D. I. & Morlock, H. C., Jr. Evoked responses to clicks and electroencephalographic stages of sleep in man. *Science*, 1962, **138**, 685–686.

Yaroush, R., Sullivan, M. J. & Enstrand, B. R. Effect of sleep on memory. II: Differential effect of the first and second half of the night. *Journal of Experimental Psychology*, 1971, **88**, 361–366.

Zung, W. W. K. & Wilson, W. P. Response to auditory stimulation during sleep. *Archives of General Psychiatry*, 1961, **4**, 548–552.

Chapter 7

Sleep Deprivation in Humans

P. NAITOH

Navy Medical Neuropsychiatric Research Unit,
San Diego, California, U.S.A.

7.1. THREE KINDS OF SLEEP DEPRIVATION

Although sleep deprivation has been known to exert detrimental influences on performance, subjective mood and other psychological activity (see Williams, Lubin & Goodnow, 1959; Wilkinson, 1965; Naitoh, in press), authors of textbooks in psychology have remained curiously silent about the topic of sleep deprivation as well as sleep in general. In Stevens' *Handbook of Experimental Psychology*, Seashore (1951) described a study of Warren and Clark (1937) to illustrate the 'extent to which the human organism can continue to perform adequately under extremely unfavourable conditions'. (p. 1358), such as sleep deprivation. However, this was the only reference to sleep deprivation in the *Handbook*. In the Woodworth and Schlosberg's *Experimental Psychology* edited by Kling and Riggs (1971), no reference could be found to sleep deprivation.

It appears that traditional psychologists have not been sensitive to the fact that sleep deprivation may muddle the effects of the experimental treatments under study, not to mention the increase in error variance that usually occurs.

Psychologists are, however, not alone in their neglect of sleep loss. Many of us have cut our regular sleep time or, in some instances, have stayed up all night, without experiencing obvious consequences on our waking behaviours. These experiences have led us to believe that we will suffer very little from sleep deprivation. This conviction, coupled with the gentle promotion by society for its member to stay awake and be productive, develops into an attitude which minimizes the effects of sleep deprivation on psychological functions. With this unconscious attitude, we become like traditional psychologists insensitive and blind to the increase in error variance that only slightly sleepy experimental subjects can introduce during some psychological experiments.

In this chapter, psychological experiments on sleep deprivation in humans are presented to show its pervasive effects in almost all aspects of psychological activity, and to provide the experimenters with knowledge which may be helpful in their recognition of sleep loss effects in given experiments.

Sleep deprivation will be discussed under three categories: (1) total sleep deprivation, (2) differential sleep stage deprivation, and (3) partial sleep deprivation.

Total or complete sleep deprivation occurs when we stay awake, voluntarily or involuntarily, through more than 24 hours. Total sleep deprivation has been most extensively studied.

Differential or selective sleep stage deprivation is a quite recent by-product of the electroencephalographic (EEG) studies of sleep. The chapter in this volume on sleep by Johnson must be consulted for a description of the sleep stages. Dement (1960) and Agnew, Webb & Williams (1967) have reported that REM sleep or stage 4 can be removed from sleeping humans without major disruption of the other sleep stages. When REM sleep (or stage 4) is removed from sleep, we have REM (or stage 4) deprivation. No other sleep stage deprivation has been attempted.

Partial sleep deprivation occurs when the customary sleep regimen is reduced from its habitual length. The timing of sleep onset or awakening is also inevitably altered from the habitual sleep pattern.

7.2. TOTAL SLEEP DEPRIVATION

Certain conceptual ambiguities still exist in specifying the amount of total sleep deprivation.

For example, if we woke up on one morning at 0700^{hr} and stayed awake until 2300^{hr} of the following day, we would have gone 40 h without sleep. During this 40-h period, however, we missed just one sleep period of, say 8 h, if we usually slept from 2300^{hr} to 0700^{hr}. To be more precise, then, we should have stated that we had experienced 40 h of continuous wakefulness, including 8 h of total sleep deprivation. In general practice, however, the hours of prior wakefulness are not distinguished from the hours of sleep deprivation, except Webb and Agnew (1971) who used the hours of prior wakefulness as a determinant of stage 4 obtained during subsequent sleep.

Another ambiguity arises from the use of the term, *total*. Sleep is a dynamic *state* of the human organism, and not a 'thing' which we can remove completely. Sleep-deprived subjects show an increasing number of brief dozing-offs or microsleeps. Polygraphic analyses of these microsleeps (Bjerner, 1949; Williams, Granda, Jones, Lubin & Armington, 1964) have shown that they are most likely stage 1, and if there is rapid intervention, they do not proceed into sleep stage 2. If we regard *sleep* stage 1 as a transitional stage or *dormiveglia* (sleep-waking, Kleitman, 1963, p. 71) then we can state that sleep deprivation would be total and complete despite microsleeps. On the other hand, if we regard stage 1 to be *real* sleep, sleep deprivation can not be total. Dement (1972) stated: 'the notion of total sleep deprivation could be somewhat illusory, and could result merely in a redistribution of activity in sleep and arousal systems in which NREM would occur in the form of hundreds of microsleeps.' (p. 337) In this chapter we will view sleep stage 1 as a transition period in which we are neither awake nor asleep. Some detailed theoretical as well as factual reasoning in this regard are given by Johnson in this volume.

What are the effects of total sleep deprivation on human subjects? We will discuss them under three broad categories: (i) task performance, (ii) psychological change and (iii) stress.

7.2.1. Task performance

7.2.1.1. Lapses

One of the main effects of total sleep deprivation (and also partial sleep deprivation) is the uneven slowing and the eventual absence of appropriate response. The slowing and absence of appropriate task-related response (that is, a pause, a blocking, or a lapse) as the major behavioural symptom of total sleep deprivation was noted by Patrick & Gilbert (1896) when they described the failure by one of their subjects to recall digits. They referred to the subject's inability to focus his attention as a kind of mental lapse.

Bjerner (1949) observed that the longer delayed reactions were usually accompanied by EEG alpha suppression, a transient fall in pulse rate and even behavioural signs of frank sleep, such as immobility, sometimes open mouth and snoring, and no reactions to weak sounds. For those delayed responses Bjerner observed a replacement of EEG alpha by EEG delta waves, sleep spindles and K-complexes. These latter EEG signs of course indicate the presence of stage 2 sleep. However, many subsequent studies have observed that the lapse in the sleep-deprived subjects is most often stage 1, and only on some occasions reaches a short period of stage 2 (Armington & Mitnick, 1959; Williams, *et al.*, 1964; Naitoh, 1969; Naitoh, Kales, Kollar, Smith & Jacobson, 1969; Naitoh & Townsend, 1970; Naitoh, Pasnau & Kollar, 1971).

The Lapse Hypothesis was formally proposed in the late 1950's by the team of researchers at the Walter Reed Hospital (Williams & Lubin, 1958; Williams *et al.*, 1959) to explain performance decrements due to total sleep deprivation.

7.2.1.2. Degradation of memory

Using a memory test of their own design, the Williams Word-Memory test, Williams, Gieseking & Lubin (1966) and Williams & Williams (1966) have reported impairment of short-term memory following total sleep loss. In the Williams Memory test, each word is announced, spelled out by the experimenter. This is followed by 10 sec of silence, during which time the subject writes down the word on paper. Immediately after a presentation of a list of the words and correction of any errors, the subject writes down all words he can recall on a blank page.

Thus, Williams and his colleagues did not believe that the impairment following to total sleep deprivation was due to a lapse or a failure to register the words. Williams & Williams (1966) concluded that 'impairment of short-term recall under sleep deprivation seems to be due to increasing difficulty with memory trace formation' (p. 173). Williams & Williams speculated further that 'sleep-loss impairment on signal detection tasks like the Pentagon Test is probably due to different mechanisms than impairment on short-term recall tests like the Word-Memory Test' (p. 173). In other studies by Wilkinson (1964), Donnell, Lubin, Naitoh & Johnson (1969) and Lubin, Moses, Johnson & Naitoh (in press) impaired short-term memory during total sleep deprivation has similarly been found.

In a recent study Vojtéchovský, Šarfatová, Votava & Feit (1971) reported impairment only in the long-term recall of 15 unfamiliar Arabian three-syllabic words. Their results indicated that acute 'sleep deprivation of 2 nights did not impair the learning ability and immediate recall in 21 subjects' but 'the retention of unusual, verbal learned material measured 8 h after the presentation was impaired already after the first night of vigil and more after the second night' (p. 144).

While the mechanisms by which total sleep deprivation impairs memory processes are still unclear, one can expect memory degradation in one form or another following sleep deprivation.

7.2.1.3. Compensatory efforts

During sleep deprivation, it is possible by expedition of extra effort for well-motivated subjects to remain awake and to maintain an acceptable level of task performance. Edwards (1941) noted that five out of 17 experimental subjects were able to hold their own in the American Council on Education Psychological Examination during 100 h of total sleep deprivation 'but obviously with only the greatest effort' (p. 90). Wilkinson (1962) reported that subjects who maintained their baseline level on an addition task during sleep deprivation showed a marked rise (probably reflecting greater effort) of electromyographic (EMG) activity in the pronator teres muscle of the inactive arm from the baseline values.

Compensatory efforts are not limited to the task situations alone. In a study by Naitoh and his group (1971), a cumulative pedometer reading was obtained from two subjects every 6 h during 171 h of sleep deprivation in one subject, and during 129 h for the second subject. As expected, the pedometer readings were significantly higher during sleep deprivation, mirroring their increased walking in an effort to stay awake.

Compensatory physiological and biochemical changes, of which the subject may be unaware, also occur during total sleep deprivation. These changes could be caused by the psychological efforts necessary to stay awake, or could be the expression of the human body's attempt to adjust to the vigil. Also, we should not regard absence of change in physiological and biochemical levels during sleep loss as indicating absence of compensation. Such an approach would be the same as regarding an unchanging level of task performance during sleep loss as a behavioural adaptation, not exploring further how this had been achieved, that is by compensatory efforts.

The studies by Brodan & Kuhn (1967) and by Brodan, Vojtchovský, Kuhn & Cepelak (1969) suggested the operation of physiological and biochemical effort during sleep deprivation, which could be observed best during recovery from sleep deprivation. Their studies used the Harvard Step Test at a fixed speed for 5 min. Average heart rate was taken during the time intervals of 1–1·5 min, 2–2·5 min and 3–3·5 min post-exercise to determine heart rate recovery, and also to derive a physical *fitness index*. The results showed a temporary but significant drop of about 5 per cent in physical fitness index during the first 48 h of sleep deprivation. However, the fitness index started to regain its loss as sleep deprivation continued, and by 120 h of sleep deprivation the fitness index was somewhat higher than the pre-deprivation level. After the first recovery sleep, the fitness index was observed to show a paradoxical sharp drop of 15 per cent from the baseline value. Brodan and his group attributed this decline in fitness index to a dominance of anabolic metabolism during the recovery days, which denied the quick energy necessary for the Harvard Step Test, although Simonson in his review (1971) implicated 'some lack of motivation' (p. 438) to explain this decline. To us, the results suggested an accumulation of physiological and biochemical cost due to continual bodily compensatory efforts to remain awake. The excessive expenditure of bodily resources was revealed only when sleep deprivation was terminated and our bodily functions were mobilized to repay the physiological and biochemical debts by, for example, stepping up anabolic metabolic processes.

7.2.1.4. Circadian effects

The early morning hours coincide with the low point of the circadian temperature cycle. They are the most probable period for potentiation of performance decrements due to sleep loss by the circadian (diurnal) cycle (Alluisi, 1969; Drucker, Cannon & Ware, 1969; Morgan, Brown & Alluisi, 1970).

7.2.2. Psychological change

7.2.2.1. Mood

Although it is widely known that total sleep deprivation alters mood (e.g., Handbook of Human Engineering Data, 1949), only recently have we realized the importance of changes in mood for detecting sleep debt (Bohlin & Kjellberg, 1973; Hendrick & Lilly, 1970; Johnson et al., in press; Lubin, et al., in press; see also Thayer, 1967). In Table 7.1 are some of the adjectives which have been found to be sensitive to one night of sleep deprivation in studies by Lubin and his associates (in press), and by Johnson and his colleagues (in press). For each adjective or phrase, the subjects are to choose one of the four answers that described their feelings best now: (1) Not at all, (2) A little, (3) Quite a bit, and (4) Extremely.

TABLE 7.1. List of adjectives believed to be sensitive to one night of sleep deprivation (Lubin et al., in press)

Active*†+	Alert*†
Carefree*++	Cheerful*
Considerate*	Efficient*
Friendly*	Full of pep*†
Good natured*	Lively*++
Relaxed*	Able to concentrate
Able to think clearly	Able to work hard
Dependable	Happy
Kind	Pleasant
Satisfied	

The starred adjectives or phrase were used in Profile of Mood States (POMS) (McNair et al., 1971). The items marked with † were used in Thayer's AD-ACL (Thayer, 1967), and those with + appeared in Hendrick and Lilly (1970).

Following sleep deprivation the feelings are less positive.

A recent study by Bohlin and Kjellberg (1973) indicated that one night of total sleep deprivation affected mood in a complex but predictable manner. They administered a Swedish version of the Thayer's Activation–Deactivation Adjective Check List (AD-ACL) (Thayer, 1967) which yielded four factors: (i) Sleep-Wakefulness, (ii) Stress, (iii) Euphoria, and (iv) Energy. The Sleep-Wakefulness and Energy factor scores were closely related to the physiological state of activation or arousal, while the Stress and Euphoria factor scores were more related to the interpretation given by the subjects to the state of activation or arousal they had felt. After one night of sleep deprivation, the Sleep-Wakefulness and Energy ratings were significantly lowered. Ratings of Stress and Euphoria were also lowered, but not significantly. Sleep deprivation could influence mood directly through changes in physiological level of activation per se, then through the subject's reaction to the changes in activation. This pattern of response is similar to the hypothesis by Schachter & Singer (1962), which specified that there were two necessary components for emotional states: Physiological arousal and Cognitive factors (or an inter-pretation of the arousal and the environmental demands).

7.2.2.2. Sleep motivation

In addition to changes in mood, alterations in 'the motive to sleep' (Murray, 1968, p. 44) have been suggested. According to Murray, we have a sleep motive. 'The term *sleep motive* is analogous to the hunger motive, the sex motive, the curiosity motive, the achievement motive, and so forth.' (Murray, 1965, p. 16) Sleep motive was defined as a disposition to sleep; it has all the necessary characteristics to qualify as a motive. It serves biological need and it has a specific goal response, as well as a specified relation to amount of deprivation and other motivating conditions. Subjectively the increase in sleep motive was experienced as an increased sleepiness or desire to sleep. An important aspect of Murray's view was that sleep deprivation resulted inevitably in a conflict between an increased strength of the sleep motive on the one hand, and biological and social motives on the other hand. Accordingly, sleep deprivation changes the relative strength of other non-sleep related motives, and also sets a familiar mechanism of frustration–aggression into motion. This means that the sleep-deprived subjects had to go through personality adjustment (Murray, 1968) to resolve this conflict between the desire to sleep and the environmental demands for them to remain awake.

7.2.2.3. Interaction of sleep loss with personality differences

In a study involving their type A and type B subjects, Meyer, DiMascio & Stifler (1970) demonstrated an interaction between the effects of sleep deprivation and personality types to drugs. Type A subjects were extroverted athletes who organized their life about the use of physical activity and self-assertiveness, while type B subjects were anxious, introverted and passive individuals who organized their life around intellectual achievement. All sub-jects underwent 20 h of wakefulness, before receiving oral dose of d-ampheta-mine (10 mg), fenocamfamin (10 or 20 mg), pentobarbital (50 mg) or placebo.

Following the sleep loss the type A subjects were not benefited by ampheta-mine at this dose level, and 'fatigue remained subjectively intolerable' (p. 99), whereas type B subjects showed a complete recovery from the detrimental effects of sleep deprivation on a Reading Comprehension task, and felt greater energy, speed, dexterity and reactivity. Only type B subjects reported relief of the clouding of thought induced by sleep deprivation, when given a 20-mg dose of fenocamfamin.

In a study of the relation of ego strength to effects of sleep loss, Strausbaugh & Roessler (1970) employed the Barron Ego Strength (Es) scale to obtain high Es and low Es subjects. They observed that high Es subjects were able to maintain performance on a meter-deflection monitoring test, but those who had low Es score deteriorated significantly. They interpreted this difference as due to ability of the high Es subjects to modulate their level of arousal in response to the demands of the environment. In support of this hypothesis was a significant rise of skin conductance level in the high Es subjects when compared to subjects with low Es score. Perhaps those with high Es score were capable of exerting greater compensatory efforts.

7.2.3. Stress

Total sleep deprivation undoubtedly causes stress and strain on physiological and biochemical functions of human subjects, although we are still uncertain how much of the strain is usually caused by total sleep deprivation in itself and how much of it is the result of the subjects' efforts to remain awake. In a recent study, Webb & Agnew (in press) have shed some light on this problem. They sleep-deprived eight subjects for two successive nights under two different deprivation conditions. In a condition of bed rest, the subjects rested in bed while being sleep deprived. In contrast to the bed rest condition, in exercise condition they pedalled, every other hour, a stationary exercise bicycle for 15 min at the speed of 20 km/h with a 2·5 kg load on the friction wheel. With this exercise load, most subjects reached near the end of endurance point. The subjects were tested with tasks under these two conditions to determine if some portion of performance decrements may be attributable to physical strains of staying awake by moving around all day long. The tasks were the Williams Word Memory Test (Williams, Gieseking & Lubin, 1966; Williams et al., 1966), the Plus Seven Task (see Johnson, Naitoh, Lubin & Moses, 1972), the Wilkinson Addition Test (Wilkinson, 1970) and the Wilkinson Auditory Vigilance Test (Wilkinson, 1970). The results showed that after sleep loss there was as much performance decrement under the bed rest condition as under the exercise condition. Thus, sleep deprivation in itself has influences on task performances. Unfortunately no biochemical data were obtained in this study.

Necessary elements of the stereotyped adaptational stress response pattern are reactions in the hypothalamo-sympathoadrenomedullary, and hypopheso-adrenocortical axis (Levi, 1972a). To these, we should add the pituitary-thyroid system for completeness of the biochemical correlates of stress (Mason, 1972). For more details, the readers are referred to the chapter by Franken-haeuser in this volume.

Recently, Fröberg, Levi and their colleagues (Levi, 1972b; Fröberg, Karlsson, Levi & Lindberg, 1972) observed that 75 h of total sleep deprivation resulted in significant increases in urinary epinephrine, urinary norepinephrine, plasma fatty acids, cholesterol, erythrocyte sedimentation rate, protein-bound iodine, and a decrease in serum iron. Kuhn and his colleagues (Kuhn, Brodan, Brodanova & Rysanek, 1969; see also Harris & O'Hanlon, 1972) likewise discovered that total sleep deprivation resulted in the increases in erythrocyte sedimentation rate, serum free fatty acids, 17-hydroxycorticosteroids (17-OHCS), vanillylmandelic acid (VMA), and a decrease in plasma iron. They also observed relative lymphopenia and relative as well as absolute neutrophilia.

Sternberg, Guggenheim, Baer & Snyder (1968) observed the excretion of epinephrine (E), norepinephrine (NE), VMA, normetanephrine, metanephrine and 17-OHCS in five male college students in four states: '8 h of sleep following 24 h of sleep deprivation; 8 h of normal sleep; 8 h of sleep deprivation with the subjects in bed; 8 h during the day with the subjects in bed awake' (p. 102). The results showed that 'wakefulness *per se* during sleep deprived night caused the increase in excretion of NE and E' (p. 107). To Sternberg and his colleagues, the increase in catecholamines excretion during sleep deprivation is attributable to wakefulness in itself, and not to stress. However, they added that it is possible that 'sleep deprivation acted as a stress or as a novel stimulus which caused an increase in the excretion of NE and E rather than the wakefulness *per se*' (p. 107).

Unfortunately not all of the studies showed the expected stress response during sleep deprivation (Fiorica, Higgins, Iampietro, Lategola & Davis, 1968; Rubin, Kollar, Slater & Clark, 1969). Rubin and his associates (1969) stated, for example, that 'modest activation of the pituitary-adrenocortical axis, and a variable increase in catecholamine biosynthesis may be associated with prolonged sleep deprivation' (p. 77), but such activation was observed only after sleep deprivation of more than 100 h.

Despite some disagreements about the circumstances and the extent of stress, the results suggest that total sleep deprivation does cause some disruption of psychoendocrine metabolism.

Not all of the stress reactions caused by total sleep deprivation are obvious. Some are very subtle. Hasselman, Schaff & Metz (1960) found that urinary epinephrine and urinary norepinephrine output during extensive bicycle ergonometric work were elevated after one night of sleep deprivation when compared to the control value. They also found, however, that a more dramatic increase in catecholamines occurred if they combined a physical work load with a physiological load, high or low ambient temperature, in the sleep deprived subjects. The urinary epinephrine and urinary norepinephrine increased by approximately 300 per cent and 200 per cent respectively under the combined loads of work and low ambient temperature in the sleep deprived subjects.

7.3. DIFFERENTIAL SLEEP STAGE DEPRIVATION

In 1960 Dement demonstrated that by waking the subjects up whenever they tried to enter REM sleep one could reduce REM sleep without seriously disturbing the other sleep stages. Four years later, Agnew and his group (1967) demonstrated that stage 4 could be similarly reduced during human sleep by repeated preventions of the subjects' attempts to enter into stage 4.

Since accurate detection of the various sleep stages requires EEG sleep recording, sleep stage deprivation takes place in its purest form in sleep laboratories. But differential sleep deprivation can occur in daily routines. When we shorten sleep duration, we tend to lose mostly REM sleep. We may lose REM sleep temporarily by sleeping in an unfamiliar bedroom for the first time. When patients take phenelzine (Nardil) or diazepam (Valium), they lose REM sleep or sleep stages 3 and 4 as long as they take these medications (Akindele, Evans & Oswald, 1970; Dunleavy & Oswald, 1973; Fisher, Kahn, Edwards & Davis, 1973; Wyatt, Kupfer, Scott, Robinson & Snyder, 1969).

Differential sleep stage deprivation is fraught with methodological problems. One of these is the difficulty of completely depriving a subject of the target sleep stage. In particular, experimenters can rarely achieve a reduction of greater than 90 per cent of REM sleep.

Another serious problem, that of the interaction of reduction of total sleep time with sleep stage deprivation, is illustrated by the celebrated case of long-term REM deprivation of three human subjects, ages 22, 21 and 26, described by Dement (1965). Dement succeeded in removing 95 per cent of REM sleep from a 22-year-old subject for eight consecutive nights without the use of any drug. But the rigorous procedure necessary to achieve the REM deprivation resulted in curtailment of total sleep time by 3 h. Dement administered Dexedrine to the second subject to block REM sleep, and sodium seconal to offset the arousing effects of Dexedrine. He achieved a 95 per cent REM deprivation over 15 consecutive nights, but the subject's total sleep time was again significantly reduced due to the frequent awakenings necessary for REM deprivation. This subject slept only 2 h 54 min on his 15th and last night of REM deprivation in contrast to his baseline sleep duration of 7 h 27 min. No data on total sleep duration were available for the last subject who was REM deprived by Dexedrine and hand-awakenings for 16 consecutive nights. Rigorous REM deprivation procedures cause sleep reduction or partial sleep deprivation after the first few nights, while sloppy REM deprivation techniques permit too much REM sleep.

Stage 4 deprivation on the other hand appears to be free from most of the above problems. Stage 4 deprivation can be performed by arousing the subject when there are two or three EEG delta waves of amplitude greater than 75 μV within 6 sec. This is usually stage 3 sleep. Since stage 4 sleep is almost always preceded by stage 3, waking the subject during stage 3 will prevent the onset of stage 4. Almost complete deprivation of stage 4 is feasible with this hand-awakening method, without undue shortening of total sleep time (see Johnson *et al.*, in press).

In stage 4 sleep deprivation, the subjects should be carefully watched, particularly in the afternoon so that they do not take afternoon naps. Karacan, Williams, Finley & Hursch (1970) found that afternoon naps significantly reduced the amount of slow-wave sleep on the night following naps.

We will discuss the overall effects of REM deprivation and stage 4 deprivation under two broad categories: (1) task performance, and (2) psychological change.

7.3.1. Task performance

The main thrust in differential sleep stage deprivation has been in the exploration of the relation of REM sleep and stage 4 to psychological and emotional disturbances. Consequently few systematic studies of the effects of sleep stage deprivation on performance have been done.

Kales, Hoedemaker, Jacobson & Lichtenstein (1964) observed that six or ten nights of REM deprivation had no effects on a digit span task and on the Stroop Colour-Word test. After three nights of REM deprivation, Sampson (1966) found no decline on digit span and on a complex serial subtraction task 'in spite of reported difficulties in attending and concentrating' (p. 313).

With respect to stage 4 deprivation, Agnew and his group (1967) applied the tasks of paced addition, grip strength, pursuit rotor and discriminated reaction time, and found that none of them deteriorated after seven nights of stage 4 deprivation.

Perhaps the two part study on total sleep deprivation, REM and stage 4 deprivation by Lubin and his group (in press) and by Johnson and his associates (in press) constitute the most extensive study of performance change. Initial results of the study by Lubin and his group were published by Johnson and his colleagues (1972). Lubin and his associates deprived subjects of all sleep for two days. As expected, task performance declined after this total sleep deprivation. Following total sleep loss they wondered whether the recovery in task performance would be differently affected by deprivation of REM sleep or stage 4 from two nights of recovery sleep? Under a working hypothesis that REM sleep (or stage 4) is necessary for performing tasks at a satisfactory level, they expected to see improved task performance if the recovery sleep following total sleep loss contained REM sleep (or stage 4).

Lubin and his group assigned subjects randomly to a control group, a REM deprivation group and a stage 4 deprivation group. The control group had uniterrupted recovery night sleep following two nights of total sleep deprivation. The REM deprivation group were denied most of their stage REM during recovery sleep. Likewise the stage 4 deprivation group was denied stage 4 during recovery sleep.

The Williams Word Memory test, the Wilkinson Addition test, the Plus Seven test, the X-crossout test, the Counting test, the Auditory Vigilance test, the Contingent Negative Variation (Naitoh, Johnson & Lubin, 1974) and the Mood test were administered to all subjects.

The results showed that recovery sleep without REM sleep or without stage 4 sleep was as recuperative as recovery sleep with no sleep stage deprivation in restoring task performance. Their conclusion was that 'other studies have shown that decreasing the *amount* of sleep certainly worsens performance. This study shows that the *kind* of sleep may not matter'.

In the second part of this study, Johnson and his group deprived subjects of REM sleep or stage 4 sleep for three consecutive nights. Then all subjects were denied total sleep for one night. This was to determine if prior sleep stage deprivation potentiated the effects of total sleep deprivation. The tests used in Part 1 and some new tests were added, such as the Davis Reading test (Davis & Davis, 1962), the Rorschach Concept Evaluation test (McReynolds, 1954), the Spielberger State-Trait Anxiety test (Spielberger, 1968), the Primary Affect Scale (Johnson & Myers, 1967) and others. No major changes in waking performance were observed after REM deprivation or stage 4 deprivation. Decrements were found following total sleep deprivation, but there were no significant between-group differences.

Thus, differential sleep deprivation did not affect most of these commonly used tasks.

Although some authors have suggested that REM sleep (or slow wave sleep) was somehow necessary for memory consolidation, experimental results have been mostly negative. Kales and his associates (1964), Greenberg, Pearlman, Fingar, Kantrowitz & Kawliche (1970), Ekstrand, Sullivan, Parker & West (1971) and Chernik (1970, 1972) observed little or no impairment in verbal learning and memory after REM deprivation in human subjects.

Feldman & Dement (1968) found a small but significant decrease in long-term memory after one night of REM deprivation, but in a subsequent study of two nights of REM deprivation Feldman did not find a memory impairment. Empson & Clarke (1970) found that 'the REM state has an important part to play in the consolidation of memories' (p. 288). But, impairment of long term recall was observed on only one of three memory tests.

Using the Zeigarnick Interrupted Task Paradigm, Grieser, Greenberg & Harrison (1972) found that REM deprivation impaired the recall of only anxiety-laden, ego-threatening materials, and not the recall of neutral materials. The results of this study should be replicated before we accept them, as Chernik (1972), using a different method, could not confirm their findings.

We have too few studies to draw any conclusion about relation of stage 4 deprivation to memory. Ekstrand & his colleagues (1971) reported no impairment of recall or relearning in the paired-associate experiment after one night of stage-4 deprivation. However, Fowler, Sullivan and Ekstrand (1973) suggested that stage 4 might be beneficial for memory consolidation.

Kopell, Zarcone, de la Pena & Dement (1972) reported that selective attention was greater following two nights of REM deprivation than after non-REM control awakenings. Selective attention was measured by the amplitude differences between the averaged visual evoked responses at the occipital lead. However, Naitoh and his colleagues (1973) did not find any significant differences in the Contingent Negative Variation amplitudes between the REM-deprived subjects and the stage 4 deprived subjects.

7.3.2. Psychological change

In the early studies, REM deprivation produced dramatic changes in psychological states (Dement, 1965; Sampson, 1966; Clemens & Dement, 1967), and it was quickly suggested that REM sleep was necessary for mental health. Subsequent studies, however, failed to confirm the inferred psychotogenic effects of REM deprivation in human subjects.

Most recent REM deprivation studies have now cast serious doubt on the occurrence of even minor psychological change in subjective mood. Kales and his group (1964) found no significant changes on the MMPI, Nowlis Adjective Check List (see Nowlis, 1965), and the Clyde Mood Scale (Clyde, 1963) following REM deprivation. Agnew and his associates (1967) reported that stage 4 deprivation produced a depressed outlook while REM deprivation caused higher irritability and lability, but these changes were not statistically reliable and remain speculative.

Chernik (1970, 1972) found no significant difference between the REM deprived subjects and their yoked controls on the Clyde Mood Scale and the McNair Mood Scale (the earlier version of the Profile of Mood States of McNair, Lorr & Droppleman, 1971).

Cartwright & Ratzel (1972), however, found significant changes in the Rorschach after REM deprivation; these changes were interpreted as *favourable*. The recent study of Johnson and his colleagues (in press) showed no significant differences between the REM deprivation group and the stage 4 deprivation group on the many psychological tests they administered.

The above results in nonclinical subjects, combined with the finding of Vogel, Traub, Ben-Horin & Meyers (1968) that REM deprivation might even be beneficial for the depressed patients, indicate that we should discard any notion that REM deprivation is severely detrimental to psychological health.

From these and other negative findings, Dement (in press) has also become critical of his earlier suggestion that adequate amounts of REM sleep were necessary for mental health. In his recent paper entitled 'The biological role of REM sleep (*circa* 1971)' (in press), Dement pointed out that, as early as 1965, he was forced to conclude that 'REM periods in the adult animal did not serve a vital function and that the organism could probably live indefinitely without them'. Citing the studies by Wyatt and his associates (1969) where prolonged abolition of REM sleep with drugs improved clinical outlook of some patients or at least do no harm, Dement (in press) recommended that we bury 'the remains of any notion that the occurrence of normal REM periods was necessary for the maintenance of more or less normal function'.

Although we have less conclusive data about stage 4, some sleep researchers believe a similar statement about the nonvital nature of stage 4 is appropriate (see also Fisher *et al.*, 1973).

In spite of the mostly negative results concerning the relation of stages of sleep to waking behaviour, most sleep researchers believe that unless sleep stages served some functions, they would not have survived in the long arduous process of evolution and natural selection. Greenberg, Pillard and Pearlman (1972) reported that REM deprivation reduced the degree of adaptation of the subjects to the second viewing of a stressful film (an excerpt from a medical film, *Basic Autopsy Procedure*). On the second viewing of the film, the REM deprived subjects were more anxious and tense than the control subjects. Perhaps such adaptation to stress could be a function of REM sleep, but the burden of proof rests on the shoulders of those who claim unique and positive effects of REM sleep (or stage 4) on psychological functions.

On the whole, as far as we are aware, differential sleep stage deprivation should be of little concern to experimenters involved with human waking behaviours (see Johnson, 1973).

7.4. PARTIAL SLEEP DEPRIVATION

Sleep reduction can be achieved in many ways, for instance, by delaying bedtime but waking up at the habitual time or by sleeping just once every 48 h (Kleitman, 1963, pp. 175–77; Meddis, 1968; Oswald, 1962, pp. 172–73).

Probably acute or chronic partial sleep deprivation is the most widely experienced type of sleep deprivation in our daily routines. It is certainly experienced by air-line employees (Atkinson, Borland & Nicholson, 1970; Harris, Pegram & Hartman, 1971; Nicholson, 1970; Preston & Bateman, 1970), astronauts (Nicholson, 1972), and medical practitioners (Friedman, Bigger & Kornfeld, 1971).

Partial sleep deprivation would thus be the type of sleep loss most likely encountered in the subjects by the experimental psychologists. Unfortunately, our information on the effects of partial sleep deprivation is incomplete. The main reasons for paucity of research data in this topic can be attributed to the difficulty in conducting experiments on chronic partial sleep deprivation, and also to the ambiguities of the results that have been reported. The confounding of the main effects of partial sleep deprivation with the effects of a few powerful nuisance variables, such as circadian rhythms, age and individual sleep habits, has contributed to much of the ambiguity.

How does the circadian rhythm contaminate the data? Shortening of sleep always involves changes in the timing of sleep. We cannot, therefore, be certain that the observed changes during partial sleep deprivation are the results of short sleep in itself, or of our imposition of wakefulness or sleep on a sensitive segment of the circadian cycle. Taub (1972) observed that disruption of the circadian cycle may account more for behavioural changes than the shortened hours of sleep.

Another complication derives from the inherent organization of sleep stages during sleep. Partial sleep deprivation results in partial differential sleep stage deprivation. Webb stated that if we reduce the usual nocturnal sleep duration from eight to four hours, we could cause a 66 per cent reduction in REM sleep, but only a 12 per cent reduction in stage 4 (Webb, personal communication).

With respect to duration of the usual sleep regimen, intuitively one would assume that subtracting a fixed amount of sleep from a group of natural short sleepers (Hartmann, Baekeland, Zwilling & Hoy, 1971; Hartmann, Baekeland & Zwilling, 1972; Webb & Agnew, 1970; Webb & Friel, 1971) may be quite different from doing the same with natural long sleepers. In addition, we may have to take into account individual differences in timing of sleep, i.e. 'morning larks' and 'night owls'. The age of the subject would undoubtedly be a factor in the response to any change in sleep regimen.

7.4.1. Task performance

The earliest study of partial sleep deprivation was conducted by May Smith (1916) who used herself as the subject. After practising on the same tasks five days a week, except during vacations, for a period of over 3 years to establish her normal variation, she reduced her customary sleep from 8 h to 1·5 h, 3·5 h and 5·5 h over three consecutive nights. She found no decrement in task performance following these reduced hours of sleep. She experienced, however, significantly large and persistent declines in performance during the recovery period from three nights of short sleep. To explain this rather paradoxical finding, she used an apt analogy: 'It is as if a man who has habitually lived on his income is suddenly confronted with an unforeseen demand for money. He may, as a solution, break into his capital, i.e. he will temporarily have command of greater resources than normally are his, but his reserve force is thereby lessened so that later less is at his command.' (p. 345)

Since this study was published, other laboratories have assessed the effects of partial sleep deprivation on human subjects (e.g., Laird & Muller, 1930; Laird & Wheeler, 1926; Freeman, 1932; Husband, 1935).

It is largely from the experimental studies by Wilkinson and his colleagues (Hamilton, Wilkinson & Edwards, 1972; Wilkinson, 1961, 1962, 1964, 1965, 1968, 1970; Wilkinson & Colquhoun, 1968) that we know now in detail what are the effects of partial sleep deprivation on the Wilkinson Addition and auditory Vigilance tasks. We know that decrements in vigilance performance occur when sleep is reduced to 1 h, or no sleep is allowed at all, just for one night, or when only 3 h of sleep (or less) are allowed over two consecutive nights, and further that this decrement will become greater as we continue the regimen of short sleep, suggesting that a cumulative deterioration occurs when only 4 h of sleep are allowed per 24 h.

The available data thus suggest that one should be sensitive to the possibility of some discernible deterioration of task performance (which would appear as lapses) if sleep is shortened to less than 4 h, from a habitual sleep regimen of 7·5 h, over five consecutive nights. This rule of thumb, however, does not mean that the effects of partial sleep deprivation can be easily seen.

To find reliable performance decrements due to partial sleep deprivation, Wilkinson and his group had to resort to test sessions which were long and boring to the subjects (Wilkinson, 1968, 1970). Their subjects underwent five 1-h vigilance sessions per day for 2 days a week, for 6 consecutive weeks, a total of 60 1-h sessions. In addition to the Wilkinson Auditory Vigilance task, the same subjects performed four 1-h Wilkinson Addition tasks per day, 2 days per week, over 6 weeks, totalling 48 1-h sessions. Only with this massive testing were Wilkinson and his associates able to detect the effects of one or two nights of short sleep.

The study by Hamilton and his associates (1972), previously mentioned, suggested that partial sleep deprivation affects the addition task more consistently than the vigilance task. In their study of auditory vigilance, they noted that the 'only real effects of $3\frac{1}{2}$ h sleep loss over 4 days is on the ability to maintain a normal rate of improvement in detection efficiency as indexed by the parameter d'' (p. 105). The parameter d' presumbly reflects the capacity of the subjects to discriminate stimulus changes, in contrast to another parameter β which represents the willingness to report the stimulus changes (see Broadbent, 1971). One of the more sensitive measures of the vigilance performance than the d', the per cent correct detection, significantly declined when sleep was reduced to 4 h over three consecutive nights. In comparison with the vigilance task, the addition task showed the effects of partial sleep loss earlier and more reliably than that of the Wilkinson Vigilance task. Accordingly, the number of additions attempted decreased significantly only after two nights of sleep reduction to 4 h per 24 h.

Johnson & MacLeod (1973) allowed three subjects to undergo scheduled gradual reduction of sleep to permit sufficient time for them to adapt to the shortened sleep, before changing to the next scheduled reduction of 30 min in sleep time. Their usual 7·5 h sleep time was therefore reduced by 30 min every 2 weeks until a 4-h schedule was reached. The subjects stayed on the 4-h sleep regime for 3 weeks. One of the subjects dropped out of the experiment at the 4·5-h schedule, thus, leaving two subjects, one male and one female. The female subject showed a decrement in level of comprehension on the Davis Reading test, and she recalled fewer words on the Williams Word Memory test when sleep was reduced to 4 h. The male subject showed a degradation of short-term memory and reduced speed of comprehension when sleep was shortened to 5·5 h. At 4-h total sleep duration, he showed a lowered level of comprehension. The male subject also completed fewer additions on the Wilkinson Addition task at 5·5 h, and his attempted additions decreased further when sleep was cut to 4 h. The female subject did not show any decrement on the addition task during the period of gradual sleep reduction.

We have been unable to find clear detrimental effects of shortened sleep on on task performance under field conditions, probably due in part to the insensitivity of our tasks used in these studies (Naitoh, in press).

7.4.2. Psychological change

A very few studies are available on changes in psychological functions due to partial sleep deprivation.

May Smith (1916) experienced muscular weariness and feelings of pain during a reduced sleep study. She also reported, however, 'the feeling of exaltation, combined with emotional belief in the power to conquer all things' (p. 342). Thus, her feelings varied from those of unpleasant muscular weariness which became at times 'positive pain' (p. 343) to ones of pleasant sensation, exaltation and power. She became emotionally labile so that she could easily burst into smiles or tears. She also experienced visual hallucinations.

In Freeman's study (1932) which involved his wife and himself as subjects, they used a schedule of four nights each of 4, 10, 8 and 6 h of sleep. The schedule was repeated seven times over a 4-week period. Freeman reported that 'one of the most interesting sidelights was the effect of sleep loss upon general and social behaviour' (p. 279). By the end of the second week, both subjects found it increasingly difficult to be sociable and 'the cantankerous outbursts which occasionally occurred between the two subjects were often quite uncivil' (p. 279). Irritability and childish behaviours persisted throughout the experiment. Halfway through their long experiment, the subjects also began to have difficulties in staying awake.

Johnson & MacLeod (1973) observed that both their subjects became less happy, less friendly, less energetic and more fatigued as total sleep times was reduced to 5 h per 24 h. Increased irritability and problems in sustaining concentration were reported by their subjects when sleep was reduced to 5 h or less.

Thus, partial sleep deprivation appears to change psychological functions in a similar manner as total sleep deprivation but to lesser extent.

Whether the deterioration in mood also lowers motivation which then results in poorer task performance remains unknown. Freeman (1932), however, remarked that he and his wife made an effort to enter the test in a 'vigorous and competitive manner.' (p. 280)

7.5. DETECTION OF EFFECTS OF SLEEP DEPRIVATION

In most psychological experiments, sleep loss effects act as noise to obscure true treatment effects. We will now proceed to illustrate briefly how sleep deprivation affects some commonly employed psychological tasks, such as reaction time, addition and vigilance. These illustrations hopefully will suggest psychophysiological methods wihich will help to identify the questionable periods during a task performance (that is, those periods contaminated by intrusions of effects of sleep loss), and enable the experimenter to exclude them from further analyses.

Figure 7.1 shows a polygraph record illustrating EEG and autonomic activity during the combined Counting task and Auditory Vigilance task (see Lubin et al., in press)

The subject assumed a reclining position, eyes closed, and was provided with a response panel with 10 keys. He was told to count by pressing the response panel keys in the order 9,8,7,6,5,4,3,2,1,9,8, etc. When the subject wished to relax for a moment, he pressed the zero key three times. The subject was also told that, while he was counting, he would hear a click. He was to press the zero key, as soon as he heard the click, and then to resume counting (the Auditory Vigilance task). The task lasted for 50 min, and 33 clicks were presented during this task. In Figure 7.1 the height of the bars on the task channel indicates which response key was pressed; the zero key had the highest amplitude, the nine key the next tallest, and the one key the shortest. The illustration was taken 4 min after the start of the Counting task, on the last of four baseline days prior to total sleep deprivation (Naitoh & Townsend, 1970).

170

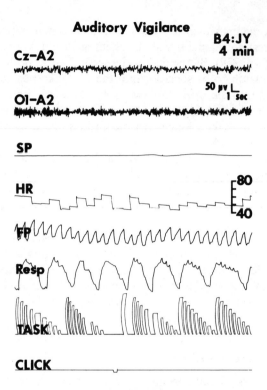

Auditory Vigilance

Cz–A2

Ol–A2

SP

HR

FP

Resp

TASK

CLICK

FIGURE 7.1. The Counting and Auditory Vigilance tasks and psychophysiological correlates. Calibration for the electroencephalograms (Cz and 01 referenced to the opposite mastoid, A2) is given in the top right corner, and for heart rate (HR) to the right in beats per minute. β4 = The last of four baseline days prior to sleep deprivation. SP = Skin potential. FP = Finger pulse. Resp. = Respiration. The subject, JY, reclined on bed, eyes closed. (Reprinted from Naitoh, P. The role of sleep deprivation research, *Human Factors*, 1970, **12**, 575–585, with permission.)

The subject's EEGs are shown on the top channels, then one channel each of skin potential (SP), heart rate (HR), finger pulse (FP), respiration, key presses and click stimulus. During this period, the subject showed an abundance of occipital EEG alpha waves (O_1–A_2), relatively small finger pulse, and regular respiration. His response to the click was fast, and his response in the Counting task was very regularly paced.

Figure 7.2 is the polygraphic record of the same subject 3·5 min after the beginning of the Counting task, but this record was taken after one night of

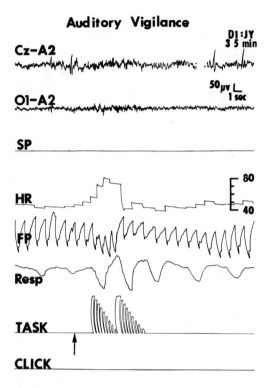

FIGURE 7.2. Psychophysiological correlates of the Counting task for subject, JY, after one night's sleep deprivation. The arrow indicates the time when the experimenter awoke subject, JY. (Reprinted from Naitoh, P. The role of sleep deprivation research, *Human Factors*, 1970, **12**, 575–585, with permission.)

total sleep deprivation. The subject was sleepy and showed a lapse. Because of this lapse, the experimenter told the subject, through an intercom, to continue counting (see the arrow in Figure 7.2). This verbal intrusion aroused the subject sufficiently for him to resume counting for about 6 sec, but he was quickly overcome by sleepiness. Except during a short period when the subject was temporarily aroused by the experimenter, his EEG indicates sleep stage 1 with vertex sharp waves and absence of occipital EEG alpha (for the electrographic details of sleep stages, see Rechtschaffen & Kales, 1968; Johnson, this volume). Autonomic responses were also indicative of drowsiness; a large, irregular finger pulse amplitude and a slow and shallow respiration pattern.

We should remember, however, that humans can become sleepy at any time, just like a cat, if the circumstances are favourable for naps, with or without sleep deprivation. Total and partial sleep deprivation simply potentiate this natural tendency to go in and out of episodic sleepiness.

Figure 7.3 illustrates this point in a subject who was performing the Counting

Auditory Vigilance

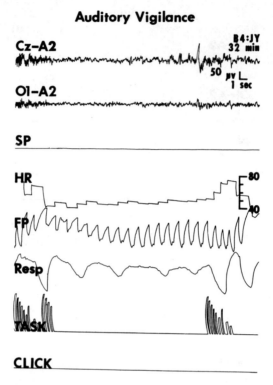

FIGURE 7.3. Psychophysiological correlates of the Counting task for the subject, JY, on the last of four baseline days (B4). See the text for the details

task. At the time this record was obtained, the subject had performed the Counting task for 32 min on the last of four baseline days (B4) prior to total sleep deprivation. The subject showed a lapse lasting about 18 sec before he aroused himself *spontaneously* to resume erratic counting, but it was only a few seconds before he again succumbed to sleepiness. The EEG alpha disappeared a fraction of a second before the subject experienced the behavioural lapse. As before, the lapse was accompanied by the appearance of vertex sharp waves, lowered heart rate, increased finger pulse amplitude, and shallower and slower respiration.

The lapse during the more complex Plus Seven task (Lubin *et al.*, in press) is quite similar to the one we have just described. The Plus Seven task is a self-paced mental addition task with a slight memory load. The task consisted of adding 7 to the starting number, e.g., 1. The subject entered the answer 8 by pressing the 8 key on the response panel which was used in the Counting task. Next the subject added 7 to 8 mentally, and pressed the keys 1 and 5. He continued in this manner, adding 7 to each previous sum. If he lost his place, he might start again at the beginning or go back to the last sum he remembered. When the sum exceeded 1000, he started again with the excess.

Figure 7.4 illustrates a polygraphic record of the EEG and autonomic activity during the Plus Seven task on the fourth and last baseline day. After 5 min in this task, the subject showed smooth and rapid mental addition as shown in the TASK channel. The subject completed six correct additions, starting from $403 + 7 = 410$. Figure 7.5 shows the polygraphic record of the same task from the same subject 5 min into the task, but after two nights of total sleep deprivation (D2). He managed to complete three correct additions. We see the lapses, and again attenuation of EEG alpha activity and slowing of heart rate are observed during the lapses.

These illustrations demonstrate clearly that some of the effects of sleep deprivation on task can be easily detected with the aid of a polygraphic record. With continuous monitoring and recording of the EEGs and autonomic variables, we can eliminate experimental segments contaminated by effects of sleep deprivation.

What if the subjects do not possess high alpha? Yoss, Moyer, Carter & Evans (1970) and other studies by Yoss and his group (Yoss, 1969; Yoss, Moyer & Hollenhorst, 1970) suggested that pupil diameter as measured by

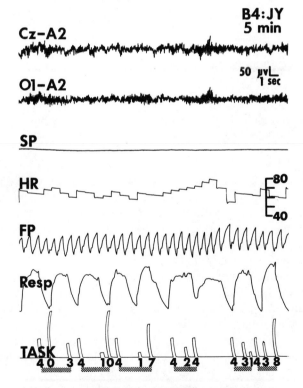

FIGURE 7.4. Psychophysiological correlates of the Plus Seven Task. The subject, JY, reclined on a bed, eyes closed. This record was taken on the last of four baseline days

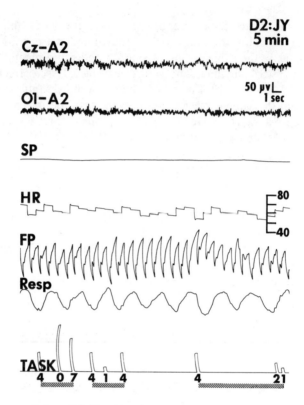

FIGURE 7.5. The Plus Seven Task and its psycho-physiological correlates after two nights' sleep deprivation in the subject, JY

infrared pupillography in the dark is a very reliable and sensitive indicator of sleepiness, and consequently of sleep deprivation. Large and stable pupils reflect an alert state, while reduced pupil diameter is seen in the drowsy state.

While the most useful indices of sleep deprivation depend on psychophysiological recordings, we can suggest some behavioural and psychological measure that are also effective indices.

Reaction time tasks are clearly influenced by the effects of sleep deprivation (e.g. Williams et al., 1959; Wilkinson, 1965; Williams et al., 1964). Williams and his group (1959) showed that the average of the 10 shortest reaction times remained virtually unchanged throughout a baseline period, three nights of sleep loss and a recovery period; but the mean reaction time of the 10 slowest responses quadrupled during three nights of sleep loss. Recently, this procedure of selecting the trials with slow reaction time was adopted by Lisper & Kjellberg (1972). They were able to detect the influence of 24 h of sleep loss with only 5 min of testing, using only the slowest 25 per cent of the reaction time. Thus, a brief reaction time task can be used before the main experiment to ascertain the presence of sleep loss in the subjects.

Another measure that may be of use in detection of sleep loss is the Adjective Check List (as shown in Table 1) which can be quickly given to the subjects at any time of the main experiment without undue interferences. The Adjective Check List is shown to be reliable in detecting sleep deprivation (Bohlin & Kjellberg, 1972; Hendrick & Lilly, 1970; Lubin *et al.*, in press).

How can we detect and remove the confounding effects of stress, compensatory efforts, and other changes present during sleep deprivation?

Unfortunately the answer to this question will not be simple, as we do not yet know the most reliable way to achieve this.

7.6. ACKNOWLEDGMENTS

The author would like to thank Dr L. C. Johnson and Dr A. Lubin for critical reading of the entire manuscript and for editorial suggestions.

This work was supported by Department of the Navy, Bureau of Medicine and Surgery. Opinions or assertions herein are the private ones of the author and are not to be construed to be official or as necessarily reflecting the views of Department of the Navy.

7.7. REFERENCES

Agnew, H. W., Jr., Webb, W. B. & Williams, R. L. Comparison of stage four and 1-REM sleep deprivation. *Perceptual and Motor Skills*, 1967, **24**, 851–858.

Akindele, M. O., Evans, J. I. & Oswald, I. Mono-amine oxidase inhibitors, sleep and mood. *Electroencephalography and Clinical Neurophysiology*, 1970, **29**, 47–56.

Alluisi, E. A. Sustained performance. In E. A. Bilodeau (Ed.), *Principles of skill acquisition.* New York: Academic Press, 1969. pp. 59–101.

Armington, J. C. & Mitnick, L. L. Electroencephalogram and sleep deprivation. *Journal of Applied Physiology*, 1959, **14**, 247–250.

Atkinson, D. W., Borland, R. G. & Nicholson, A. N. Double crew continuous flying operations: A study of aircrew sleep patterns. *Aerospace Medicine*, 1970, **41**, 1121–1126.

Bjerner, B. Alpha depression and lowered pulse rate during delayed actions in a serial reaction test: a study in sleep deprivation. *Acta Physiologica Scandinavia*, 1949, **19**, No. 65.

Bohlin, G. & Kjellberg, A. Self-reported arousal during sleep deprivation and its relation to performance and physiological variables. *Scandinavian Journal of Psychology*, 1973, in press.

Brodan, V. & Kuhn, E. Physical performance in man during sleep deprivation. *Journal of Sports Medicine and Physical Fitness*, 1967, **7**, 28–30.

Brodan, V., Vojtěchovský, M., Kuhn, E. & Čepelák, J. Changes of mental and physical performance in sleep deprived healthy volunteers. *Activitas Nervosa Superior*, 1969, **11**, 175–181.

Broadbent, D. E. *Decision and stress.* London: Academic Press, 1971.

Cartwright, R. D. & Ratzel, R. W. Effects of dream loss on waking behaviors. *Archives of General Psychiatry*, 1972, **27**, 277–280.

Chernik, D. A. W. The effect of REM sleep deprivation on learning and memory. Unpublished doctoral dissertation, University of Texas at Austin, 1979.

Chernik, D. A. Effect of REM sleep deprivation on learning and recall by humans. *Perceptual and Motor Skills*, 1972, **34**, 283–294.

176

Clemens, S. & Dement, W. Effect of REM sleep deprivation on psychological functioning. *Journal of Nervous Mental Disease*, 1967, **144**, 485–491.

Clyde, D. J. *Clyde mood scale manual*. Coral Gables: University of Miami Biometrics Laboratory, 1963.

Davis, F. B. & Davis, C. C. *Davis Reading Test*. New York: Psychological Corporation, 1962.

Dement, W. The effect of dream deprivation. *Science*, 1960, **131**, 1705–1707.

Dement, W. C. Studies on the function of rapid eye movement (paradoxical) sleep in human subjects. In M. Jouvet (Ed.), *Aspect anatomofonctionnels de la physiologie du sommeil*. Paris: Centre National de la Recherche Scientifique, 1965. pp. 572–611.

Dement, W. C. The biological role of REM sleep (*circa* 1971). In W. Webb (Ed.), *The physiology of sleep and dreams*, in press.

Dement, W. C. Sleep deprivation and the organization of the behavioral states. In C. D. Clemente, D. P. Purpura & F. E. Mayer (Eds.), *Sleep and the maturing nervous system*. New York: Academic Press, 1972, pp. 319–355.

Donnell, J., Lubin, A., Naitoh, P. & Johnson, L. Relative recuperative value of sleep stages after total sleep deprivation; a progress report. *Psychophysiology*, 1969, **6**, 239–240.

Drucker, E. H., Cannon, L. D. & Ware, J. R. The effects of sleep deprivation on performance over a 48-hour period. Alexandria, Va.: Human Resources Research Office, George Washington University. *Technical Report No. 69–8*, 1969.

Dunleavy, D. L. F. & Oswald, I. Phenelzine, mood response, and sleep. *Archives of General Psychiatry*, 1973, **28**, 353–356.

Edwards, A. S. Effects of the loss of one hundred hours of sleep. *American Journal of Psychology*, 1941, **54**, 80–91.

Empson, J. & Clarke, P. Rapid eye movement and remembering. *Nature*, 1970, **227**, 287–288.

Ekstrand, B., Sullivan, M. J., Parker, D. F. & West, J. N. Spontaneous recovery and sleep. *Journal of Experimental Psychology*, 1971, **88**, 142–144.

Feldman, R. & Dement, W. C. Possible relationships between REM sleep and memory consolidation. *Psychophysiology*, 1968, **5**, 243.

Fiorica, V., Higgins, E. A., Iampietro, P. F., Lategola, M. T. & Davis, A. W. Physiological responses of men during sleep deprivation. *Journal of Applied Physiology*, 1968, **24**, 167–176.

Fisher, C., Kahn, E., Edwards, A. & Davis, D. M. A psychophysiological study of nightmares and night terrors. *Archives of General Psychiatry*, 1973, **28**, 252–259.

Fowler, M. J., Sullivan, M. J. & Ekstrand, B. R. Sleep and memory. *Science*, 1973, **179**, 302–304.

Freeman, G. L. Compensatory reinforcements of muscular tension subsequent to sleep loss. *Journal of Experimental Psychology*, 1932, **15**, 267–283.

Friedman, R. C., Bigger, J. T. & Kornfeld, D. S. The intern and sleep loss. *New England Journal of Medicine*, 1971, **285**, 201–203.

Fröberg, J., Karlsson, C.-G., Levi, L. & Lindberg, L. Circadian variations in performance, psychological ratings, catecholamine excretion, and diuresis during prolonged sleep deprivation. *International Journal of Psychobiology*, 1972, **2**, 23–36.

Greenberg, R., Pearlman, C., Fingar, R., Kantrowitz, J. & Kawliche, S. The effects of dream deprivation: implications for a theory of the psychological function of dreaming. *British Journal of Medical Psychology*, 1970, **43**, 1–11.

Greenberg, R., Pillard, R. & Pearlman, C. The effect of dream (stage REM) deprivation on adaptation to stress. *Psychosomatic Medicine*, 1972, **34**, 257–262.

Grieser, C., Greenberg, R. & Harrison, R. H. The adaptive function of sleep: the differential effects of sleep and dreaming on recall. *Journal of Abnormal Psychology*, 1972, **80**, 280–286.

Hamilton, P., Wilkinson, R. T. & Edwards, R. S. A study of four days partial sleep deprivation. In W. P. Colquhoun (Ed.), *Aspects of human efficiency*. London: English Universities Press, 1972, pp. 101–113.

Handbook of human engineering data. Medford, Mass.: Tufts College, 1949.

Harris, W., & O'Hanlon, J. F. A study of recovery functions in man. Santa Barbara Research Park, Goleta, Calif.: Human Factors Research, Inc. *Technical Memo No. 10–72* from US Army Human Engineering Laboratories, Aberdeen Proving Ground, Md., 1972.

Harris, D. A., Pegram, G. V. & Hartman, B. O. Performance and fatigue in experimental double-crew transport missions. *Aerospace Medicine*, 1971, **42**, 980–986.

Hartmann, E., Baekeland, F., Zwilling, G. & Hoy, P. Sleep need: How much sleep and what kind? *American Journal of Psychiatry*, 1971, **127**, 1001–1008.

Hartmann, E., Baekeland, F. & Zwilling, G. R. Psychological differences between long and short sleepers. *Archives of General Psychiatry*, 1972, **26**, 463–468.

Hasselman, M., Schaff, G. & Metz, B. Influences respectives du travail, de la temperature ambiante et de la privation de sommeil sur l'excrétion urinaire de catécholamines chez l'homme normal. *Comptes Rendus des Séances de la Société de Biologie*, 1960, **154**, 197–201.

Hendrick, C. & Lilly, R. S. The structure of mood: A comparison between sleep deprivation and normal wakefulness conditions. *Journal of Personality*, 1970, **38**, 453–465.

Husband, R. W. The comparative value of continuous versus interrupted sleep. *Journal of Experimental Psychology*, 1935, **18**, 792–796.

Johnson, E., III & Myers, T. I. The development and use of the Primary Affect Scale (PAS). Naval Medical Research Institute, Bethesda, Md. *Research Report No. 31*, 1967.

Johnson, L. C. Psychological and physiological changes following total sleep deprivation. In A. Kales (Ed.), *Sleep: physiology and pathology*. Philadelphia: Lippincott, 1969, pp. 206–220.

Johnson, L. C. Are states of sleep related to waking behavior? *American Scientist*, 1973, **61**, 326–338.

Johnson, L. C. & MacLeod, W. L. Sleep and awake behavior during gradual sleep reduction. *Perceptual and Motor Skills*, 1973, **36**, 87–97.

Johnson, L. C., Naitoh, P., Lubin, A. & Moses, J. Sleep stages and performance. In W. P. Colquhoun (Ed.), *Aspects of human efficiency*, London: English Universities Press, 1972, pp. 81–100.

Kales, A., Hoedemaker, F. S., Jacobson, A. & Lichtenstein, E. L. Dream deprivation: an experimental reappraisal. *Nature*, 1964, **204**, 1337–1338.

Karacan, I., Williams, R. L., Finley, W. W. & Hursch, C. J. The effects of naps on nocturnal sleep: Influence on the need for stage 1 REM and stage 4 sleep. *Biological Psychiatry*, 1970, **2**, 391–399.

Kleitman, N. *Sleep and wakefulness*. (2nd ed.) Chicago: University of Chicago Press, 1963.

Kling, J. W. & Riggs, L. A. (Eds) *Woodworth and Schlosberg's Experimental Psychology*. (3rd ed.) New York: Holt, Rinehart & Winston, 1971.

Kopell, B. S., Zarcone, V., de la Pena, A. & Dement, W. C. Changes in selective attention as measured by the visual averaged evoked potential following REM deprivation in man. *Electroencephalography and Clinical Neurophysiology*, 1972, **32**, 322–325.

Kuhn, E., Brodan, V., Brodanova, M. & Rysanek, K. Metabolic reflection on sleep deprivation. *Activitas Nervosa Superior*, 1969, **11**, 165–174.

Laird, D. A. & Muller, C. G. *Sleep, why we need it and how to get more of it*. New York: The John Day Co., 1930.

Laird, D. A. & Wheeler, W. What it costs to lose sleep. *Industrial Psychology*, 1926, **1**, 694–696.

Lisper, H. O. & Kjellberg, A. Effects of 24-hour sleep deprivation on rate of decrement in a 10-minute auditory reaction time task. *Journal of Experimental Psychology*, 1972, **96**, 287–290.

Levi, L. (Ed.) *Stress and distress in response to psychosocial stimuli.* Oxford: Pergamon Press, 1972(a).

Levi, L. Psychological and physiological reactions to and psychomotor performance during prolonged and complex stressor exposure. In L. Levi (Ed.), *Stress and distress in response to psychosocial stimuli.* Oxford: Pergamon Press, 1972, pp. 119–139(b).

Lubin, A., Moses, J., Johnson, L. C. & Naitoh, P. The recuperative effects of REM sleep and stage 4 sleep on human performance after complete sleep loss: Experiment 1. *Psychophysiology*, in press.

Mason, J. W. Organization of psychoendocrine mechanisms. A review and reconsideration of research. In N. S. Greenfield & R. Sternbach (Eds.), *Handbook of psychophysiology.* New York: Holt, Rinehart and Winston, 1972, pp. 3–91.

McNair, D. M., Lorr, M. & Droppleman, L. F. *Profile of Mood States.* San Diego, Calif.: Educational and Industrial Testing Service, 1971.

McReynolds, P. Rorschach concept evaluation technique. *Journal of Projective Techniques*, 1954, **18**, 60–74.

Meddis, R. Human circadian rhythms and the 48 hour day. *Nature*, 1968, **218**, 964–965.

Meyer, R. E., DiMascio, A. & Stifler, L. Personality differences in the response to stimulant drugs administered during sleep-deprived state. *Journal of Nervous and Mental Disease*, 1970, **150**, 91–101.

Morgan, B. B., Jr., Brown, B. R. & Alluisi, E. A. Effects of 48 hours of continuous work and sleep loss on sustained performance. University of Louisville, Kentucky: Performance Research Lab. *Interim Tech. Rep ITR-70–16*, 1970.

Murray, E. J. *Sleep, dreams, and arousal.* New York: Appleton-Century-Crofts, 1965.

Murray, E. J. Sleep deprivation and personality adjustment. In L. E. Abt & B. F. Riess (Eds.), *Progress in clinical psychology.* New York: Grune & Stratton, 1968.

Naitoh, P. Sleep loss and its effects on performance. *Navy Medical Neuropsychiatric Research Unit Tech Rep. No. 68–3*, 1969.

Naitoh, P. *Sleep-loss in man.* Springfield, Ill.: Charles C. Thomas, in press.

Naitoh, P., Johnson, L. C. & Lubin, A. The effect of selective and total sleep loss on the CNV and its psychological and physiological correlates. *Electroencephalography and Clinical Neurophysiology*, in press.

Naitoh, P., Kales, A., Kollar, E. J., Smith, J. C. & Jacobson, A. Electroencephalographic changes after prolonged sleep loss. *Electroencephalography and Clinical Neurophysiology*, 1969, **27**, 2–11.

Naitoh, P., Pasnau, R. O. & Kollar, E. J. Psychophysiological changes after prolonged deprivation of sleep. *Biological Psychiatry*, 1971, **3**, 309–320.

Naitoh, P. & Townsend, R. E. The role of sleep deprivation research in human factors. *Human Factors*, 1970, **12**, 575–585.

Nicholson, A. N. Sleep patterns of an airline pilot operating world-wide East-West routes. *Aerospace Medicine*, 1970, **41**, 626–632.

Nicholson, A. N. Rest and activity patterns of prolonged extraterrestrial missions. *Aerospace Medicine*, 1972, **43**, 253–257.

Nowlis, V. Research with the mood adjective check list. In S. S. Tomkins & C. E. Izard (Eds.), *Affect: measurement of awareness and performance.* New York: Springer, 1965. pp. 352–389.

Oswald, I. *Sleeping and waking.* Amsterdam: Elsevier, 1962.

Patrick, G. T. W. & Gilbert, J. A. On the effects of loss of sleep. *Psychological Review*, 1896, **3**, 469–483.

Preston, F. S. & Bateman, S. C. Effect of time zone changes on the sleep patterns of BOAC B. 707 crews on world-wide schedules. *Aerospace Medicine*, 1970, **41**, 1409–1415.

Rechtschaffen, A. The control of sleep. In W. A. Hunt (Ed.), *Human behavior and its control*. Cambridge, Mass.: Schenkman Press, 1971, pp. 75–92.

Rechtschaffen, A. & Kales, A. (Eds) *A manual of standardized terminology, techniques and scoring system for sleep stages of human subjects*. Washington, D. C.: Public Health Service, US Government Printing Office, 1968.

Rubin, R. T., Kollar, E. J., Slater, G. G. & Clark, B. R. Excretion of 17-Hydroxycorticosteroids and vanillylmandellic acid during 205 hours of sleep deprivation in man. *Psychosomatic Medicine*, 1969, **31**, 68–79.

Sampson, H. Psychological effects of deprivation of dreaming sleep. *Journal of Nervous and Mental Disease*, 1966, **143**, 305–317.

Schachter, S. S. & Singer, J. E. Cognitive, social, and physiological determinants of emotional state. *Psychological Review*, 1962, **69**, 379–399.

Seashore, R. H. Work and motor performance. In S. S. Stevens (Ed.), *Handbook of experimental psychology*. New York: Wiley, 1951.

Simonson, E. Sleep deprivation. In E. Simonson (Ed.), *Physiology of work capacity and fatigue*. Springfield, Ill.: Charles C. Thomas, 1971. pp. 437–439.

Smith, May. A contribution to the study of fatigue. *British Journal of Psychology*, 1916, **8**, 327–350.

Spielberger, C. D. *The Spielberger State-Trait Anxiety Inventory*. Palo Alto, Calif.: Consulting Psychologists Press, 1968.

Sternberg, H., Guggenheim, F., Baer, L. & Snyder, F. Catecholamines and metabolites in various states of arousal. *Journal of Psychosomatic Research*, 1968, **13**, 103–108.

Strausbaugh, L. J. & Roessler, R. Ego strength, skin conductance, sleep deprivation, and performance. *Perceptual and Motor Skills*, 1970, **31**, 671–677.

Taub, J. M. Psychobehavioral effects of sleep pattern variation. Unpublished doctoral dissertation, University of California, Santa Cruz, 1972.

Thayer, R. E. Measurement of activation through self-report. *Psychological Reports*, 1967, **20**, 663–678.

Vogel, G. W., Traub, A. C., Ben-Horin, P. & Meyers, G. M. REM deprivation. II. The effects on depressed patients. *Archives of General Psychiatry*, 1968, **18**, 301–311.

Vojtěchovský, M., Šafratová, V., Votava, Z. & Feit, V. The effect of sleep deprivation on learning and memory in healthy volunteers. *Activitas Nervosa Superior*, 1971, **13**, 143–144.

Warren, N. & Clark, B. Blocking in mental and motor tasks during a 65-hour vigil. *Journal of Experimental Psychology*, 1937, **21**, 97–105.

Webb, W. B. & Agnew, H. W. Jr. Sleep stage characteristics of long and short sleepers *Science*, 1970, **168**, 146–147.

Webb, W. B. & Agnew, H. W. Jr. Stage 4 sleep: Influence of time course variables. *Science*, 1971, **174**, 1354–1356.

Webb, W. B. & Agnew, H. W. Jr. Effects on performance of high and low energy expenditure during sleep deprivation. *Perceptual and Motor Skills*, In press.

Webb, W. B. & Friel, J. Sleep stage and personality characteristics of 'natural' long and short sleepers. *Science*, 1971, **171**, 587–588.

Wilkinson, R. T. Interaction of lack of sleep with knowledge of results, repeated testing, and individual differences. *Journal of Experimental Psychology*, 1961, **62**, 263–271.

Wilkinson, R. T. Muscle tension during mental work under sleep deprivation. *Journal of Experimental Psychology*, 1962, **64**, 565–571.

Wilkinson, R. T. Effect of up to 60 hours of sleep deprivation on different type of work. *Ergonomics*, 1964, **7**, 175–186.

Wilkinson, R. T. Sleep deprivation. In O. G. Edholm and A. L. Bachrach (Eds), *The Physiology of human survival*. New York: Academic Press, 1965, pp. 399–430.

Wilkinson, R. T. Sleep deprivation: Performance tests for partial and selective sleep deprivation. In L. E. Abt & B. F. Riess (Eds), *Progress in clinical Psychology*, New York: Grune & Stratton, 1968, pp. 28–43.

Wilkinson, R. T. Methods for research on sleep deprivation and sleep function. In E. Hartmann (Ed.), *Sleep and dreaming*. Boston: Little, Brown and Co., 1970, pp. 369–381.

Wilkinson, R. T. & Colquhoun, W. P. Interaction of alchohol with incentive and with sleep deprivation. *Journal of Experimental Psychology*, 1968, **76**, 623–629.

Williams, H. L., Gieseking, C. F. & Lubin, A. Some effects of sleep loss on memory. *Preceptual and Motor Skills*, 1966, **23**, 1287–1293.

Williams, H. L., Granda, A. M., Jones, R. C., Lubin, A. & Armington, J. C. EEG frequency and finger pulse volume as predictors of reaction time during sleep loss. *Electroencephalography and Clincial Neurophysiology*, 1964, **16**, 269–279.

Williams, H. L. & Lubin, A. Effects of acute sleep loss on performance. Talk given to Neuropsychiatry Division, Psychology Department, Walter Reed Army Institute of Research, Washington, D.C., Jan. 8, 1958.

Williams, H. L., Lubin, A. & Goodnow, J. J. Impaired performance with acute sleep loss. *Psychological Monograph*, 1959, **73**, No. 14 (Whole No. 484).

Williams, H. L. & Williams, C. L. Nocturnal EEG profiles and performance. *Psychophysiology*, 1966, **2**, 164–175.

Wyatt, R., Kupfer, D., Scott, J., Robinson, D. & Snyder, F. Longitudinal studies of the effect of monoamine oxidase inhibitors on sleep in man. *Psychopharmacologia* (Berlin), 1969, **15**, 236–244.

Yoss, R. E. The sleepy driver: A test to measure ability to maintain alertness. *Mayo Clinics Proceedings*, 1969, **44**, 769–783.

Yoss, R. E., Moyer, N. J., Carter, E. T. & Evans, W. E. Commercial airline pilot and his ability to remain alert. *Aerospace Medicine*, 1970, **41**, 1339–1346.

Yoss, R. E., Moyer, N. J. & Hollenhorst, R. W. Pupil size and spontaneous pupillary waves associated with alertness, drowsiness and sleep. *Neurology* (Minneapolis), 1970, **20**, 545–554.

Chapter 8

Psychophysiology of the Menstrual Cycle

BRIAN BELL

Psykologisk Institut, Psykiatrisk afdeling, Kommunehospitalet, Øster Farimagsgade 5, 1399 Copenhagen, Denmark

MARGARET J. CHRISTIE

St. Mary's Hospital Medical School, and Bedford College, University of London, Regent's Park, London NW1 4NS

and

PETER H. VENABLES

Department of Psychology, University of York, Heslington, York YO1 5DD

8.1. INTRODUCTION

Placed as it is in the 'state' section of the book this chapter aims to describe the (relatively small amount of) research on the psychophysiology of the menstrual cycle; such findings as there are suggested the need for greater awareness on the part of experimental psychologists of not only between-sex differences in psychophysiological parameters, but also of between-menstrual-cycle-phase difference within the female subject population.

Some researchers are already aware that '...it would be grossly erroneous to mix men and women subjects where psychophysiological measures are being obtained...' (Shmavonian, Yarmat & Cohen, 1965), and that there is a need to employ some sort of experimental control. A survey (Bell, 1973) of the experimental studies on normal subjects reported in the journal, *Psychophysiology*, for the years 1964–1970 is summarised in Table 8.1; this table

TABLE 8.1. Sex of subjects as reported in two psychological journals

Subject information	Psychophysiology	Journal of Experimental Psychology
No sex stated (%)	14·3	3·6
Male and female (%)	24·2	71·1
All male (%)	54·5	19·3
All female (%)	7·0	6·0
Experiments with control for the menstrual cycle (%)	2·6	Not given

[a]*Psychophysiology*, 1964–1970, Vols. 1–6.
[b]*Journal of Experimental Psychology*, 1966–1967, Vols. 71–75 (After Schultz, 1969).

includes also Schultz's (1969) data, and shows that 54·5 per cent of studies were on all-male subjects, while all-female studies represented only 7 per cent of the total number of investigations. Of these latter studies only 2·6 per cent reported that testing of female subjects was restricted to a particular phase of the cycle. It might be expected that failure to control for cycle phase could introduce avoidable variance into the data, and this suggestion is perhaps supported by findings such as those of Korn & Moyer (1968) and Johnson (1963). The latter worker employed 60 female subjects in a study of decision-making and physiological arousal, no mention being made of cycle phase control. The author commented on the amount of variability in resting heart rate; if the menstrual cycle systematically affects cardiovascular function, and if no control of cycle phase is included in the design, such variability could be expected. Obviously, though, considerable work on the psychophysiology of the menstrual cycle needs to be undertaken before the nature and extent of essential control can be specified: the recent most comprehensive coverage of *Biorhythms and Human Reproduction* (Ferin, Halberg, Richart & Vande Wiele, 1974) gives a very useful overview, and subsequent sections of this chapter describe some of the work ongoing in this area of research.

8.2. DIRECTIONS TO RESEARCH ON THE MENSTRUAL CYCLE

8.2.1. A biological rhythm

Cyclical phenomena are of increasing importance in physiological research (Conroy & Mills, 1970; Sollberger, 1965; Wolf, 1962) and have been reviewed for psychophysiology by Brozek (1964). Thus, the menstrual cycle may be considered within the general context of biorhythms, and attention given to questions of its intrinsic and extrinsic aspects. Although much of the internal mechanism which underlies the human menstrual cycle is reasonably defined there is considerable doubt as to the *external* influences which may be involved. Suggestions range from a lunar mediate (Bramson, 1929; Menaker, 1959) to the role of pheromones (McClintock, 1971). In the latter case, this influence is proposed as an explanation for coincident cycles (Kleitman & Ramsaroop, 1948) and the menstrual synchrony common among friends who spend considerable time in close proximity. Tragakis & Morton (1974) have recently reported a study of ultradian psychophysiological rhythms in both male and female subjects and suggest that there may be some periodicity in both sexes.

8.2.2. A medical problem

In 1953 Greene and Dalton wrote the first article for the British medical press on the subject, but in the subsequent two decades the syndrome of psychological phenomena such as irritability, depression and lethargy, together with physiological aspects such as increased blood pressure and oedema, has become increasingly well-documented. Dalton's (1964) review of the *cause* of the premenstrual syndrome links mood changes, water retention, etc., with an insufficiency of progesterone during the pre-menstrum, and a subsequent depletion of 'raw materials' for the production of adrenal corticosteroids. She posits a temporary imbalance of corticosteroids, dysfunction of mineralo-corticoids leading to a temporary disruption of normal sodium (Na^+), potassium (K^+), and water metabolism. That electrolyte disturbances may be linked with mood shifts in *clinical* conditions is apparent from workers such as Coppen (1967), Bunney, Goodwin and Murphy (1972), and Maas (1972), but only recently has interest in the association between electrolytes and mood been examined in non-psychiatric populations. Janowsky, Berens & Davis (1973) have, for example, reported their correlations between mood, weight, and electrolytes during the menstrual cycle in 11 female college volunteers and have developed a renin–angiotensin–aldosterone hypothesis of pre-menstrual tension. Further consideration of electrolyte status in menstrual cycle phases is presented in Sections 8.3.3 and 5.

Parlee (1973) has recently presented an extensive review of the premenstrual syndrome, commenting on problems of methodology.

8.2.3. An occupational hazard

Dalton (1970) has described the cyclical fluctuations in many aspects of 'efficiency' at work, ranging from skewed distributions of academic examination results to industrial accidents. More recently, Redgrove (1971) reviewed relations between menstrual cycles and human performance in the industrial setting. She interprets the evidence concerning changes in performance as suggesting that there may be significant daily changes which are hidden if the cycle is dealt with in over-large units, and that there are individual differences in the effects of cycle phase. Further, Redgrove (1971) invokes motivation, suggesting that (rather like problems of assessing performance after sleep deprivation, e.g. Wilkinson, 1965; Oswald, 1963) the menstrual cycle does appear to affect the capacity to carry out certain tasks, but the extent to which the effects are manifest depends on the extent to which increased effort can (or is?) able to offset cyclical effects. She concludes with a suggestion that more research should be directed toward a better understanding of the cycle and its effects. A recent review by Sommer (1973) has examined cognitive function and perceptual motor behaviour during the cycle. One of her earlier findings with the Watson–Glaser Critical Thinking Appraisal Test was that there was no systematic relation between cycle phase and performance, but that subjects taking oral contraceptives showed a significantly higher level of performance!

8.2.4. An aspect of female sexuality

In work on relationships between the menstrual cycle and psychological phenomena there is one approach which Redgrove (1971) links particularly with psychoanalysis, and its emphasis on sexual feelings and orientation. She cites early studies by Benedek & Rubenstein (1939) who related psychodynamic processes to ovarian activity. A more recent publication (Diamond, Diamond & Mast, 1972), reports visual detection thresholds to be lowest around the time of ovulation in women not taking steroidal contraceptives, though cyclical variation was not found in male subjects, or in females on oral contraception. They interpret their findings in terms of the role of vision on sexual arousal, and suggest that the greater sensitivity around ovulation, in modalities mediating sexual receptivity, would increase the probability of copulation and hence conception. Wynn (1973) reported a bimensual rhythm in pitch perception in a single subject study. A teleological approach to studies of the menstrual cycle is fairly rare, but one is suggested in the concluding section of this chapter.

Having briefly mentioned approaches to menstrual cycle work in terms of biological rhythm research, its medical problems, its industrial aspect, and its relation to female sexuality, the discussion focuses in more detail on studies from psychophysiologists, after an outline of cycle stages and physiological mechanisms.

8.3. PHYSIOLOGY OF THE MENSTRUAL CYCLE

8.3.1. The normal menstrual cycle

The normal menstrual cycle consists of a series of physiological events related to the process of reproduction. It is conventionally defined as the time interval between the onset of one period of uterine bleeding to the start of the next uterine blood flow (Grossman, 1967). Smith (1968) prefers to regard the flow as symptomatic of the end of the cycle. The time interval ranges from 20–35 days, both across and sometimes within individuals; the median interval is 28 days.

The sequence of physiological and hormonal events which comprises the menstrual cycle involves three main 'target' organs: the uterus, ovary, and pituitary. The hypothalamus has been suggested as a central control mechanism operating by means of the release of two specific neurohumours, namely, follicle-stimulating hormone releasing factor (FSHRF) and luteinizing hormone releasing factor (LHRF). Structural or morphological changes taking place within the reproductive tract are dependent on the nature of inter-relations between pituitary and ovarian hormones, themselves influenced by FSHRF and LHRF; the whole cycle can be pictured as a sensitive feedback system such as is shown in a figure of Langley (1966).

The menstrual cycle can be considered as a number of distinct phases having morphologic and associated hormonal characteristics; for example, five phases are clearly distinguishable by histological and biological assessment:

(1)	Menstruation	—	uterine bleeding (Days 1–4)
(2)	Preovulation	—	formation of follicles in the ovulatory oestrogen phase, under the primary influence of follicle-stimulating-hormone (FSH). As follicles mature oestrogen is secreted, causing the endometrium to thicken, inhibiting FSH, but stimulating release of luteinizing hormone (LH). (Days 5–13)
(3)	Ovulation	—	One or two mature follicles ovulate, become vascularized and form a corpus luteum. This is in effect a temporary endocrine organ which secretes progesterone. (Day 14).
(4)	Postovulation	—	(Days 15–25)
(5)	Premenstruation	—	if fertilization does not ensue, the corpus luteum regresses to the corpus albicans and there is a sharp reduction in the secretion of oestrogen and progesterone. There is progressive degeneration of the endometrium, leading to phase 1, and the loss of sloughed off tissue and blood in the menstrual flow. (Days 26–28)

(Day numbers refer to a 28-day cycle.)

Langley's (1966) figure summarizes the hormonal variations in successive phases of the cycle, showing a double oestrogen peak at approximately days 14–21, and a single progesterone peak around day 21.

Oestrogen and progesterone are also secreted by the adrenal cortex, and though the reproductive tract is the target area mainly associated with their activity, there is increasing evidence that these hormones have effects outside the reproductive system. Much of the evidence comes from work on animal preparations, but some is available from human studies, suggesting that primary or secondary effects of hormonal state are being reflected in other than the reproductive system.

8.3.2. Central effects of menstrual cycle phases

Laidlaw (1956) observed a significant decrease in the frequency of epileptic attacks reported by women undergoing progesterone therapy, and Morrell (1959) found that administered oestrogen precipitated a seizure, these being more frequent in the pre-menstrual phase when progesterone level falls steeply. Variations in the human female electroencephalogram (EEG) have been related to menstrual cycle phase: Matousek, Volavka & Roubicek (1967) reported increased theta during menstruation, and increases in both alpha and theta were reported by Roubicek, Tachezy & Matousek (1969); Gautry (1969) compared EEGs from normally cycling females with those of treated anovulatory patients. In both normal and restored cycles theta waves predominated prior to ovulation and declined in the post-ovulatory phase. Alpha increased during menstruation and in the pre-menstrual phase, in comparison with the rest of the cycle. Margerison, Anderson & Dawson (1964) suggest that variation in EEG may relate to plasma Na^+ concentrations, and Margerison, St. John-Loe & Binnie (1967) suggest that one might reasonably anticipate EEG changes in conditions likely to influence membrane potentials in the brain.

8.3.3. Menstrual cycle phases and mineralocorticoid function

Reich (1962) indicated that aldosterone secretion varies throughout the menstrual cycle, reporting a slight mid-cycle elevation of urinary aldosterone excretion followed by a luteal rise peaking at premenstruum and falling before, or at, the onset of menses. Gray, Strausfield, Watanabe, Sims & Soloman (1968) also reported increased aldosterone secretory rates during the luteal phase (i.e., second half) of the cycle. However, progesterone is said to act as an aldosterone antagonist (Landau and Lugibhil, 1961; Landau, Lugibhil, Bergenstal & Dimick, 1957) and it is difficult, at present, to pinpoint exactly the mechanism whereby Na^+ and water are retained during the premenstruum. Despite difficulties of interpreting the results there does seem to be some hormonal mediation of electrolyte balance during the menstrual cycle, and there are indications of reciprocity between ovarian steroids and adrenocorticoids. Further, the mineralocorticoids appear to be differentially affected by progesterone and oestrogen at different phases of the cycle.

A recent report (Janowsky, Berens & Davis, 1973) concerns correlations between mood, weight, and electrolytes during the menstrual cycle, and offers a renin–angiotensin–aldosterone hypothesis of pre-menstrual tension. The authors include a comprehensive bibliography covering the electrolyte/mood aspects of menstrual cycle phenomena, and suggest that although there is to date no direct evidence in humans for angiotensin effects on behaviour, it is reasonable to consider the possibility that premenstrual–menstrual emotional upset reflects and effect of angiotensin. Their data show increases in negative affect, weight and urinary K/Na ratios in the luteal/pre-menstrual phases of the cycle. Puskulian (1972) reported an increase in salivary Na^+ during the pre-menstrual phase, and a mid-cycle decrease in Na^+ accompanied by a decrease in the Na/K ratio. De Marchi (1973) has reported significant menstrual increases in salivary Na^+ and decreases in K^+, together with marked K^+ increases at ovulation together with Na^+ decreases. A significant aspect of De Marchi's finding is the fact that flow rates were constant through the cycle (see Chapter 10).

Another interesting finding, though at present its causative mechanism is uncertain, is the reported increase in human uterine fluid K^+ concentration $[K^+]$ during the luteal phase of the menstrual cycle (Clemetson, Kim, De Jesus, Mallikarjuneswara & Wilds, 1973). These authors reported that mean $[K^+]$ rose from 17·9 mEq/l in the follicular phase to 33·7 mEq/l in the luteal ($p<0·001$). However the K^+ *content* of fluid was not increased, suggesting movements of Na^+ and water rather than of K^+. These authors note that high $[K^+]$ in uterine fluid would reduce the membrane potential of the endometrium and so facilitate blastocyst-endometrial contact, bringing a possible teleology to studies of luteal/pre-menstrual phase phenomena which has been noticably lacking up to now (Bell, 1973). Thus, if electrolyte and water shifts during the luteal phase are at all related to provision of optimal conditions for implantation and survival of a fertilized ovum, one might reasonably view associated mood changes in this light also: perhaps a transient 'negative affect' is highly effective in repelling the male at a time when the physiological activity of orgasm might jeopardize the chances of blastocyst-endometrial adhesion?

Conner & Miller (1973) have reported studies of uterine fluid $[Na^+]$ and $[K^+]$ in rats. Their findings were that in ovariectomized rats there is a positive relation between oestradiol dose and $[K^+]$. In their study $[Na^+]$ decreased concomitantly and the authors argue the case that their findings support the suggestion of an active transport process under the influence of oestrogen.

Turning now to consideration of autonomic nervous system (ANS) function in relation to the menstrual cycle, the following section considers the reflection of this in heart rate (HR) measures, and evidence relating to electrodermal activity and its underlying eccrine sweat glands. Little & Zahn (1974) have recently noted that examination of cyclical changes in ANS activity seems incomplete: in their study they recorded skin temperature, skin resistance, respiration rate (RR), HR, and finger pulse volume. The last named data were not presented in the report; their finding of a significant luteal rise in respiration rate is noted here, and the remainder of their results is presented in Section 3.4.

8.3.4. Menstrual cycle phases, autonomic function, and metabolism

There are known body temperature changes through the cycle, notably a rise after ovulation; and there are known thermal influences on cardiac function, but no *consistent* finding that heart rate changes parallel cyclical temperature shifts. It may, however, be that the luteal rise in body temperature underlies some observed variation in, for example, respiration and HR, and that more sophisticated statistical analysis such as that of a double analysis of covariance as used by Zahn (personal communication) is required to demonstrate the phenomenon. The present chapter focuses more on electrolyte than on temperature/ANS parameters, and the role of luteal increases in body temperature is not considered further.

Evidence for some covariance comes from Kleitman & Ramsaroop (1948), who found two cyclical increases in heart rate coinciding with the two peaks in oestrogen secretion. Clinical data (Dalton, 1964) indicate cyclic variations in blood pressure, but the precise nature of relationships between hormone secretion and cardiovascular function during the cycle has not been defined.

Reinke, Ansah & Voigt (1972), with a series of investigations on hormonal contraception, gestation, and the puerperium, examined the effect of the menstrual cycle on carbohydrate and lipid metabolism in normally cycling females. The only significant change in values was an increase of free fatty acid values in blood in association with the increased progesterone levels of the luteal phase.

Russell (1972) has reviewed relations between psychological and nutritional factors in disturbances of menstrual function and ovulation, noting that although in anorexia nervosa feeding disorders and emaciation are usually the most conspicuous clinical features, cessation of menstruation may be the first event in the onset of the illness (Kay & Leigh, 1954).

Recently Crisp, Mackinnon, Chen & Corker (1973) reported relations between improved clinical condition in anorexia nervosa and changes in hormonal state.

Wineman (1971) reviews previous studies of autonomic nervous system (ANS) status in normal women through the menstrual cycle. She interprets previous work in terms of reduced sympathetic nervous system (SNS) function during periods of high oestrogen levels, and bases her investigation on use of the $\bar{A}$ score (Wenger, 1948) of autonomic balance. The variables reported by Wineman (1971) were sub-lingual temperature, heart period, diastolic blood pressure, palmar and volar conductance, salivary volume and conductance change. There were significant phase differences in $\bar{A}$ scores and sub-lingual temperature, with $\bar{A}$ being high (i.e., SNS dominance lower) during menses and follicular and ovulatory phases. During the luteal phase $\bar{A}$ scores were lowest.

Little & Zahn (1974) examined ANS activity and mood ratings in five young (18–24 years) and 7 older (27–42 years) women during a complete menstrual cycle. During the ovulatory phase there were significant increases in autonomic responsivity, as shown in SC and HR data, and in the luteal phase there were, in addition to the increases in RR, increases in HR, body temperature and SR. Older women had a higher basal body temperature, less HR variability and higher SR, particularly in the luteal phase of the cycle. These workers have focused on progesterone activity as a possible factor determining age differences: a subsequent study of theirs examined the effect on male subjects of an oral intake of 10 mg/day of Provera (medroxyprogesterone acetate). The authors found a significant rise in temperature and reaction time and a decrease in HR variability during the drug intake. There were significant decreases in SC level and increases in the 'sluggishness' of SCRs. At this point, however, it must be noted that one cannot necessarily extrapolate from findings in studies with *synthetic* materials to phenomena in normally cycling subjects which may be determined by naturally occurring progesterone.

Some account of palmar eccrine sweat glands and electrodermal activity is available in Venables & Christie (1973): sufficient evidence has now accrued to suggest that skin conductance and resistance phenomena are dependent in a major way on eccrine sweat gland activity, but that the negativity of skin potential level (SPL) may be determined by both sweat gland function and external/internal electrolyte concentration gradients. The extent to which one or other determinant dominates is apparently dependent on the level of arousal in which the subject is examined. Considering here the evidence of palmar eccrine sweat gland variation through the menstrual cycle, Mackinnon (1954) reported a significant fall in the number of active glands after ovulation, this reduction being maintained until menstruation; such a fall is suggested by Little & Zahn (1974) as being of relevance to their observed luteal increase in SR.

Evidence relating to cyclical changes in electrodermal activity has, in the past, been inconclusive: some evidence of this, and of recent ongoing work is presented in Section 8.4, which considers more recent work, undertaken by psychophysiologists, where the menstrual cycle, and its phases, is the experimental variable, and associated changes in behaviour and physiological state of major interest. Two general trends can be seen in such studies, one broadly determined by consideration of 'arousal' and performance, and one influenced by ideas regarding electrolyte shifts and mood. Before examining studies subsumed under these two headings, however, some general treatment of methodological problems associated with menstrual cycle research is presented.

8.4. PSYCHOPHYSIOLOGICAL INVESTIGATION OF MENSTRUAL CYCLE PHENOMENA

8.4.1. Methodological difficulties

A constantly-recurring theme through this chapter is the dearth of unequivocal evidence, and the need for further study. One major barrier to progress must be the difficulties associated with research in this area, which range from problems, for psychologists working in a non-medical environment, of accurately determining cycle stages in individual subjects, to the inevitable reticence which, even in this day and age, surrounds this topic of menstruation. Redgrove (1971), for example, describes her doubts about the reliability of data from one '... very self-conscious girl ...' who, it was possible, '... felt reluctant to disclose the dates of her menstrual periods' (1971, p. 221). Also, Dalton (1970) writes on a '... blinkered attitude to menstruation' ... which is ... 'utterly Victorian'. So, given such reticence, there will be problems in recruiting subjects, and when they do volunteer for a study, it is increasingly difficult to find a normally cycling subject not taking oral contraceptives. Having found such subjects it is still a demanding process for subject and experimenter to arrange repeated testing which can accommodate the idiosyncracies of individual cycles. The existence of inter- and intra-subject variability in cycle length exacerbates the problem of adequately defining its phases. The mid-cycle shift toward an increase in the awakening basal body temperature has been used for years as a fairly reliable indicator of ovulation (Rubenstein, 1937; Hartman, 1965), but the mechanism of this action is still unknown (Moore, 1966).

Ideally, the phases should be defined by their hormonal and morphological characteristics, but this involves techniques of biochemical, cytological and histological investigation not normally available to the psychologist. The precision with which phases can be identified probably determines the research strategy used in any investigation of menstrual cycle phenomena. Bearing in mind Redgrove's (1971) warning about the loss of less robust phenomena in over-gross temporal sampling, one can range (depending on the experimenter/subject staying power) from daily sampling to a gross division into menstrual, follicular and luteal phases. Bell (1973) has, with apparent value, divided the cycle into low and high hormonal periods, and compared psychophysiological data which had been collected daily from these two phases: further details are given in Section 8.5. The strategy adopted determines the form of data treatment: Reynolds (1942) proposed that separate cycles can be standardized on a percentile basis, data from each observed day being multiplied by the reciprocal of total cycle length × 100. Dalton (personal communication) has made the following suggestions for division of menstrual cycle data:

'1. *Seven 4-day phases:*

Days 1– 4	menstruation	low oestrogen no progesterone
Days 5– 8	postmenstruation	rising oestrogen no progesterone
Days 9–12	pre-ovulation	high oestrogen no progesterone

Days 13–16	ovulation	falling oestrogen peak F.S.H. and L.H.
Days 17–20	postovulation	rising oestrogen and progesterone
Days 21–24	early premenstruum	high oestrogen and progesterone
Days 25–28	late premenstruum	falling oestrogen and progesterone

This breakdown can be used retrospectively when the first day of the last menstruation is known, or prospectively by asking the subject to post a stamped-addressed form when menstruation starts.

Ovulation does not always occur precisely on Day 14, especially in long and short cycles. By using the phase to cover the four days 13–16, most women's ovulation would be included, and these are the days when peak plasma levels of F.S.H. and L.H. are observed.

If basal temperature records are used to accurately pinpoint ovulation then the other days of the cycle can be adjusted by adding or subtracting days in the preovulation of postovulation phase.

2. *Three phases*: uses only the 4 days immediately before menstruation as the "Premenstrual Phase"; the first four days of menstruation as the "Menstrual Phase", and all the other days of the cycle are included in the "Intermenstrual Phase". This division emphasizes the effect of the rapid fall in oestrogen and progesterone in the premenstruum, and low oestrogen and no progesterone in menstruation. This division can be used regardless of cycle length, and is useful in an unprepared population who cannot accurately remember the date of the last menstruation, but can confirm whether or not they are menstruating on the day of interview and can then be questioned again 4 or 7 days later.'

However, treatment of data from menstrual cycle research is a problem which has not yet received a satisfactory solution. Problems associated with *analysis* of data from repeated testing have been examined by Mefferd in Chapter 2, and problems associated with its *collection*, which involve consideration of increasing *habituation* and its psychophysiological concomitants, and possible increases in *practice* and its effect on performance, are implicit in Chapter 3. One may not always be able to recruit a population of habituated subjects (Christie & Venables, 1971a) for repeated study, nor can one always have subjects with an acquired competence such as used by Redgrove (1968) in her examination of cyclical differences in the typing performance of office secretaries, or by Johnson (1932) in his study which employed tight-rope walkers!

8.4.2. Arousal and performance through menstrual cycle phases

Kopell, Lunde, Clayton & Moos (1969) cite evidence of progesterone's anaesthetic effects when given intravenously to animals (Selye, 1941) and humans (Merryman, Boiman, Barnes & Rothchild 1954). Oestrogen lowers seizure thresholds in rats (Wolley & Timiras, 1962) and progesterone has the opposite effect (Selye, 1941); as has previously been mentioned, female epileptics have a high incidence of seizures in the premenstruum, and progesterone therapy is said to have value in lowering their incidence (Greene & Dalton, 1953; Logothetis, Harner, Morrel & Torres, 1959). The general subject of progesterone–CNS relationships is reviewed by Hamburg (1966).

Kopell *et al.* (1969) studied putative indices of arousal through the menstrual cycles of eight women, measuring two-flash thresholds (2FTs), reaction time (RT), skin potential level and time estimation, in conjunction with plasma cortisol estimation and mood assessment. There were significant phase effects on time estimations, which were longer in the premenstruum. There was an increase in 2FT in this phase, which approached significance, and significant correlations between time estimation and 2FT which varied from 0·220 to 0·438. There was also a significant inverse correlation between cortisol levels and 2FTs ($r = 0·286$). The authors discussed their results in terms of two possible explanations: a distorted time sense as part of a mild, transient, confusional state when progesterone is withdrawn, or changes in the state of arousal which may be secondary to hormonal variations. De Marchi & Tong (1972) also examined 2FT, and Tong, De Marchi, Wilson & Wong (1973) reported that temporal judgment showed a steady rise in scores from Day 4, and that there was a significant increase in temporal production scores just prior to or at menstruation. They note the problems associated with interpreting time judgment data, but suggest the value of the concept of arousal in studying the psychophysiology of the menstrual cycle. Section 8.5 reports recent work by Bell, where studies of arousal were combined with investigations of mood and electrolytes.

8.5. THE BIRMINGHAM STUDIES

8.5.1. Overview

These studies were carried out by Bell (1973) who explored the effects of menstrual cycle phase, in both pill-users and normally-cycling females, on a range of psychophysiological measures. They included assessment of autonomic and electrolyte status, of performance, and of mood. Two studies were carried out in a controlled laboratory environment similar to that described by Christie & Venables (1971a) to examine both tonic and phasic activity and the 'basal' (Christie & Venables, 1971a) state. The first study sampled data at four points of the cycle, and in the second study each subject was tested every day through a complete cycle. Mood assessment was undertaken in the second study using the Thayer (1967) Activation–Deactivation Check-

List (AD–ACL), and in a third study a postal questionnaire provided further AD–ACL data from 171 subjects. Studies 1 and 2 were carried out on nulliparous subjects: Dalton (personal communication) has noted that one cannot necessarily extrapolate from findings on nulliparous to multiparous subjects.

8.5.2. Study No. 1

Sampling in this study was undertaken at four points of the cycle, namely, around menstruation, ovulation, in the post-ovulation, and in the postmenstrual phases. Given a 28-day cycle the sampling would be on days 3, 14, 21 and 27, but adjustments were made for cycles which deviated from a 28-day pattern; siting of the initial test-session was systematically rotated to control for possible sequence effects.

Subjects were eight nulliparous females with no history of gynaecological disorder, and ages ranged from 18·2–21·6 years (mean = 19·4). Cycle lengths ranged from 24 to 25 days (mean = 29·8), and each subject maintained a record of oral temperature, recorded each evening throughout the study. Each of the four test sessions for all subjects was comprised of an orientation period with the stimulus being a light flash of 0·10 sec. and a rise time of 50 msec, and a digit transformation task (after Tursky, Schwarz & Crider, 1970); during each session electrocardiogram (ECG) and skin potential responses and levels (SPRs, SPLs) were recorded by means of a Beckman polygraph. Skin temperature was also recorded at this time, and resting values for the autonomic indices were collected during the periods preceding and following each task.

8.5.2.1. Findings

Examination of the data collected during orienting showed no systematic variation which could be attributed to the menstrual cycle phase, but there was a significant increase in the frequency of non-specific electrodermal responses during the early part of the cycle.

During the digit-transformation task there were no significant findings associated with the ECG, but SPL change exhibited a significant interaction effect between cycle phase and task difficulty. Thus, the easier transformation was associated with a larger SPL change in the pre-menstrual phase, but the more difficult one was associated with a smaller one.

Examination of resting values showed no evidence of a cycle effect in the ECG but a significant main effect was seen in the electrodermal data, with the lowest SPL recorded during menstruation and the highest premenstrually.

Tentative conclusions from these data could be that perhaps the electrodermal rather than the cardiovascular changes suggest the value of further examination, and that apart from the finding of significant phase differences in non-specific responses, tonic rather than phasic values seem a more profitable field for exploration.

8.5.3. Study No. 2

One major difference between this and the first study was the more intensive examination of the subjects: testing was carried out at the same time on every day between 11.00 and 14.00 hours at a time convenient to the subject. Thus, for each subject, a complete cycle was examined on a daily basis and data were available from 245 sessions. As in the first study no gynaecological disorder was reported, and the mean age of subjects was 20·4 years (range $= 18·7$–$21·7$); cycle lengths ranged from 27–33 days, with a mean value of 29·3 days.

Another major difference was in the use of 'basal' skin potential levels (BSPL) in contrast to the SPLs of Study 1: no stimulus trials were included, and each test session lasted for 1 h, with subjects relaxing in bed-rest conditions. In contrast to Study 1 skin potentials were recorded with 0·5 per cent potassium chloride (KCl) following the recommendations of Venables & Christie (1973). The difference between 'resting' and 'basal' SPL has been described by Christie & Venables (1971a, 1972, 1974). In the 'basal' state palmar eccrine sweat glands are relatively quiescent and the value of the potential recorded in this condition appears to be determined by a non-sudorific factor, namely the K^+ concentration gradient between the electrode (containing 0·5 per cent KCl jelly) and the epidermis (Christie & Venables, 1971b). A more detailed account of BSPL is given in Chapter 10 and two points only need to be made here: first, that with a constant value of $[K^+]$ in the external KCl it becomes possible, on the basis of a Nernstian model, to examine individual differences in epidermal $[K^+]$ by means of differences in recorded BSPL. Such values of epidermal $[K^+]$ may be regarded as reflecting not some purely local condition but a general status of extracellular fluid (ECF) (Christie & Venables, 1971c).

Secondly, there are individual differences in the time taken to reach the point of relaxation which is sufficient for recording of a 'basal' SPL (Christie & Venables, 1974), thus a comparison of resting data across a group of subjects is more appropriate when such data are sampled at each individuals' 'basal' point rather than after some constant temporal interval. For example, ECG sampled around the point of BSPL can provide adequate comparison of subjects' resting heart period (HP) from a 10-cycle length of record (Christie & Venables, 1971c).

In this second study skin potential and ECG were monitored, and palmar surface film (Bell, Christie & Venables, 1975) collected for analysis of Na^+ and K^+. A count of active palmar eccrine sweat glands was made from the middle finger of the dominant hand, by the method of Sutarman & Thomson (1952), at the end of each resting session. At its beginning subjects completed the Thayer AD–ACL.

8.5.3.1. Study No. 2—findings

A significant cycle effect was found in all the variables, namely BSPL, ECG, palmar surface electrolytes and mood. Discussion of these is centred on data sampled at the 'basal' point, on sweat gland activity, palmar surface electrolytes, and on mood.

Data were found to be most usefully examined after grouping into two phases, namely, the 'low hormonal' (LHP), and the 'high hormonal' (HHP). In a 28-day cycle these phases would be equivalent to the days shown in Table 8.2.

TABLE 8.2. Breakdown of the days and phases based on a 28-day cycle

Days-1	Phase	Period
26–28	Late premenstrual	Low hormonal
1–2	Early menstrual	
3–5	Late menstrual	
6–8	Early postmenstrual	
9–11	Late postmenstrual	
12–14	Early ovulatory	High hormonal
15–16	Late ovulatory	
17–19	Early postovulatory	
20–22	Late postovulatory	
23–25	Early premenstrual	

8.5.3.1.1. Data sampled at the 'basal' point. Examining first the BSPL values, there was evidence of a significant cycle effect which was particularly apparent during the low hormonal phase, i.e. from Day 27 to Day 12. LHP data showed a cycle phase effect significant at less than the 0·01 level of probability: the mean BSPL was 13·87 mV at the beginning, and increased to 16·73 mV in the early post-menstruum, after which there was a subsequent reduction in the late post-menstruum. The BSPL changes in the HHP were not statistically significant, but lowest values were recorded around ovulation (13·08 mV). This low negitivity of BSPL at this time is paralleled by reports (Burr & Musselman, 1938; Barton, 1940a,b) of large positive potentials at ovulation, and by findings of increases in the positivity of electrovaginal potentials reported by Lemon & Mozden (1965).

Individual differences in the time to reach BSPL were compared through the low and high hormonal phases. It has previously been reported (Christie & Venables, 1974) that in subjects who are habituated to an experimental environment such times have a relative intra-subject constancy. Significant differences in the mean times to BSPL were noted in the HPP ($F = 3·82$, $P < 0·025$) with the time being reduced to 10·66 min in the early post-ovulatory time, and increased to 15·35 min in late postovulatory periods. Such differences in the subjects of Study 2, who would be well habituated after their repeated testing, may be attributed to within cycle changes in whatever components of 'arousal' are implicated in the process of relaxation to BSPL. A similar increase in time to BSPL is seen in subjects relaxing to a point of BSPL after having been exposed to 10 min of noise avoidance (Christie & Venables, 1974).

Turning now to data sampled from the ECG records, i.e. from 10 cycles of ECG around the point of BSPL: HR was examined, and exploratory investigations were undertaken with the amplitudes of both the T and QRS complexes. As was seen in examination of BSPL data, significant variations in HR were seen in the LHP: HR increased from 73·89 to 79·82 after menstruation ($F = 9·0°$, $P<0·025$). Mean HR in the LHP was 76·04 beats/min and in the HHP this was 77·51 beats/min this was not quite significant, but heart period (HP) *was* significantly reduced ($t = 2·41$, $P < 0·05$). Similar findings are those reported by Little & Zahn (1974) who showed HR to be increased in the luteal phase.

Further examination of the ECG records involved measurement of the amplitude of both T and QRS complexes. Details of such measurement are given by Christie & Venables (1971c), and apart from a report of Venables & Christie (1974) these aspects of the ECG have been neglected by psychophysiologists. It has, however, been reported by Papadimitriou, Roy & Varkarakis (1970) that T-amplitude measurement gives a useful indication of ECF (i.e., plasma) [K^+]: further details are given in Chapter 10. Virtually nothing has been reported on similar electrolyte mechanisms associated with QRS amplitude, though Kernan (1965) discusses the dependence of the amplitude of muscle action potential on the intra- to extracellular distribution of Na^+. The amplitude of this is reduced when intracellular [Na^+] is increased, and Bell (1973) suggests that R-wave amplitude should be increased at points in the menstrual cycle when Na^+ reabsorption is increased.

There were found to be highly significant differences in R-wave amplitude in both LHP and HHP ($F = 4·50$, $P<0·01$ and $F = 2·68$, $P<0·05$ respectively). R-amplitude was at its maximum in the late menstrual phase of the LHP, and in the HHP there was a saw-toothed variation with a maximum in the early post-ovulatory period. At this point there was a marked decrease in T-wave amplitude: variation was significant in the HHP ($F = 3·14$, $P< 0·025$) though not in the LHP. If the QRS and T-wave amplitudes reflect in any way the pattern of Na^+ and K^+ shifts in ECF the early post-ovulatory period may be one in which [Na^+] is increased and [K^+] reduced.

8.5.3.1.2. Palmar eccrine sweat gland activity. Again, it was found that in the low rather than the high hormonal phases the greatest cyclical effect was shown: there was increased sweat gland activity [as evidenced by the Sutarman and Thomson (1952) technique] in the menstrual phases, and no significant differences in the HHP. The finding of increased sudorific activity during menstruation is in marked contrast to the report of Mackinnon (1954). Bell (1973), however, notes that Mackinnon's samples were collected in the early morning, and in a hospital environment, and suggests that much more information is needed regarding diurnal variation in palmar eccrine sweating before adequate comparison is made. It may be that, Mackinnon having examined her subjects when skin conductance values (and therefore palmar eccrine sweat gland activity) are known to be low, and Bell when they are at a zenith, cyclical differences in the *patterning* of sweat gland activity could account for the different findings.

8.5.3.1.3. Palmar surface electrolytes. The interest in electrolytes noted in Sections 8.2.2 and 8.3.2 has tended to focus more on Na^+ than K^+ : the neglect of the latter ion may, however, be an unfortunate omission, and the present finding do suggest that K^+ rather than Na^+ changes are the ones showing significant cyclical differences. Once more the statistically significant differences were found in the low rather than high hormonal phase. There was, in the LHP, a continuous and significant ($F = 3.18$, $P < 0.05$) decline in $[K^+]$ from 24.64 mEq/l in the late pre-menstrual to 14.03 mEq/l in the late post-menstrual phase. In the HHP there was a rise to 24.08 mEq/l in the late post-ovulatory phase, but this was not statistically significant. A comparison, however, of $[K^+]$ for the two phases showed that the concentration was significantly ($t = 2.43$, $P < 0.05$) greater (20.40 mEq/l) in the HHP than in the LHP (18.18 mEq/l).

In the HHP there was a significant cycle effect on Na/K ratio ($F = 2.73$, $P < 0.05$) with a reduction in the early post-ovulation stage.

An overall comparison of data with that for male subjects reported by Christie and Venables (1971b) showed that there were no major differences: Bell's values for $[K^+]$, Na/K ratio, and weight were 19.49 mEq/l, 2.11, and 47.25 mg, as compared with the male values of 18.17 mEq/l, 2.14 and 47.51 mg. The finding of higher $[K^+]$ in female subjects together with their lower BSPL values is support for the hypothesized inverse relation between ECF $[K^+]$ and recorded BSPL. The relation between $[K^+]$ and BSPL through the cycle only holds in the LHP, however, and it may be that some other determinant is responsible for the low BSPLs of ovulation. One possibility is that of some relation between potential and temperature.

8.5.3.2. Interim summary

An interim summary of the findings from Study No. 2 can be presented in terms of a number of pointers indicating possible directions for much-needed research into the psychophysiology of the menstrual cycle, and in terms of the need for an adequate model with which to relate an otherwise inchoate set of apparently useful data.

First, it may be suggested that approaches via exploration of cation (and especially of K^+) shifts may be particularly useful. It may be that a suitable model with which to approach such cyclical changes is a teleological one as suggested by the findings of Clemetson, Kim, De Jesus, Mallikarjuneswara and Wilds (1973) in their report of production of higher uterine $[K^+]$ in the luteal phase as a means of lowering endometrial potentials and ensuring blastocyst adhesion in the event of an ovum being fertilized. Thus, it may be that uterine $[K^+]$ changes in the luteal phase are the end point of a number of related physiological changes which are ongoing during the low hormonal phase of the cycle. Surprisingly little is known about the extra-renal controlling (see Chapter 10) mechanisms involved in maintenance of appropriate $[K^+]$ in various organ systems. But it is possible that measurment of T- and QRS-amplitudes, of BSPL, and of palmar surface electrolytes, is capable of giving some insight into the organism's management of K^+ movements, and that the significant variations in the LHP reflect changes appropriate to preparation of optimal uterine conditions for the post-ovulatory luteal phase.

How the heart rate changes, reported by Bell (973) and by Little and Zahn (1974), are integrated into management of K^+ shifts can only be speculated upon, perhaps with reference to relations between ANS transmitters (Ross, 1962).

One final point of current interest relates to the possible relation between epidermal hydration, poral closure, and a reduction in the negativity of SPL. Palmar surface fluid weight is increased in the HHP which, although not significantly so, suggests the possible value of the method for examination of skin hydration phenomena and associated menstrual cycle changes such as exacerbation of acne (Williams & Cunliffe, 1973), poral closure, and reduced SPL.

8.5.4. Mood changes

Returning now to another aspect of Study 2, namely that of the assessment of cyclical differences in mood as measured by Thayer's AD–ACL. This method of mood assessment was also used in a subsequent postal questionnaire, detailed later.

A brief outline only of the results from this aspect of the studies is presented here: greater detail may be found in Bell (1974).

There is a quite extensive literature dealing with fluctuations in mood and affect during the menstrual cycle. In general, studies have dealt either with the delineation of symptomatology associated with the pre-menstrual syndrome (Sutherland & Stewart, 1965; Moos, 1968; Reeves, Garvin & McElin, 1971; Moos, Kopell, Melges, Yalom, Lunde, Clayton & Hamburg, 1969) or with affective changes associated with ovulation (Ivey & Bardwick, 1968). While there is considerable agreement that changes in mood and affect do take place, there is much less concensus of opinion with regard to their aetiology and the temporal patterning of change during the cycle. Ivey and Bardwick's (1968, p. 344) assertion that the menstrual cycle presents itself 'as an arena for the physical acting out of psychological conflicts' represents one current school of thought in which psycho-analytical interpretation of cycle symptomatology is foremost. In contrast, the work by Janowsky, Gorney, and Mandell (1967) and Moos (1969) has concentrated on the likelihood of some kind of somatic determinant of behavioural variation during the cycle.

A variety of test instruments has been employed in investigations of mood characteristics of the cycle: these include the Nowlis Mood Adjective Checklist (Nowlis, 1965) used by Little & Zahn (1974) and previously by Moos *et al.* (1969), and relatively unstructured interview procedures (Ivey & Bardwick,

1968). The use of the Nowlis MACL and Moos' (1968) Menstrual Distress Questionnaire are of particular relevance in the present context, since both instruments provide information on what might be described variously as an 'arousal' or 'activation' factor. Activation, indexed by ratings on the MACL adjectives (active, energetic, vigorous), was found to be significantly increased in the ovulatory phase and lowest both premenstrually and menstrually by Moos, Kopell, Melges, Yalom, Lunde, Clayton & Hamburg (1969). Little & Zahn (1974) report a similar mid-cycle peak in positive activation using the MACL, but failed to find any evidence for changes in negative activation. Moos (1969) employed a Menstrual Distress Questionnaire in which an arousal factor was included; adjectives and statements comprising this factor were mainly of positive-affect connotation (affectionate, orderliness, excitement, feelings of well-being, bursts of energy). The questionnaire was administered to 839 subjects; there were indications that responses on the questionnaire depended to some extent on whether the respondent could be classified clinically as suffering from pre-menstrual depression. In general, the study found arousal to be low both at menstruation and at the pre-menstrual phase. There appears to have been relatively little other research in which arousal or activation as measured by self-report questionnaires has been used.

Self-estimates of mood and alertness made on graphic scales were obtained in the study by Patkai, Johansson & Post (1971). Two factors showed significant variation: the lowest estimates for 'restlessness' were found during the post-ovulation period and higher scores were produced premenstrually. 'Apprehensiveness' exhibited a post-menstural peak. In contrast, Kyger & Webb (1972) failed to find overall significant variation in mood states of a group of normal subjects tested with a battery of test insturments including the Tennessee Self Concept Scale.

Thayer (1967, 1970) has described the development and use of an adjective checklist designed specifically as a self-report measure of levels of activation. The initial factor analytic study yielded four Activation–Deactivation (AD–ACL) factors: Deactivation–Sleep, High Activation, General Deactivation, and General Activation. The adjectives associated with each factor are given in Table 8.3. A later study in which the AD–ACL was administered to a group of male subjects (Thayer, 1967), with concomitant monitoring of heart rate and skin conductance, resulted in substantial correlations between the ACL factors and the physiological parameters. Skin conductance was positively correlated with General Deactivation and High Activation; a similar positive relationship was found for heart rate and these factors. Heart rate was also correlated with the Deactivation–Sleep factor. Confirmation of these relationships was made in a later study which used female college students. Significant differences in factor scores were found in a study concerning diurnal variation in activation (Thayer, 1967) with the deactivation factors showing large increases in the late evening which were matched by decreases in the activation factors.

In Study 2 the AD–ACL dimensions of Deactivation–Sleep (DS) and

TABLE 8.3. Major Factors of the Activation-Deactivation Checklist

Activation–deactivation adjective checklist (AD–ACL) factor	Adjective
Deactivation–Sleep (DS)	Sleepy Tired Drowsy
High Activation (HA)	Clutched-up Jittery Stirred up Fearful Intense
General Deactivation (GD)	At rest Still Leisurely Quiescent Quiet Calm Placid
General Activation (GA)	Lively Active Full of pep Energetic Peppy Vigorous Activated

General Activation (GA) showed significant variation during the LHP: the late menstrual phase score for DS was 1·48 and there was a menstrual increase to 2·24. GA showed a corresponding decrease, but there was no significant variation in HA or GD. Correlations between the AD–ACL factors and physiological variables are shown in Table 9.4.

Study 3 was a postal investigation. Respondents to an advertisement placed in the MENSA monthly newsletter were sent two copies of the AD–ACL to be completed during their premenstrual and menstrual phases at a fixed time during the day (between 11.00 a.m. and 1.00 p.m.). A total of 171 respondents completed and returned the questionnaire. An additional group of 11 replies was excluded on the grounds that they did not meet the age criterion (between 18–38 years), or indicated cycle irregularities, or did not have satisfactorily completed forms. The respondents were subdivided into pill or non-pill groups, and married and single groups, prior to analysis. A significant cycle effect was found for each AD–ACL factor. Both DS and GD showed an increase between the premenstruum and menstruation, while HA and GA showed a

TABLE 8.4. Correlation (rho) between physiological parameters and AD–ACL factors

	AD–ACL factor			
	DS	HA	GD	GA
BSPL	0·292*	−0·199	0·271	−0·252*
SPL change	−0·048	−0·023	−0·197	−0·082
BSPL time	0·042	0·050	0·146	0·123
Heart rate	0·031	0·129	−0·178	−0·094
Heart period	0·217	−0·050	0·249*	0·161
T-wave	0·084	−0·179	−0·270*	−0·158
R-wave	0·226*	0·194	−0·040	0·114
K$^+$	0·146	0·648***	−0·209	0·107
Na/K	0·209	−0·021	0·334**	−0·126
Active sweat glands	0·265*	−0·040	−0·059	−0·047

*$P < 0.05$
**$P < 0.01$
***$P < 0.001$

decrease. The relation between DS and GA scores in this study parallels that found in the laboratory study. Additionally, a significant main effect for use of oral contraceptive was found for the DS factor—the scores for subjects taking the pill were reduced when compared with those obtained by non-pill subjects. Further, the GA factor showed an interaction effect for pill-usage and cycle phase: the premenstrual and menstrual score for the contraceptive group remained almost unchanged, the score for the non-pill group showed a decline during the menstrual phase.

8.5.5. Future work: a cross-cultural perspective

The studies which have been described have dealt exclusively with subjects drawn from Western cultures. While a large body of research has been carried out with an emphasis on the cross-cultural aspects of the menarche, there appear to have been little or no studies dealing with the psychophysiological concomitants of cycle function in non-Western subject samples. As an initial step towards the investigation of menstrual cycle parameters in such groups a study is now being implemented in Mauritius using Moos' (1969) Menstrual Distress Questionnaire. It is planned to administer English, Creole and French language versions of this instrument to samples drawn from the island's main ethnic groups: namely, Hindu, Moslem, Creole and Franco-Mauritian. The data obtained from this normative study are expected to indicate the extent to which cultural factors influence distress symptoms. Anecdotal evidence that symptoms such as pre-menstrual tension and depression together with menstrual cramps are common in women from various tribes in equatorial West Africa has been provided for the authors by a Dutch midwife* who worked in a development hospital serving a largely rural area in the Ivory Coast. Once it became known in the area that the hospital was able to provide

*We are indebted to Mathilde Sergeant for this information.

medication which tends to alleviate distressing menstrual symptoms (either through a course of oral contraceptives or by simple analgesic dosage) large numbers of women travelled to attend the daily outpatient clinic. Many of these women had apparently walked considerable distances and most were prepared to wait several days for a consultation.

Hamburg (1966) indicated that the differential effects of progesterone in cycle function may in part be genetically determined. Again, it would seem that the hereditary components of menstrual typology have received scant attention from investigators. It may well be that the extension of the classic twin method to psychophysiological studies of the menstrual cycle would provide useful information: the employment of such a methodological approach within a cross-cultural context would be of obvious value.

8.6. CONCLUSIONS

This chapter has attempted to present some account of research into psycho-physiological aspects of the menstrual cycle. One general conclusion which can be drawn is that experimental psychologists may need to take account of cyclical variation when designing studies which involve female subjects. A more specific conclusion is that there is scope for a range of fundamental research on psychophysiological aspects of the menstrual cycle. Such research has its methodological problems, but these can be dealt with, given ingenuity... and persistence! Finally, models are lacking, with which to systematize the findings gradually accumulating from a number of research activities: one approach is via the possible adaptive function of cation shifts in the luteal phase in preparation for blastocyst adhesion in the uterus.

Another approach, and one which has not been examined in any detail in this chapter, is via the well-documented change in body temperature which characterizes ovulation. It is perhaps less easy to find a teleological explanation for this phenomenon, but it may be that a temperature change underlies the changes in recorded variables such as HR and RR, and determines the changes temporal judgment. However, it must be obvious that there is scope for pursuit of a number of research interests within the field of work on the menstrual cycle.

8.7. ACKNOWLEDGMENTS

This work was undertaken during tenure of a Medical Research Studentship in the Department of Psychology at the University of Birmingham, and thanks are due to Dr Phil Feldman and Dr Tony Carr for their advice and encouragement. Dr Anne Broadhurst helped in the contact of subjects. The Department of Mineral Engineering, University of Birmingham, provided facilities for the analysis of electrolyte samples. The chapter was prepared while Dr Bell was a Royal Society Fellow in Denmark.

The chapter was written during the tenure of a grant from the Social Science

Research Council to the second and third authors and while they were in the Department of Psychology, Birkbeck College, University of London.

The authors are indebted to Dr Katharina Dalton for her invaluable comments on the chapter.

8.8. REFERENCES

Barton, D. S. Electrical correlates of the menstrual cycle in women. *Yale Journal of Biology and Medicine*, 1940, **12**, 335–344(a).

Barton, D. S. A study of temperature and electrical potentials in the menstrual cycle. *Yale Journal of Biology and Medicine*, 1940, **12**, 503–524(b).

Bell, B. Psychophysiological studies of the menstrual cycle. Unpublushed Ph.D. thesis, 1973, University of Birmingham, England.

Bell, B. Self-reported activation during the menstrual cycle. In preparation for *Journal of Interdisciplinary Cycle Research*, 1974.

Bell, B., Christie, M. J. & Venables, P. H. Menstrual cycle variation in potassium. *Journal of Interdisciplinary Cycle Research*, 1975. (In press).

Benedek, T. & Rubenstein, B. B. The correlation between ovarian activity and psychodynamic processes: menstrual cycle phase. *Psychosomatic Medicine*, 1939, **1**, 461–485.

Bramson, J. Statisch onderzoek naar de correlatie tusschen mannphase en menstruatie bij 10,000 vrouwen. *Psychologische en neurologische bladen*, 1929, **1**, 63–76.

Brožek, J. Psychorhythmics: a special review. *Psychophysiology*, 1964, **1**, 127–141.

Bunney, W. E., Goodwin, F. K. & Murphy, D. L. The 'switch process' in manic-depressive illness. III. Theoretical implications. *Archives of General Psychiatry*, 1972, **27**, 312–317.

Burr, H. S. & Musselman, L. K. Bioelectric correlates of the menstrual cycle in women. *American Journal of Obstetrics and Gynecology*, 1938, **35**, 743–751.

Christie, M. J. & Venables, P. H. Characteristics of palmar skin potential and conductance in relaxed human subjects. *Psychophysiology*, 1971, **8**, 523–532(a).

Christie, M. J. & Venables, P. H. Sodium and potassium electrolytes and 'basal' skin potential levels in male and female subjects. *Japanese Journal of Physiology*, 1971, **21**, 659–668(b).

Christie, M. J. & Venables, P. H. Basal palmar skin potential and the electrocardiogram T-wave, *Psychophysiology*, 1971, **8**, 779–786(c).

Christie, M. J. & Venables, P. H. Site, state, and subject characteristics of resting skin potential. *Psychophysiology*, 1972, **9**, 645–649.

Christie, M. J. & Venables, P. H. Mood changes in relation to age, EPI scores, time, and day. *British Journal of Social and Clinical Psychology*, 1973, **12**, 61–72.

Christie, M. J. & Venables, P. H. Change in palmar skin potential level during relaxation after stress. *Journal of Psychosomatic Research*, 1974, **18**, 301–306.

Clemetson, C. A. B., Kim, J. K., De Jesus, T. P. S., Mallikarjuneswara, V. R. & Wilds, J. H. Human uterine fluid potassium and the menstrual cycle. *Journal of Obstetrics and Gynaecology of the British Commonwealth*, 1973, **80**, 553–561.

Conner, E. A. & Miller, J. W. The sodium and potassium content of rat uterine luminal fluid. *Journal of Endocrinology*, 1973, **59**, 181–182.

Conroy, R. & Mills, J. *Human Circadian Rhythms*. London: Churchill, 1970.

Coppen, A. The biochemistry of affective disorders. *British Journal of Psychiatry*, 1967, **113**, 1237–1264.

Crisp, A. H., MacKinnon, P. C. B., Chen, C. & Corker, C. S. Observations of gonadotrophic and ovarian hormone activity during recovery from anorexia nervosa. *Postgraduate Medical Journal*, 1973, **49**, 584–590.

Dalton, K. Similarity of symptomotology of premenstrual syndrome and toxaemia of pregnancy and their response to progesterone. *British Medical Journal*, 1954, **2**, 1071.

204

Dalton, K. Menstruation and accidents. *British Medical Journal*, 1960, **2**, 1425–1426.

Dalton, K. Menstruation and crime. *British Medical Journal*, 1961, **2**, 1752–1753.

Dalton, K. *The premenstrual syndrome*. London: Heineman, 1964.

Dalton, K. *The menstrual cycle*. Harmondsworth: Penguin, 1970.

De Marchi, G. W. Personal communication, 1973.

De Marchi, G. W. & Tong, J. E. Menstrual, diurnal, and activation effects in the resolution of temporally paired flashes. *Psychophysiology*, 1972, **9**, 362–367.

Diamond, M., Diamond, A. L. & Mast, M. Visual sensitivity and sexual arousal levels during the menstrual cycle. *Journal of Nervous and Mental Disease*, 1972, **155**, 170–176.

Edelberg, R. Biopotentials from the skin surface: the hydration effect. *Annals of the New York Academy of Sciences*, 1968, **148**, 252–262.

Ferin, M., Halberg, F., Richart, R. M. & Vande Wiele, R. L. *Biorhythms and human reproduction*, New York: Wiley, 1974.

Fowles, D. C. & Venables, P. H. The effects of epidermal hydration and sodium reabsorption on palmar skin potential. *Psychological Bulletin*, 1970, **73**, 363–378.

Gautry, J. P. Quantitative analysis of EEG variations during spontaneous or restored menstrual cycle. *Neuroendocrinology*, 1969, **5**, 368–373.

Gray, J. A., Strausfield, K., Watanabe, M., Sims, E. & Solomon, S. Aldosterone secretory rates in the normal menstrual cycle. *Journal of Clinical Endocrinology*, 1968, **28**, 1269–1275.

Greene, R. & Dalton, K. The premenstrual syndrome. *British Medical Journal*, 1953, **1**, 1007–1013.

Grossman, S. P. *A textbook of physiological psychology*. London: Wiley, 1967.

Hamburg, D. A. Effects of progesterone on behavior. Association for Research into Nervous and Mental Diseases, *Endocrinology and the Central Nervous System*, 1966, **43**, 251–265.

Hartman, C. Wanted: an easily detected sign of impending or just completed ovulation. In Keefer, C. S. (Ed.), *Human ovulation: A symposium*. London: Churchill, 1965, 21–45.

Ivey, M. E. & Bardwick, J. M. Patterns of affective fluctuation in the menstrual cycle. *Psychosomatic Medicine*, 1968, **30**, 336–345.

Janowsky, D. S., Berens, S. C. & Davis, J. M. Correlations between mood, weight, and electrolytes during the menstrual cycle: a renin–angiotensin–aldosterone hypothesis of premenstrual tension. *Psychosomatic Medicine*, 1973, **35**, 143–154.

Janowsky, D. S., Gorney, R. & Mandell, A. J. The menstrual cycle. Psychiatric and ovarian-adrenocortical hormone correlates: case study and literature review. *Archives of General Psychiatry*, 1967, **17**, 445–469.

Johnson, G. B. The effect of periodicity on learning to walk a tight wire. *Journal of Comparative Psychology*, 1932, **13**, 133–141.

Johnson, H. J. Decision-making, conflict and physiological arousal. *Journal of Abnormal and Social Psychology*, 1963, **67**, 114–124.

Kay, D. & Leigh, D. The natural history, treatment, and prognosis of anorexia nervosa, based on a study of 38 patients. *Journal of Mental Science*, 1954, **100**, 411–431.

Kernan, R. P. *Cell K*. Washington: Butterworths, 1965.

Kessell, N. & Coppen, A. The prevalence of common menstrual symptoms. *Lancet*, 1963, **2**, 61–64.

Kleitman, N. & Ramsaroop, A. Periodicity in body temperature and heart rate. *Endocrinology*, 1948, **43**, 1–20.

Kopell, B. S., Lunde, D. T., Clayton, R. B. & Moos, R. H. Variations in some measures of arousal during the menstrual cycle. *Journal of Nervous and Mental Diseases*, 1969, **148**, 180–187.

Korn, J. H. & Moyer, K. E. Effects of set and sex on the electrodermal orienting response. *Psychophysiology*, 1968, **4**, 453–459.

Kyger, K. & Webb, W. W. Progesterone levels and psychological state in normal women. *American Journal of Obstetrics and Gynecology*, 1972, **112**, 759–762.

Laidlaw, J. Catamenial epilepsy. *Lancet*, 1956, **2**, 1235–1237.

Landau, R. L. & Lugibihl, K. The catabolic and natriuretic effects of progesterone in man. *Recent Advances in Hormone Research*, 1961, **17**, 249–292.

Landau, R. L., Lugibihl, K., Bergenstal, D. M. & Dimick, D. F. The metabolic effects of progesterone in man: dose response relationships. *Journal of Laboratory and Clinical Medicine*, 1957, **50**, 613–620.

Langley, L. L. *Homeostasis*. London: Chapman and Hall, 1966.

Lemon, H. M., & Mozden, P. J. Vaginal potential and total estrogen excretion during normal menstruation, postcastration and hormonal therapy. In Keefer, C. S. (Ed.), *Human ovulation. A symposium*. London: Churchill, 1965, 132–159.

Little, B. C. & Zahn, T. P. Changes in mood and autonomic functioning during the menstrual cycle. *Psychophysiology*, 1974. In press.

Logothetis, J., Harner, R., Morel, F. & Torres, F. The role of estrogens and catamenial exacerbation of epilepsy. *Neurology*, 1959, **9**, 352–360.

McClintock, M. K. Menstrual synchrony and suppression. *Nature*, 1971, **229**, 244–245.

MacKinnon, P. C. B. Variations in the number of active palmar digital sweat glands during the human menstrual cycle. *Journal of Obstetrics and Gynaecology of the British Empire*, 1954, **61**, 390–393.

Maas, J. W. Adrenocortical steriod hormones, electrolytes, and the disposition of catecholamines with particular reference to depressive states. *Journal of Psychiatric Research*, 1972, **9**, 227–241.

Margerison, J. H., Anderson, W. McC. & Dawson, J. Plasma sodium and the EEG during the menstrual cycle of normal females. *Electroencephalography and Clinical Neurophysiology*, 1964, **17**, 540–544.

Margerison, J. H., St. John-Loe, P. & Binnie, C. D. Electroencephalography. In, Venables, P. H. & Martin, I. (Eds.), *A manual of psychophysiological methods*. Amsterdam: North-Holland, 1967.

Matoušek, M., Volavka, J. & Roubíček, J. Elektroencefalogram u normální populace. II. Vliv fyziologíckych xmén na EEG. *Československa psychiatrie*. 1967, **63**, 73–78.

Menaker, M. Lunar periodicity in human reproduction: a likely unit of biological time. *American Journal of Obstetrics and Gynecology*, 1959, **77**, 905–914.

Merryman, W., Boiman, R., Barnes, L. & Rothchild, I. Progesterone 'anesthesia' in human subjects. *Journal of Clinical Endocrinology*, 1954, **14**, 1567–1569.

Moore, W. W. The adrenal cortex. In Selkurt, E. E. (Ed.), *Physiology*. Boston: Little, Brown, 1966.

Moos, R. H. The development of a menstrual distress questionnaire. *Psychosomatic Medicine*, 1968, **30**, 853–867.

Moos, R. H. Typology of menstrual cycle symptoms. *American Journal of Obstetrics and Gynecology*, 1969, **103**, 390–402.

Moos, R. H., Kopell, B. S., Melges, F. T., Yalom, I. D., Lunde, D. T., Clayton, R. B. & Hamburg, D. A. Fluctuations in symptoms and moods during the menstrual cycle. *Journal of Psychosomatic Research*, 1969, **13**, 37–44.

Morrell, F. The role of oestrogens in catamenial exacerbation of epilepsy. *Neurology*, 1959, **9**, 352–360.

Nowlis, V. Research with the MACL. In Tomkins, S. S. & Izard, C. E. (Eds.), *Affect, cognition and personality*. New York: Springer, 1965.

Oswald, I. Reaction time and menstruation. *British Medical Journal*, 1963, **1**, 1019.

Papadimitriou, M., Roy, R. R. and Varkarakis, M. Electrocardiographic changes and plasma potassium levels in patients on regular dialysis. *British Medical Journal*, 1970, **2**, 268–269.

Parlee, M. B. The premenstrual syndrome. *Psychological Bulletin*, 1973, **80**, 454–464.

206

Patkai, P., Johansson, G. & Post, B. Variations in physiological and psychological functions during the menstrual cycle. *Reports from the Psychological Laboratories, University of Stockholm*, 1971, 340.

Puskulian, L. Salivary electrolyte changes during the normal menstrual cycle. *Journal of Dental Research*, 1972, **51**, 1212–1216.

Redgrove, J. A. *Work and the menstrual cycle*. Unpublished Ph.D. thesis, University of Birmingham, 1968.

Redgrove, J. A. Menstrual cycles. Chapter 6, In W. P. Colquhoun (Ed.), *Biological rhythms and human performance*. London: Academic Press, 1971.

Reeves, B. D., Garvin, J. E. & McElin, T. W. Premenstrual tension, symptoms, and weight changes related to potassium therapy. *American Journal of Obstetrics and Gynecology*, 1971, **109**, 1036–1041.

Reich, M. The variation in urinary aldosterone levels of normal females during their menstrual cycle. *Australasian Annals of Medicine*, 1972, **11**, 41–49.

Reinke, V., Ansah, B. & Voigt, K. D. Effect of the menstrual cycle on carbohydrate and lipid metabolism in normal females. *Acta Endocrinologica*, 1972, **69**, 762–768.

Reynolds, S. R. M. A method for correlating data from menstrual cycles of different lengths. *American Journal of Obstetrics and Gynecology*, 1952, **44**, 151–152.

Ross, E. J. Biological properties of aldosterone. *British Medical Bulletin*, 1962, **18**, 164–169.

Roubiček, J., Tachezy, R. & Matoušek, M. Electricka cinnost mozkova u probehu menstrucniho cyklu. *Ceskoslovenska psychiatrie*, 1969, **64**, 90–94.

Rubenstein, B. S. The relationship of cyclic changes in human vaginal smears to body temperatures and basal metabolic rates. *American Journal of Physiology*, 1937, **119**, 635–641.

Russell, G. F. M. Psychological and nutritional factors in disturbances of menstrual function and ovulation. *Postgraduate Medical Journal*, 1972, **48**, 10–13.

Schultz, D. P. The human subject in psychological research. *Psychological Bulletin*, 1969, **72**, 214–228.

Selye, H. Studies concerning anesthetic action of steroid hormones. *Journal of Pharmacology and Experimental Therapeutics*, 1941, **73**, 127–141.

Shmavonian, B. M., Yarmat, A. J. & Cohen, S. I. Relationships between the autonomic nervous system and central nervous system in age differences in behavior. In A. T. Welford Z J. E. Birren (Eds.), *Behavior, Aging and the Nervous System*. Springfield, Thomas, 1965.

Smith, A. *The body*. London: Allen and Unwin, 1968.

Sollberger, A. *Biological Rhythm Research*, New York: Elsevier, 1965.

Sommer, B. The effect of menstruation on cognitive and perceptual-motor behaviour: A review. *Psychological Medicine*, 1973, **35**, 515–534.

Sutarman, & Thomson, M. L. A new technique for enumerating active sweat glands in man. *Journal of Physiology*, 1952, **117**, 51P–52P.

Sutherland, H. & Stewart, I. A critical analysis of the premenstrual syndrome. *Lancet*, 1965, **1**, 1180–1183.

Thayer, R. E. Measurment of activation through self-report. *Psychological Reports*, 1967, **20**, 663–678.

Thayer, R. E. Activation states as assessed by verbal report and four psychophysiological variables. *Psychophysiology*, 1970, **7**, 86–94.

Tong, J. E., De Marchi, G. W., Wilson, M. & Wong, S. Arousal and the biological clock: Menstrual diurnal and activation effects on temporal judgment, 1973. In press.

Tragakis, C. & Morton, A. Sex differences in sensorimotor, cognitive and affective ultradian psychological rhythms: A preliminary report. *Journal of Interdisciplinary Cycle Research*, 1974, **4**. In press.

Tursky, B., Schwarz, G. E. & Crider, A. Differential patterns of heart rate and skin resistance during a digit-transformation task. *Journal of Experimental Psychology*, 1970, **83**, 451–457.

Venables, P. H. & Christie, M. J. Mechanisms, instrumentation, recording techniques, and quantification of responses. Chapter 1, In W. F. Prokasy & D. C. Raskin (Eds.), *Electrodermal Activity in Psychological Research*, New York: Academic Press, 1973.

Venables, P. H. & Christie, M. J. Neuroticism, physiological state and mood: An exploratory study of Friday/Monday changes. *Biological Psychology*, 1974, **1,** 201–211.

Wenger, M. A. Studies of autonomic balance in Army Air Force personnel. *Comparative Psychology Monographs*, 1948, **19,** No. 4.

Wilkinson, R. T. Sleep deprivation. Chapter 14, In O. G. Edholm & A. L. Bacharach (Eds.), *The Physiology of Human Survival*. London: Academic Press, 1965.

Williams, M. & Cunliffe, W. J. Explanation for pre-menstrual acne. *Lancet*, 1973, **2,** 1055–1057.

Wineman, E. W. Autonomic balance changes during the human menstrual cycle. *Psychophysiology*, 1971, **8,** 1–6.

Wolf, W. (Ed.) Rhythmic functions in the living system. *Annals of the New York Academy of Sciences*, 1962, **98,** 753–1326.

Wolley, D. & Timiras, P. The gonad-brain relationship: effects of female sex hormones on electroshock convulsion in the rat. *Endocrinology*, 1962, **70,** 196–209.

Wynn, V. T. Absolute pitch in humans, its variations and possible connections with other known rhythmic phenomena. Chapter 4, In G. A. Karkut & J. W. Phillis (Eds.), *Progress in Neurobiology*, Vol. 1, Part 2, Oxford: Pergamon, 1973.

Chapter 9

Pleasure

ROBERT M. STERN, JO-ANN H. FARR and WILLIAM J. RAY

The Pennsylvania State University

9.1. INTRODUCTION

9.1.1. Defining pleasure

We included in our working definition of pleasure the observation, participation or imagination of activities or objects that are sought out by the individual. When talking about humans and probably other organisms, it would be too restrictive to limit the definition to consumatory behaviour alone, i.e. sex, eating and drinking. We also examined in addition to these obvious pleasurable states, sports, exercise and recreation, aesthetic experiences, altered states of consciousness and humour.

One immediate problem with this definition is this: should we include as pleasurable states those that are sought out by some individuals but are at the same time destructive of bodily tissue? Examples include masochism, some forms of drug addiction, alcoholism, etc. A closely related problem is the matter of the inclusion as pleasurable of states that the individual is compelled to seek out, e.g. the compulsive eater, drinker, gambler, jogger, etc.

In order to gain a better understanding of pleasure, it appeared advantageous to examine the concept of pain. Sternbach (1968) defines pain as 'an abstract concept that refers to (1) a personal, private sensation of hurt; (2) a harmful stimulus which signals current or impending tissue damage; (3) a pattern of responses which operate to protect the organism from harm' (p. 12).

Adapting Sternbach's definition to pleasure one can indeed say that pleasure is an abstract concept, and that it refers to a personal private sensation. It is however, difficult to determine the advantage to the organism of pleasure. One could argue as Plato did that the function of pleasure is to tell the organism when he is growing correctly; but even this has certain limited utility since pain may accompany growth, as in the case of a muscle's becoming stronger. Also, pleasure may accompany activities that are harmful overall to the body, as in overeating or the taking of certain drugs. A possible role of pleasure would be to achieve on an individual level those activities which are necessary for the species as a whole. That is, where eating itself or sex itself not pleasurable, then there would be few organisms that would freely enter into these activities for the good of the species. By seeking pleasure, which of course is connected with the reduction of tension in most individuals, individuals carry on the preservation of the species as a seemingly natural process without any awareness of purpose or consequences.

Pleasure in the above definition represents a state of balance of normal functioning. It is not seen in this definition so much as a state which has specific physiological manifestations as it is a condition of general well being and balance. This is the early Greek position concerning pleasure. Whereas pleasure to Plato had been a satisfactory fulfilment of a need, Aristotle added to this by including the pursuit of the Good as being pleasurable. There was a distinction made between higher cognitive functioning and lower bodily sensations. Emotions were said to be associated with the intellect whereas passions were connected with lower bodily processes. Feelings were believed to be attached to all kinds of sensations as well as to higher cognitive functioning. Similar to this was Plato's statement that pains and pleasures arise from the mind, from the body, or from both.

Beebe-Center (1932) in his book *Pleasantness and Unpleasantness* makes the distinction that 'pleasant' refers to concrete objects, to the things themselves, whereas 'pleasantness' is an abstract term referring to a quality of a substance, not the substance itself. The same is true of 'unpleasant' and 'unpleasantness'. It might be added to this that pleasure is a state of the person observing, experiencing, or imagining the object or activity and thus not always directly related to the object itself—one man's pleasure is another man's pain. Whereas pleasantness and unpleasantness are on a continuum of abstract qualities; if something is less pleasant, then it is more unpleasant in comparison. However, the same cannot be said of pleasure and pain. That is, not to have pleasure or not to be in a pleasurable state is not the same as experiencing pain and vice versa.

9.1.2. The literature search

Having agreed upon our admittedly shaky definition of pleasure, we searched for psychophysiological research using J. Stern's (1964) broad definition: 'any research in which the dependent variable is a physiological measure and the independent variable a behavioral one' (p. 90).

In our search of the literature we relied heavily on *Psychological Abstracts*, *Psychophysiology*, *Journal of Psychosomatic Research*, *Psychosomatic Medicine* and specialized journals and texts in the subareas covered. The pattern of use of 'Pleasure' as a subject heading in the indexes of *Psychological Abstracts* is thought to be revealing of interest in this area. 'Pleasure' or 'Pleasantness' appears as a heading from 1927 to 1943 with the exception of 1934. 'Pleasure' reappears in 1949 and 1950, disappears in 1950 and returns in 1954 and remains as a heading until 1961. From 1962 to 1968 neither 'Pleasure' nor any related form of the word appears as a heading. In 1969 and until January 1973 seekers of 'Pleasure' are referred to 'Emotions'. In February 1973, 'Pleasure' returned to the *Psychological Abstracts*.

As the reader will see below, we found relatively few articles to review with the exception of the area of sex. Why has there been so little research devoted to the psychophysiology of pleasure in comparison with the psychophysiology of pain or unpleasantness? Practical considerations have probably contributed greatly to this situation. What is a pleasurable stimulus that can be easily brought into the laboratory? How do we quantify it? Will it be pleasurable for all subjects? And studying the psychophysiology of pleasure in the real world requires expensive telemetry equipment and entails all of the problems that go with the lack of control inherent in field research.

A desire on the part of most psychophysiologists to record from subjects in 'extreme' states has left a large gap in our knowledge of pleasure. For example, no studies were found in which the subject drank two beers and enjoyed an hour's conversation with friends while the experimenter recorded psychophysiological changes. Instead, one finds psychophysiological studies of intoxication. One does not find psychophysiological reactions to eating Thanksgiving dinner in the literature or, more to the point, reactions to eating a normal pleasurable meal. Even in the area of sexual responses, in which much literature is available, we found that most studies deal with orgasms. We did not find any studies in which psychophysiological responses were recorded from a young couple while they sat holding hands on the rocks overlooking the ocean and watching the sun go down.

9.1.3. Historical background

Beebe-Center (1932) and Ruckmick (1936), two of the most complete sources of early work in the area of the psychology of pleasure, agree that Mosso's treatise, concerning the *Circulation of Blood in the Human Brain*, which appeared in 1880, described the first use of the expressive procedure in the study of emotions and feeling. The expressive procedure, according to

Ruckmick, refers to the recording of bodily changes to affective stimuli. Mosso measured blood volume changes in exposed human brains and in the periphery in response to pleasant and unpleasant stimuli.

Following Mosso's pioneering work, two influences served to stimulate a large number of studies in the general area of the psychophysiology of pleasure. The first was Darwin's *Expression of the Emotions in Man and Animals* (1872) and the related theories of emotion of James (1884) and Lange (1885). The second was Wundt's tri-dimensional theory of feeling which appeared in 1896.

9.1.3.1. Pleasurable emotions

It has been suggested that Darwin's (1872) theory offered a basis for examining emotions as an organic process, a process which should be as much within the domain of physiologists as that of philosophers. Darwin himself approached the area of pleasure as an ethologist and attempted to discuss those activities associated with the emotions. He observed joy to be associated with an increase in 'various purposeless movements—to dancing about, clapping the hands, stamping' (p. 196). An increased flow of blood is also associated with the 'excitement of pleasure'. Darwin states, 'from the excitement of pleasure, the circulation becomes more rapid; the eyes are bright, and the colour of the face rises' (p. 210).

Whereas Darwin sought to determine the purpose of a particular emotion for the organism, James cautioned against pushing our explanations...too far in the teleological direction. As is well known, James (1884) stated, 'that our feelings of the same *bodily* changes as they occur is the emotion' (p. 13, author's italics).

Work on the question of pleasure and pain was also being developed in terms of the philosophical implications. Trigg (1970) suggested that the approach of looking at pain and pleasure as the opposite of each other was philosophically characteristic of the end of the nineteenth century. The underlying assumption was that pain and pleasure were to be treated in the same fashion. Trigg suggested that the period directly following took the 'common sense' approach of which pain was viewed as a sensation and pleasure as an emotion. That is, an individual generally feels the sensation of pain and this sensation is located in a specific area of the body. Pleasure, on the other hand, represents a more global state. For example, one does not say 'my hand feels pleasant' in the same manner as one says 'my hand hurts'.

However, most psychologists continued to view pleasure and pain as emotions. Allport (1924) suggested that the two antagonistic branches of the autonomic nervous system (ANS), cranio-sacral (parasympathetic) and the sympathetic could be paired with 'two groups of emotions having opposed qualities of feeling, pleasant and unpleasant, respectively' (p. 86). Functions which appear as part of eating are parasympathetically governed and the related sensations are usually pleasurable. Also certain muscle responses prior to orgasm are parasympathetic in nature. There are, however, exceptions to this formulation (Gellhorn & Loofbourrow, 1963). Some of these are (1) Sadness causes crying through parasympathetic impulses; (2) bad odours as well as good ones elicit parasympathetic activity such as salivation; and (3) fear and anxiety may activate the bladder through the parasympathetic nervous system. Current textbooks in physiological psychology that deal with the topic of pleasure (e.g., Morgan, 1965) still refer to pleasant emotions or activities as being linked to the parasympathetic system and unpleasant to the sympathetic.

9.1.3.2. Simple affective stimuli

Commencing at the beginning of this century, Wundt and his followers conducted a long series of experiments relating cardiovascular and respiratory responses to hedonic tone. In 1901, Brahn, working in Wundt's laboratory, examined the relationship of pleasant versus unpleasant feeling to vasomotor activity. His basic finding was that pleasant feeling is accompanied by vasodilation and a slowed pulse. Beebe-Center (1932) pointed out, however, that Orth in 1903 and Alechsieff in 1907 criticized Brahn's study because of the lack of instrospective data. On the other hand, Alechsieff obtained similar physiological responses to pleasant feelings: vasodilation and a slowed pulse. He also reported finding 'weakened' breathing. Perhaps one of the more consistent findings and one with implications for a current theoretical controversy was that heart rate seemed to decrease in response to pleasant stimuli and increase to unpleasant stimuli.

In the 1930's the galvanic skin response (GSR) was first put to common use in the study of bodily responses to pleasant stimuli. Dysinger (1931) presented 150 words to his subjects and recorded their GSRs as they rated each word on a five-point scale from 'very pleasant' to 'very unpleasant'. The smallest response was seen for indifferent words. The size of the response increased with either pleasantness or unpleasantness. Shock & Coombs (1937) recorded GSRs of children as they rated 16 odours on a similar five-point scale. The girls, again, showed low responding to the indifferent stimuli and larger GSRs to both extremely pleasant and unpleasant stimuli. The boys, on the other hand, showed equally small responses to indifferent and pleasant odours. Lanier (1941) showed words to his subjects and recorded their GSRs as they rated each word 'Indifferent,' 'Pleasant,' 'Unpleasant,' or 'Mixed'. His results supported his hypothesis that the response to 'Mixed' words would show the greatest GSRs. He discusses the results in terms of 'affective conflict'.

9.2. SEX

For the purposes of this discussion, psychophysiological responsiveness during sexual arousal will be divided into two major categories. First, those reactions which have been recorded during human coitus (and masturbation to orgasm) will be discussed, and, second, those reactions which are seen to take place in response to psychological stimulation of a milder nature such as erotic films and pictures will be covered.

9.2.1. Physiological responses during human coitus

As early as 1896 an intrepid investigator, G. Kolb, was interested in undertaking scientific experiments concerned with sexual intercourse. His attempts to measure heart rate during sexual activity are the earliest psychophysiological references in the literature of this subject (Fox, 1970a). The increases in heart rate, he reported, approximately 150 bpm in both male and female during peak arousal periods, were supported by the findings of Boas & Goldschmidt (1932).

Of historic interest are the experiments of Reich (1942) with electrodermal measurements which led to his postulation of an elaborate theory of the function of the orgasm. He recorded skin potential from vaginal mucosa, anal mucosa, lips, tongue, nipples, earlobes, forehead, penis and palm of the hand, areas which Reich defined as 'erogenous zones'. He concluded that erogenous areas had higher skin potentials than nonerogenous areas and that pleasure resulted in a rise in skin potential while displeasure produced drops in potential.

Multiple physiological measures were first recorded by Klumbies & Kleinsorge in 1950, and they reported blood pressure increases in the female of 50 Torr (1 Torr is approximately equal to 1 mmHg), and in the male of 130 Torr, with the peak at the moment of orgasm (Kinsey, Pomeroy, Martin & Gebhard, 1953).

The study of reactions in the CNS during orgasm was first attempted by Mosovich & Tallaferro (1954). Measurement was undertaken with scalp EEG during self-stimulation to orgasm. The records showed three phases common in all subjects: (1) sudden increase in rapid activity, particularly from the temporal lobe, with sudden rise of muscle action potentials superimposed on all cortical areas recorded, (2) slowing of electrical activity with increased voltage until there were paroxysmal waves (3 per sec) mixed with alternating rhythmic muscular discharges which persist and are followed by, (3) depression of the electrical activity with alternating, clonic muscular discharges. The question of contamination of the EEG data due to the presence of muscle artifacts in this study appears obvious.

Bartlett (1956) reported marked fluctuations in HR in both sexes during foreplay and prior to intromission. Constant acceleration of heart rate to orgasm was apparent after intromission. The peak at orgasm was 170 bpm; a sharp decrease then occurred. Marked hyperventilation also occurred following intromission, with respiration rates fluctuating before this point and then constantly accelerating to peaks of 20–70 during orgasm.

Masters & Johnson (1966) must·be largely credited with providing the scientific basis for much of our understanding of the anatomical and physiological aspects of sexuality. Changes in sexual anatomy and physiology during auto-stimulation and coitus have been observed by physical examination, bio-chemical methods, and cinematography. An artificial penis was constructed through which colour photographic records could be made throughout the entire female sexual response cycle. This device is powered by an electric motor and the woman can control the speed and depth of its movements so as to imitate coitus. Four phases of sexual arousal have been isolated and defined by these investigators: excitement, plateau, orgasm and resolution.

Typical reactions found for males during the excitement phase include: tumescence of the penis and thickening and tensing of the scrotal integument due to vasocongestion, contraction of smooth muscles of the dartos layer, elevation of testes due to shortening of spermatic cords, and increase in testicle size. Excitement phase reactions in the female include increase in breast size, nipple erection, tumescence of clitoral glans and shaft, production of vaginal lubrication (11–30 sec after the initiation of effective sexual stimulation), involuntary expansion and lengthening of the inner two-thirds of the vaginal barrel, thickening of the vaginal walls and elevation of majora labia.

The plateau phase is characterized by sympathetic responses such as pronounced tachycardia and elevations in blood pressure and hyperventilation. During the plateau phase rates of 110–175 + bpm have been recorded in both males and females, peaking at 180 + bpm during orgasm. The slower the initial heart rate at resting level, the lower the rate during sexual stimulation. Systolic blood pressure increases 30–80 mmHg during plateau phase and 20–60 mmHg during orgasmic phase in females and increases 40–100 mmHg for males. Diastolic blood pressure elevations during the same periods ranged 20–40 mmHg in females and 20–50 mmHg in males. Respiratory rates over 40/min have been recorded during orgasm in both sexes. Bartholin and Cowper gland secretary activity, in females and males respectively, takes place during plateau phase. Sex tension flush may also be observed in 75 per cent of females and 25 per cent of males during this stage as well as creation of orgasmic platform in the outer two-thirds of the vaginal barrel. Significant increase (50–100 per cent) is also observed in the uterus in females during plateau state.

Involvuntary muscular spasms of genitals and secondary sex organs as well as the external sphincter of the rectum mark the orgasmic phase. Full elevation of the uterus in females is seen in late plateau stage with constant increase in corpus irritability until identifiable contraction pattern indicates the onset of orgasm. The average is five to eight vigorous contractions accompanied by similar contractions in orgasmic platform. In the male, regularly recurring contractions of sphincter urethrae, bulbospongiosus, ischiocavernosus, and perineal muscles produce the ejaculatory reaction. After the first three to four contractions at intervals of 0·8 sec, the penile contractions reduce markedly in force and frequency. In both sexes, vasocongestion and muscular tension gradually diminish during resolution phase. Sympathetic responses (hyperventilation, heart rate, and blood pressure) drop rather sharply, generally to slightly below resting levels, before returning to resting levels. The sweating response is seen in 30–40 per cent of subjects, and this occurs coincident with the fading of the sex tension flush.

Fox & Fox (1969) report changes in blood pressure and respiratory patterns similar to findings of Bartlett (1956) and Masters & Johnson (1966). These experiments were conducted with an individual married couple with 11 years of mutual coital experience. They took place in complete privacy and in the familiar surroundings of their own bedroom. Their results showed that blood pressure rose from 120 mmHg to 175 mmHg at the moment of onset of ejaculation in the male, while the female peaked at 200 mmHg during orgasm. Blood pressure was then seen to drop sharply to below resting level during resolution or post-orgasmic phase and then return to normal.

Somewhat different breathing patterns were discussed for each sex by these investigators. In the male the typical pattern of hyperventilation in late plateau was recorded with respiration rates of 40/min at orgasm decreasing to 30/min afterward, while volume of air breathed was 39 litre/min before ejaculation and 51 litre/min afterward. Baseline respiration average was 20/min and volume was 10/min. The female exhibited a breathing pattern marked by periods of apnea (breath holding) before hyperventilation began at the onset of orgasm. Rates of 16/min and volume of 13 litre/min before late plateau increased to 35/min with volume of 44 litre/min at orgasm. These investigators hypothesize, as did Masters & Johnson, that the exertion of intercourse is not seen as sufficient to produce either the respiratory or blood pressure changes recorded. Alternatively, they suggested that a combination of hormonal factors, heart rate increases and muscular tension is responsible.

Intravaginal and intrauterine pressure changes in female during coitus were measured by Fox, Wolfe & Baker (1970). Rather than employing abdominal and intrauterine electrodes as did Masters & Johnson, they favoured the use of a pressure sensitive radio-pill. Results showed negative pressure in vagina during intromission and male orgasm but positive pressure during female orgasm. Uterine pressures were minimal during male orgasm but increased markedly during female orgasm to a positive pressure of 40 cmH$_2$0, followed by a sharp fall to negative 26 cmH$_2$0. The suggestion from these measures is that a pressure gradient exists between the vagina and the uterus, a possible factor in sperm transport.

Heath (1972) has supplied data obtained from both deep and surface EEG recordings during sexual arousal which culminated in orgasm. Data is provided on two subjects, one male undergoing treatment for severe behavioural disorders and one female undergoing treatment for intractable epilepsy. Changes in recordings from deep structures were significant and consistent. Most marked was the appearance of spike and slow-wave activity with superimposed fast activity from the septal region during orgasm. Occasional minor reflections of activity in amygdala were noted. EEG returned to baseline as orgasm and sexual arousal subsided. Both patients displayed the same pattern during orgasm. Little or no change was reflected in surface EEG recordings during these periods. This appears to further support other reports of no correlates between sexual orgasm and scalp EEG. An exception to this is the study cited earlier by Mosovich & Tallaferro suggesting that scalp recording over occipital cortex during orgasm might reflect activity in amygdala providing that problems of muscle artifact can be dealt with effectively.

9.2.2. Physiological responses during exposure to erotic stimuli

An immediate problem encountered in a review of the psychophysiological recording of responses to erotic stimuli is the fact that some investigators appear to implicitly assume that stimuli such as discrete nude slides and erotic motion pictures will be equally sexually arousing across and within both individuals and sexes. Yet there is good reason to suspect that the stimuli sufficient to titillate a male may differ significantly from that to which a female is responsive. Kinsey *et al.* (1953) reported, for instance, that females do not find pictures of nude males arousing. In the case of males, many subjectively report more sexual arousal to pictures of females nudes which more closely approximate what is available to them in their own environment than to the 'Playboy' nude who is magnificently endowed and generally unavailable. One might also suspect a difference in reaction to discrete slides versus films of erotic events.

Further, unless masturbatory activity is included in the experimental design, it might logically be predicted that subjects would not get beyond the excitement phase of sexual arousal where parasympathetic responsiveness has been found to be dominant. It should be noted, however, that most of the physiological measures commonly recorded have been sympathetic, e.g. GSR, vasomotor activity.

One of the earliest accounts of an attempt to explore patterns of somatic responses to sexual stimuli was by Davis & Buchwald (1957). Eleven variables were monitored. The stimuli presented consisted of 12 slides, including two pictures in each of six categories: horror, fear, cartoons, landscapes, female nudes and geometric abstractions. Subjects included 12 males and 12 females. Pictures of female nudes elicited greater combined responses for both sexes that did other pictures. The authors concluded that males responded distally while females evidently responded axially, that pictures of female nudes had high stimulating value, and that GSR appeared to offer a highly reliable way to assess arousal to visual stimuli. At no point did they state that the arousal produced was sexual in nature. Subjective reports could have been helpful to shed light on this factor.

Koegler & Kline (1965) recorded palmar skin resistance, GSR lability (number of fluctuations), heart rate, finger pulse volume and respiration rate in response to six films, including two sexual films. All male subjects subjectively reported enjoyment of and sexual arousal to the heterosexual film. Their autonomic reactions were similar to those of females watching a circumcision film. The conclusion of the authors was that positive and negative affect states were indistinguishable.

Wenger, Averill & Smith (1968) also recorded autonomic activity during sexual arousal. They chose as their erotic stimuli sexually arousing reading material and compared reactions on eight physiological variables to those obtained while reading neutral material. The resulting pattern of physiological responsiveness to erotic passages included increases in both systolic and diastolic blood pressure in palmar skin conductance, and in the number of GSRs. Both heart rate and respiration rate remained relatively constant. Finger temperature showed a significant decrease during the reading of erotic material, while face temperature yielded no significant difference between erotic and control material. Subjective reports of the sexual arousal value of the erotic material indicated that the erotic passage was quite effective in producing sexual excitement. One S reported attaining a full erection. The authors point out that it may be very important to look at both the qualitative and the quantitative stages of the development of an emotional state. There may well be significant variance of autonomic response patterns as a function of intensity of emotion. The type of responses elicited in this study appear to be characteristic of Masters & Johnson's first or excitement phase of sexual arousal.

Corman (1968) compared responses to 50 control slides, 15 Playboy nude slides and an erotic film of coitus without explicit views of genitalia. Soft music was added to enhance the experimental set. Both systolic and diastolic blood pressure increased significantly in going from control to nude slides, further significant increases accrued in going from nude slides to erotic films. Heart rate did not increase significantly in going from control to Playboy slides. However, an increase of + 5 bpm was observed during the most arousing scene of the movie. Respiration rate and variability remained relatively stable. Although face temperature was unaffected, finger temperature decreased significantly during the motion picture, but not during slides of nudes. This supports Wenger *et al.* (1968) findings about finger temperature drop.

Romano (1969), with a subject population of 39 married males utilizing the same erotic film as Corman (1968) plus a neutral and a concentration camp film in counterbalanced design, found that both the erotic and the atrocity film produced significant increases in spontaneous GSRs relative to the control condition, but the erotic and atrocity conditions did not differ significantly from each other. Although significant blood pressure changes comparable to Corman's findings to the erotic film were observed, they occurred during the atrocity film also. Changes in heart rate were not significantly different from control during either film, in contrast to Corman's heart rate findings. No respiratory effects were observed, and no significant changes occurred in finger, face or chest temperatures. Subjective reports of positive affect to the sex film and negative affect to the concentration camp film were elicited.

Hain & Linton (1969), using slides of male and female nudes as visual sexual stimuli and all male subjects, failed to find differences in GSRs or respiration, even though semantic differential ratings produced large differences. This finding differs from that of Loisselle & Mollenauer (1965), who found that females produced more GSRs to slides of nude males than to slides of nude females and more spontaneous GSRs to nude slides than to those of clothed figures.

The importance of a difference in experimental set in such testing situations was pointed out by Martin (1964). He compared changes in skin conductance from beginning to end of an entire series of pictures including one set of six Playboy slides and six landscapes and a second set of 12 landscapes. For one half of the subjects, stimulus presentation was preceded by a permissive set, in the rest by an inhibitory set. Less drop in skin conductance was found when nudes were being shown and this difference was even greater after an inhibitory set.

Roessler & Collins (1970) made continuous recordings of the heart rate, skin conductance and respiratory responses of 20 males while they were shown a sexual and a neutral film in a counterbalanced design. Skin conductance responses were significantly higher to the sexual film than to the neutral film. Significantly greater increases occurred in heart rate and pulse amplitude due to the erotic film than due to the neutral film. A comparison of heart rate and skin conductance data indicated that when skin conductance increased, heart rate was found to decrease, and the points at which this phenomena occurred were the same as those points in the film rated as most arousing. Respiration rate was greater to the erotic film than to the control film.

In a study marred by lack of counterbalanced stimulus presentation, Bernick, Kling & Borowitz (1971) compared heart rate responses of nine males to neutral slides, to two stag films (one hetero- and one homosexual), and to an Alfred Hitchcock suspense film. Increases over baseline were significant for the heterosexual stag and suspense films. However, they did not differ significantly between films.

The latest study available involving the measurement of physiological responses to sexual films is composed of two separate experiments by Adamson, Romano, Burdick, Corman & Chebib (1972). In the first experiment, comparing responding to erotic films and slides, significant differences occurred in heart rate, systolic and diastolic blood pressure and finger temperature, with heart rate and both blood pressure measures being greater during the film and finger temperature decreasing during the film. The heart rate increases in this and other studies using erotic films (Corman, 1968; Roessler & Collins, 1970) is in contrast to relatively stable heart rate findings of Wenger et al., 1968 and Romano, 1969.

In the second experiment, viewing both the erotic film and an unpleasant film resulted in a significant increase in systolic and diastolic blood pressure and number of GSRs and significant decreases in palmar skin resistance and finger temperature. Heart rate was significantly increased by the erotic film only and the average decrease in finger temperature was about equal for each stimulus.

A study by Fisher & Osofsky (1968) sought to examine physiological correlates of sexual responsiveness in females. Three conditions were compared (1) a control session (2) a session where a gynaecologist made 'touch threshold' determinations and examined electrodes on breast and labia and (3) a session consisting of a standard gynaecological examination. Heart rate, GSR, skin resistance (hand, breast, labia and ankle) and skin temperature (hand, rectum, vagina and ankel) were recorded. Physiologic data seem inconclusive as to whether sexual arousal was in evidence or not.

Not only has no single response in the studies so far reviewed shown reliability as an indicant of sexual arousal, but no pattern of responses has revealed itself either. Since first stage or excitement phase of sexual arousal as defined by Masters & Johnson (1966) is characterized by vasocongestion in erogenous areas, it would appear fruitful to concentrate efforts of measurement of response changes in these areas.

Freund (1963) developed a penis plethysmograph for measuring changes in penile volume during sexual arousal in an attepmt to devise a laboratory method for diagnosing the predominance of homosexual versus heterosexual interest in the male. Subjects included 58 homosexuals and 65 heterosexuals whose penile volume was recorded while they viewed slides of nude males and of nude females of five different age categories. Summed reactions correctly identified all 65 heterosexuals and 48 of the homosexuals. Significant agreement also occurred in age preference of the sexual object.

Freund, Sedlacek & Knob (1965) presented a modification of the original plethysmograph utilizing a simpler transducer. The technique of measuring the volume of the male genital has been extended to successful diagnosis of sex and age preference of sexual object in hetero- and homosexuals and pedo-philiacs (Freund 1965, 1967a, 1967b, 1970). A similar device was described by McConaghy (1967) in a study where the data showed differential responding by 22 male homosexuals and 11 male heterosexuals to movies of nude males and females.

Bancroft, Jones & Pullan (1966) have also described a simple transducer for measuring penile erections consisting of silicone rubber tubing filled with mercury and fitted with platinum electrodes. Problems with movement artifact were reported absent with this new device.

In an investigation of autonomic correlates of penile erection, Bancroft & Mathews (1972) recorded heart rate, forearm blood pressure, and skin con-ductance of 10 normal male subjects. In the first part of the experiment the subject was asked to look at a series of 10 coloured slides of naked or partially clad women and to rate them for sexual interest. In the second part of the experiment each subject was required to look at three additional slides but to avoid mental imagery as far as possible. During the third phase each subject was given instructions to fantasize. Three fantasies were requested: (1) sexual intercourse with an attractive woman; (2) as sexually exciting a situation as possible; (3) reading a newspaper. Data showed that the only physiological variable which successfully discriminated between sexual and non-sexual stimuli was erectile change. There was a strong indication that visual stimuli without accompanying visual imagery may not be as successful in producing erectile responses as are erotic fantasies.

Another unique attempt at recording sexual arousal reactions has been reported by Zuckerman (1971). He described Bell & Stroebel's attempts to record scrotal and testicular reactions. Activity in dartos and cremaster muscles is measured with a scrotal strain gauge placed around the neck of the scrotum. Preliminary results suggest that elevation of the testicles may take place in states of stress as well as in sexual arousal.

Measurement of blood flow and temperature changes in the female genitals has also been undertaken. Shapiro, Cohen, Di Bianco & Rosen (1968) report the use of a thermal flowmeter designed to measure changes in blood flow in the vaginal wall. Results indicate that the blood flow technique is sensitive to reported changes in arousal. Tart (1973) described a clitorolplethysmograph to measure changes in blood flow in the clitoris and blood flow and temperature changes in the vaginal barrel. A modified form of Tart's device has been used by Fisher & Davis (1973) using a vaginal photoelectric cell.

Bardwick & Behrman (1967) have attempted to investigate effects of anxiety, sexual arousal and menstrual cycle on uterine contractions. The measuring device consisted of a balloon attached to a thick polyethylene tube and inserted into the uterus and filled with water. Measures included tonus, amplitude, and number and duration of contractions. Data showed that the uterus responded to both sexual stimulation and anxiety with increased amplitude and amplitude variance of contraction. No significant differences in uterine motility were found in pooled data between sessions in which stimuli had been presented and those in which content was neutral. There are problems with this technique since the balloon was expelled frequently and some women reported pain during its use. The telemetry technique of Fox (1970a) appears to hold more promise.

Jovanovic (1971) reviewed five objective methods for observing physiological responses of sexual organs in humans to erotic and non-erotic stimuli. These methods have been chiefly used in sleep research, where penile erection is seen to occur during dream phases of sleep (Fisher, Gross & Zuch, 1965). Jovanovic presented three new devices for use in recording genital arousal in humans: a phallograph to record erections in males, a kolpograph to measure vaginal contractions, and a clitorograph to record erections of the clitoris. No data were presented to evaluate the usefulness of these new techniques.

9.2.3. Drugs and hormonal changes

The demonstrated rise in systolic blood pressure during orgasm has become a matter of concern to those specialists advising and treating persons with cardiovascular disease. Recent work by Fox (1970b) has shown that the ingestion of 120–160 mg of β-adrenergic blocking agent causes a significant reduction in the rise of systolic blood pressure during human coitus. Tachycardia was also reduced.

Research on another aspect of the use of drugs (Everett, 1972) concomitant with coitus has revealed that amyl nitrite ('poppers') inhaled prior to orgasm produces subjective reports of increased awareness, intensified and prolonged orgasm and an increased sense of involvement and excitement.

However, dangerous side effects, physiologically substantiated, include increased tachycardia, increased ocular pressure, and profound vasodilation of coronary blood vessels with a drop in peripheral blood pressure and intense headaches.

Fox (1970a) in reviewing the physiology of coitus discussed the role of hormones in sexual intercourse. At present this is an area of great mystery. Research has shown that oxytocin is detectable in the blood stream of females but not of males immediately after orgasm. It disappears 3 to 4 min after its release. A series of samples must be collected as it is released in spurts. Oxytocin has also been detected in the blood stream of mothers during breast feeding.

Interest in the role of neuro-chemicals in sexual arousal began with the work of Clark & Treichler (1950). They showed that psychic stimulation of the prostate caused the release of urinary acid phosphatase (AP) into the urethra. Gustafson, Winokur & Reichlin (1963) collected data which supported Clark & Treichler's hypothesis. When a group of subjects were shown an erotic film a significant mean increase in AP was found in males but not in females when urine samples collected pre- and post- to the film showing were analysed. Barclay (1970) found no significant difference in pre- and post-AP levels when pictures of female nudes were used as arousal stimuli. However, when subjects were shown an erotic film, significant differences seemingly related to the amount of sexual experience of the subject occurred. Those who had no experience (had never engaged in coitus) had little or no AP in urine following the movie, while those with experience had significant increases. Separating high 'sexual drive' (based on number of self-reported orgasms per month) from low 'sexual drive' individuals showed that there was a significantly lower amount of AP in urine of low drives after the film.

Levi (1969) has examined urine of subjects for possible catecholamine excretions following different types of arousal. In response to a 'high quality love film' (no genitalia in evidence), adrenaline and noradrenaline reactions were minimal or absent in the urine of 15 females. The effects of a blatantly erotic film on 57 females and 50 males was quite different. Both males and females showed a significant increase in adrenaline, with the increase in males being greater than that in females. Although differences in the amounts of noradrenaline also occurred in both sexes, they were not statistically significant. A significant increase in urine volume also occurred in both sexes. Males rated the films as more arousing than did females, and this appeared to be paralleled by corresponding differences in excretion levels and increases over control levels in males. The author discussed his results in terms of a possible explanation of the Kinsey hypothesis that men are more prone to sexual arousal from visual stimuli than are females.

Bernick, Kling & Borowitz (1968) measured plasma 17 hydroxocorticoid levels in blood samples of males after they viewed a heterosexual stag film, a homosexual stag film and a suspense film. Samples were drawn 10 min before the film, 10 min after the film, and 1 h after the film. Changes in steroid levels were insignificant. The lack of a difference in response to the erotic film is surprising after the Levi (1969) findings and is perhaps explained by differences in sample collection techniques. As Fox (1970a) points out, serial samples may be very important, since certain types of neuroendocrine release are being found to take place in spurts. Thus, more sophisticated collection and analyses techniques may produce different results.

9.3. EATING, DRINKING AND ODOURS

Not one article was found in which pleasure was somehow manipulated or measured in terms of food and physiological responses recorded.

In his handbook chapter, *Human Food Attitudes and Consumption*, Pilgrim (1967) reviewed many studies and papers (e.g., Gottlieb & Rossi, 1961) which dealt with the pleasantness of various foods, but not one involved physiological recording. The title of Young's (1967) chapter in the same volume, *Palatability: The Hedonic Response to Foodstuffs*, encouraged the present writers, but the material therein dealt with consumatory behaviour in rats.

What about articles dealing with physiological responses to food regardless of pleasantness of the stimuli? There are, of course, the several volumes entitled 'Alimentary Canal' in the *Handbook of Physiology*. However, there is almost no mention of ANS responses other than those directly involved in the process of digestion.

One study is known to the present authors in which ANS responses to eating a normal meal were recorded in human subjects (Christie & Venables, *in preparation*). However, in terms of relevance to this chapter, this study is only a preliminary step. That is, Christie and Venables are not dealing with the pleasantness of the food their subjects eat, but their results will give us some idea of the pattern and magnitude of ANS changes that can be expected when food is ingested. One example of a non-digestive ANS change that takes place after eating is the depression of the T wave in the electrocardiogram (EKG). Taylor, Kerwin & Franks (1958) and Sears & Manning (1959) studied the EKGs of hundreds of air force cadets and observed the lowering of the T wave after eating, which they attributed to alterations in potassium metabolism. Drinking orange juice, which is rich in potassium, increased the amplitude of the T wave.

The literature on the pleasurable effects and psychophysiology of drinks such as ethyl alcohol is also very sparse. One could go to a standard reference book such as Goodman & Gilman (1965) to determine the effects of alcohol on the nervous system. But would this be relevant to a chapter on the psychophysiology of pleasure? We think not. The literature on the influence of alcohol on subjective reactions has been reviewed by Carpenter (1962) and Wallgren & Barry (1970). Myrsten, Hollstedt & Holmberg (1972) studied the effects of a moderate amount of whisky (0·72 g/kg body weight) on mood, catecholamine excretion, and heart rate in males and females. Maximum blood-alcohol values, rate of alcohol elimination, and adrenaline excretion were significantly higher for the females. Pleasurable subjective reports were more pronounced in the males. Heart rate increased for males and females in response to alcohol.

The final study to be mentioned in this section is a recent investigation of the relationship of pleasantness and unpleasantness of odours to salivation. Pangborn & Berggren (1973) measured parotid secretion in 12 subjects to three pleasant and three unpleasant, among other, odours. Their conclusions were that parotid secretion is not related to the pleasantness or unpleasantness of olfactory stimuli.

9.4. SPORTS, EXERCISE AND RECREATION

Unfortunately, this section must begin much like the last—not one article was found which dealt with *both* the pleasurable aspects of sports, exercise or recreation and with psychophysiological responses.

The pleasurable side of these activities has been neglected in the literature until fairly recently. Of late, however, various theories such as stress-seeking have been used to account for man's participation in sports. Two recent collections of relevant papers have been edited by Klausner (1968) and Lunchen (1970).

Maslow (1954) has expressed his views in terms of his theory of self-actualization about the distorted way in which most of us view these activities.

'As excellent illustration of the way in which our culture is unable to take its end experiences straight may be seen in fishing, hunting, golfing, etc.

'Generally, these activities are extolled because they get people into the open, close to nature, out into the sunshine, or into beautiful surroundings. In essence, these are ways in which what *should be* unmotivated end activities and end experiences are thrown into a purposeful, achieving, pragmatic framework in order to appease the Western conscience' (p. 299).

The self-actualizing person would be one who participates in sports, exercise and recreation simply because of the pleasure. Maslow has stated, however, that he has found relatively few self-actualizing people. Interestingly enough, a recent report from the President's Council on Physical Fitness and Sports (1973) indicates that only 12 per cent of people who take part in sports and/or exercise reported that they do so primarily for pleasure.

Physiological data related to sports and exercise are plentiful. Standard textbooks which devoted numerous chapters to this subject include Johnson (1960), Jokl & Simon (1964). No studies were found, on the other hand, in which physiological measures were recorded during recreational activities, e.g. camping, boating, gardening.

9.5. AESTHETICS

The topics included here are the psychophysiology of music and colour. Two general bibliographies of the psychology of aesthetics are by Hammond (1933) and Chandler & Barnhart (1938).

Although a large number of studies sought to examine the relationship between music and physiological functioning, few made distinctions that would allow their results to be included in a section on pleasantness. There was in general a confounding of 'preference' with 'pleasantness' and little if any experimental control for attention or general state of the subject before he began the experiment.

Pythagoras is said to have analysed the quality of tones that he found in a blacksmith's shop. His emphasis was on the ratios he found between the tones and in turn the effects of these ratios on the emotions. The underlying assumption here is that emotionality may follow naturally from the combining of certain tonal relationships. In a sense, Pythagoras was seeking to establish objective relationships between the emotions and external stimuli. Thus, the implicit assumption was that the individual could be viewed as a passive respondent who was influenced by the natural properties of the music.

Diserens (1923) reviewed the literature of reactions to musical stimuli and concluded that music could furnish the basis for the genesis of emotion according to the James–Lange theory.

A few researchers did discuss the pleasantness aspect of music. For example, Ortman (1922) concluded that musical stimuli are most pleasant when moderate in pitch, and duration. Hyde (1924) suggested that the effects of music are related to an interest in the music and that these effects are strongest in those individuals 'that found pleasure in the song'.

The pleasantness of different colours was also a topic of interest to psychology, with research dating back to Wundt's laboratory (see Chandler, 1934; and Kreitler & Kreitler, 1972 for reviews). Kreitler & Kreitler concluded:

'Many investigators share the explicit or implicit assumption that preferences express the pleasure or displeasure evoked by a colour and thus reflect the affect or emotion attending the perception of colours. Yet, judgments of preference do not tend to be accompanied by any of the usual manifestations of emotions (p. 66)'.

After reviewing the work on aesthetics for this chapter, it can be concluded that the time in which music and colour studies were most popular did not correspond with an interest in or equipment to perform psychophysiological studies. Thus, there is a dearth of studies examining in a systematic fashion aesthetics, the nature of the stimuli, and psychophysiology.

9.6. ALTERED STATES OF CONSCIOUSNESS

As was suggested in the introduction to this chapter, there are two approaches to defining pleasure. The first is that pleasure is the opposite of pain and the the second definition refers to a certain heightened sensation when the body is working properly. Both of these uses of the word pleasure are apparent in the employment of meditation and relaxation for the seeking of pleasure. That is, in the first sense of the word, both meditation and relaxation have been utilized for escaping the present existence that an individual finds himself faced with; they are also used in the second sense to establish balance within a person.

9.6.1. Meditation

Although there is ample classification of different forms of meditation (*cf.* Naranjo & Ornstein, 1971), there is a tendency for meditation to be covered as an unitary topic. The research is similar to that in the beginning of sleep studies before stages of sleep were developed. Those studies that have differentiated have done so on the basis of the tradition from which the meditation developed (e.g., Zen *vs* Buddhist) rather than on characteristics of the meditation itself. Those studies in which psychophysiological measures have been taken did not attempt to ascertain the feeling state of the subjects involved. The best sources of material in this area are Tart's (1969) *Altered States of Consciousness* and the *Biofeedback and Self-Control* annuals (Barber, DiCara, Kamiya, Miller, Shapiro & Stoyva, 1971; Stoyva, Barber, DiCara, Kamiya, Miller & Shapiro, 1973; Shapiro, Barber, DiCara, Kamiya, Miller & Stoyva, 1973) which include Timmons & Kamiya's 1970 bibliography of meditation.

Concerning psychophysiological changes, Bagchi & Wenger (1957) reported that there were no consistent heart rate or respiration patterns across all the yogi they examined during meditation. They did report that electrical resistance of the skin was always found to increase during meditation. They concluded that yogic meditation involved deep relaxation of a certain aspect of the autonomic nervous system without drowsiness or sleep and a type of cerebral activity without highly accelerated electrophysiological manifestation. Anand, Chhina & Singh (1961) examined the EEG changes during yogic meditation. These authors were interested in the psychophysiology of the state of *samadhi*, a state which they described as 'ecstasys'. Alpha was found to be most predominant during *samadhi* and at this time could not be blocked by sensory stimuli, whereas alpha was easily blocked for the same subjects during periods of nonmeditation. Kasamatsu & Hirai (1966) looked at EEG changes during Zen meditation. These authors were the first to begin describing stages of meditation as reflected by psychophysiological changes. The four stages differentiated by EEG patterns were: (1) appearence of alpha with eyes open (eyes were open and looking about a yard in front of the person throughout meditation); (2) increase in amplitude of persistent alpha; (3) decrease of alpha; and (4) appearance of theta. According to the authors, this last stage did not always occur and was associated with the length of time an individual had been involved in Zen meditation. The authors also noted that the EEG changes present in Zen meditation were not the same as those of hypnotic states.

Wallace (1970) and Wallace & Benson (1972) have examined the physiological correlates of transcendental meditation. They reported that during meditation oxygen consumption and heart rate decreased and skin resistance increased.

There was an EEG pattern of intensification of alpha with occasional theta. It is interesting to note that these authors conclude that there is little resemblance between the physiological changes found during meditation and those usually observed during sleep and hypnosis.

It has been suggested that autogenic training may be viewed as a form of meditation. However, as described by Luthe (1963), the technique may be more similar to autosuggestion. This makes the problem of psychophysiological studies of pleasantness more difficult because, like hypnosis, if the person is to tell himself for example, that his hands are warm or his heart rate is decreasing, and if the specific change does take place, it is difficult to differentiate the physiological changes that were related to the autosuggestion from those that were related to the pleasantness of being able to control one's physiology.

9.6.2. Relaxation

The study of relaxation may offer more illumination into the physiological aspects of pleasantness since the task is that of becoming relaxed. The psycho-physiological correlates of relaxation have been generally researched in terms of behavioural therapies. However, there was some work around the turn of the century concerning pleasure and muscle activity.

In relation to muscular activity Kulpe stated that pleasurable states were regularly accompanied by an increase of the force of voluntary muscular action, and unpleasurable states as regularly by its diminution. In 1901, Titchener suggested that when a *very pleasant* stimulus is applied the curve drops a little, and then rises again, to a point above the level of the normal. He concluded that the pleasant stimulation makes us stronger, the unpleasant makes us weaker. These clear-cut distinctions were later found to be wanting.

Surprisingly enough, studies in which subjects were requested to relax did not always produce consistent and significant changes in physiological variables. Simpson, Dansereau and Giles (1971) reported that although there were physiological changes, it was difficult to ascribe these to the technique *per se*. There authors divided their subjects into three experimental groups, one that practised meditation, one that practised relaxation, and a control group. Although they found physiological changes similar to those reported by Wallace using transcendental meditation, these authors concluded that Wallace's findings do not appear to be very different from those observed in their experiment, even in comparison to the untrained control group.

Research with the systematic desensitization technique which has relaxation at its core is also inconclusive as to the role of physiological mechanisms. In fact, it has been argued (Rachman, 1968) that what has been called relaxation refers to a feeling of calmness as opposed to a state of reduced muscle tension. Thus even those areas of research that claim to modify muscular behaviour directly are faced with a cognitive-somatic problem which remains ambiguous at this time.

9.7. HUMOUR

As Berlyne (1972) has pointed out, humour is unique in that it signifies pleasure in all cases and for everyone, unlike some of the other states discussed in this chapter. Art is not always pleasurable, neither is sports, eating, sex, etc.; but humour, we would all agree, is by its unstated definition pleasurable. At least four reviews of the psychology of humour (Perl, 1933; Treadwell, 1967; Berlyne, 1969; Goldstein & McGhee, 1972) have appeared, the last including a bibliography with almost 400 items. However, there has been very little work on the psychophysiology of humour.

One of the first papers in this area was published by Martin (1905). She found that when Ss reported cartoons to be funny, their respiration and pulse rate increased. No statistics are reported. Spencer (1916) reported that when his Ss were amused, respiration became deeper and faster, pulse rate increased and muscle potential increased. No data are presented. Wolff, Smith & Murry (1934) measured laughter and GSRs to race-disparagement jokes; however, they failed to report the physiological data.

Schachter & Wheeler (1962) conducted a study to see the effects of epinephrine and chlorpromazine on behavioural measures of amusement while their Ss watched a slapstick film. In general, their results showed that the stimulant epinephrine increased amusement, but not all of the crucial differences were significant.

Films have been used by other investigators to examine differential physiological patterns. Sternbach (1962) showed the film *Bambi* to 8-year-olds while recording several ANS measures. The children indicated which scene was for them the saddest, scariest, nicest and funniest. Unfortunately, there was no consistent pattern of ANS responding for the funny scenes. Averill (1969) showed films depicting sadness and mirth to college males and recorded ANS changes. He reported that sympathetic activation was common in both with cardiovascular changes more prominent during the sad film and respiratory changes more noticeable during the comedy film. Levi (1965) examined urinary output of adrenaline and noradrenaline while female office clerks watched, among others, an agitating and aggression-provoking film and a comedy film. Again, sympathetic activation was common to both. Viewing of both both films resulted in similar and significant increases in adrenaline excretion and similar adrenaline/noradrenaline ratios.

Fry (1963) in his book *Sweet Madness: A Study of Humor* stated: '...it is not yet possible to demonstrate the electrochemical events that are stimulated in human physiology and result in the subjective experiencing of humor' (p. 138). He has, however, presented two papers since then (Fry, 1969; Fry & Stoft, 1971) attempting to uncover a physiological basis of humour.

Berlyne (1972) related the pleasurable aspect of humour to changes in arousal. Either of two mechanisms can give rise to pleasure according to his theory. One is an 'arousal boost,' which is a moderate rise in arousal, the other an 'arousal/jag,' the reduction of arousal after it has climbed to an uncomfortably high level.

In the introduction to their paper, Langevin & Day (1972) describe the results of a study that they conducted in which 16 adults were shown 10 slides of cartoons which they rated for humour while the Es recorded GSR and heart rate. The results indicated that there was a positive correlation between the amplitude of GSRs and heart rate increase, and how humorous the cartoons were rated. Langevin & Day sum up the state of our knowledge in this field: 'Thus while anecdotal and suggestive evidence of physiological correlates of humour appreciation can be found in the literature, there does not seem to be a single definitive study to show the correlation of humor appreciation with physiological measures' (p. 131).

9.8. SUMMARY AND CONCLUSIONS

There have been very few empirical studies concerned with the psychophysiology of pleasure. That is, very few papers were found which included subjective report data relevant to the Ss' pleasure state *and* psychophysiological data. The majority of studies reviewed in this chapter deal with the psychophysiology of sexual responding. But even these articles, strictly speaking, should not have been included because they fail to report subjective data. It was assumed that sexual activities were pleasurable and the psychophysiological responses were examined. In the other areas reviewed, the psychophysiological literature was so sparse that even if the present authors were willing, in the absence of subjective report data, to accept the activities, e.g. eating, sports, etc., as pleasurable, there were very few relevant studies.

Why is it the case that psychophysiologists have almost completely ignored man's pleasurable states? Some practical considerations were mentioned in introduction. It is difficult to quantify and bring into the laboratory most pleasurable stimuli. It is also difficult to equate a pleasurable stimulus across Ss. A more general consideration is that at the time psychologists were interested in pleasure and related concepts, the end of the nineteenth century, there was very little psychophysiological equipment available for recording. And now psychophysiology is flourishing, but few psychophysiologists seem interested in questions related to pleasure. Another more theoretical factor mentioned previously is that psychophysiologists generally record from Ss in 'extreme' states, e.g. stress. If we accept the early Greek definition of pleasure as a state of balance and general well-being, then it is not surprising, although unfortunate, that psychophysiologists have almost completely ignored this area.

The present authors felt that regardless of one's theoretical orientation there is a great deal to be gained from the study of the psychophysiology of pleasure. In addition to filling a gap in our basic knowledge of behaviour, there is the possibility that such studies will have clinical applications. That is, if a clinician knew his client's typical ANS pleasure pattern(s), perhaps the client's current deviation from this pattern could be used for diagnostic purposes to determine the manner in which the person's physiology is imbalanced.

9.9. REFERENCES

Adamson, J. D., Ramano, K. R., Burdick, J. A., Corman, C. L. & Chebib, F. Physiological responses to sexual and unpleasant film stimuli. *Journal of Psychosomatic Research*, 1972, **16**, 153–162.

Allport, F. H. *Social psychology*. Boston: Houghton-Mifflin, 1924.

Anand, B. K., Chhina, G. S. & Singh, B. Some aspects of electroencephalographic studies in yogis. *EEG and Clinical Neurophysiology*, 1961, **13**, 452–456.

Averill, J. R. Autonomic response patterns during sadness and mirth. *Psychophysiology*, 1969, **5**, 399–414.

Bagchi, B. K. & Wenger, M. A. Electrophysiological correlates of some yogi exercises. *EEG and Clinical Neurophysiology*, 1957, Supplement **7**, 132–149.

Bancroft, J. & Mathews, A. Autonomic correlates of penile erection. *Journal of Psychosomatic Research*, 1972, **16**, 153–162.

Bancroft, J. H., Jones, H. G. & Pullan, B. P. A simple transducer for measuring penile erection with comments on its use in treatment of sexual disorders. *Behavior Research and Therapy*, 1966, **4**, 239–241.

Barber, T. X., DiCara, L. V., Kamiya, J., Miller, N. E., Shapiro, D. & Stoyva, J. (Eds) *Biofeedback and self-control, 1970*. Chicago: Aldine-Atherton, 1971.

Barclay, A. M. Urinary acid phosphatase secretion in sexually aroused males. *Journal of Experimental Research in Personality*, 1970, **4**, 233–238.

Bardwick, J. M. & Behrman, S. J. Investigation into effects of anxiety, sexual arousal, and menstrual cycle phase on uterine contractions. *Psychosomatic Medicine*, 1967, **29**, 468–482.

Bartlett. Physiologic responses during coitus. *Journal of Applied Physiology*, 1956, **9**, 469–472.

Beebe-Center, J. G. *The psychology of pleasantness and unpleasantness*. New York: Van Nostrand, 1932.

Berlyne, D. E. Laughter, humor and play. In G. Lindzey & E. Aronson (Eds.), *Handbook of Social Psychology*. (2nd ed.), Vol. 3. Reading, Mass.: Addison-Wesley, 1969.

Berlyne, D. E. Humor and its kin. In J. H. Goldstein & P. E. McGhee (Eds.), *The psychology of humor*. New York: Academic Press, 1972.

Bernick, N., Kling, A. & Borowitz, G. Pupil size, heart rate and plasma steroids during sexual arousal and anxiety. *Psychophysiology*, 1968, **4**, 502. (Abstract).

Bernick, N., Kling, A. & Borowitz, G. Physiologic differentiation of sexual arousal and anxiety. *Psychosomatic Medicine*, 1971, **32**, 341–351.

Boas, E. P. & Goldschmidt, E. F. *The heart rate*. Springfield, Ill.: Thomas, 1932.

Carpenter, J. A. Effects of alcohol on some psychological processes. *Quarterly Journal of Studies on Alcohol*, 1962, **23**, 274–314.

Chandler, A. *Beauty and human nature*. New York: Appleton-Century, 1934.

Chandler, A. and Barnhart, E. *A bibliography of psychological and experimental aesthetics 1864–1937*. Berkeley, Cal.: University of California Press, 1938.

Christie, M. J. & Venables, P. H. Personal communication, 1973.

Clark, L. C. & Treichler, P. Psychic stimulation of prostatic secretion. *Psychosomatic Medicine*, 1950, **12**, 261–263.

Corman, C. Physiologic response to sexual stimulus. Unpublished bachelor's thesis, University of Manitoba, Canada, 1968.

Darwin, C. *Expression of the emotions in man and animals*. London: Murray, 1872.

Davis, R. C. & Buchwald, A. M. An exploration of somatic response patterns: Stimulus and sex differences. *Journal of Comparative and Physiological Psychology*, 1957, **50**, 44–52.

Diserens, C. M. Reactions to musical stimuli. *Psychological Bulletin*, 1923, **20**, 173–199.

Dysinger, D. W. A comparative study of affective responses by means of the impressive and expressive methods. *Psychological Monographs*, 1931, No. 187.

230

Everett, G. M. Effects of amyl nitrite ('poppers') on sexual experience. *Medical Aspects of Human Sexuality*, Dec. 1972, 146–151.

Fisher, C. & Davis, D. M. Personal communication, 1973.

Fisher C., Gross, J. & Zuch, J. Cycle of penile erection synchronous with dreaming (REM) sleep. *Archives of General Psychiatry*, 1965, **12**, 29–45.

Fisher, S. & Osofsky, H. Sexual responsiveness in women, physiological correlates. *Psychological Reports*, 1968, **22**, 215–226.

Fox, C. A. Physiology of coitus. *Science Journal*, June 1970, 80–84(a).

Fox, C. A. Reduction in the rise of systolic blood pressure during human coitus by the β-adrenergic blocking agent, propanol. *Journal of Reproduction and Fertility*, 1970, **22**, 587–590(b).

Fox, C. A. & Fox, B. Blood pressure and respiratory patterns during human coitus. *Journal of Reproduction and Fertility*, 1969, **19**, 405–415.

Fox, C. A., Wolfe, H. S. & Baker, J. A. Measurement of intra-vaginal and intra-uterine pressures during human coitus by radio-telemetry. *Journal of Reproduction and Fertility*, 1970, **22**, 243–251.

Freund, K. A laboratory method for diagnosing predominance of homosexual and heterosexual erotic interest in the male. *Behavior Research and Therapy*, 1963, **1**, 85–93.

Freund, K. Diagnosing heterosexual pedophilia by means of a test of sexual interest. *Behavior Research and Therapy*, 1965, **3**, 229–234.

Freund, K. Diagnosing homo and heterosexuality and erotic age preference by means of a psychophysiological test. *Behavior Research and Therapy*, 1967, **5**, 209–228(a).

Freund, K. Erotic preference in pedophilia. *Behavior Research and Therapy*, 1967, **5**, 339–348(b).

Freund, K. The structure of erotic preference in the nondeviant male. *Behavior Research and Therapy*, 1970, **8**, 15–20.

Freund, K., Sedlacek, E. & Knob, K. A simple transducer for mechanical plethysmography of the male genital. *Journal of Experimental Analysis of Behavior*, 1965, **8**, 169–170.

Fry, W. F., Jr. *Sweet madness: A study of humor*. Palo Alto: Pacific Books, 1963.

Fry, W. F., Jr. Humor in a physiological vein. *Beckman Instruments News latter*, 1969.

Fry, W. F., Jr. & Stoft, P. Mirth and oxygen saturation levels of peripheral blood. *Psychotherapy and psychosomatics*, 1971, **19**, 76–84.

Gellhorn, E. & Loofbourrow, G. N. *Emotions and emotional disorders*. New York: Hoeber, 1963.

Goldstein, J. H. & McGhee, P. E. An annotated bibliography of published papers on humor in the research literature and an analysis of trends: 1900–1971. In J. H. Goldstein and P. E. McGhee (Eds.), *The psychology of humor*. New York: Academic Press, 1972.

Goodman, L. S. & Gilman, A. The pharmacological basis of therapeutics (3rd ed.). New York: Macmillan, 1965.

Gottlieb, D. & Rossi, P. H. *A bibliography and bibliographic review of food and food habit research*. Chicago: Quartmaster Food and Container Institute, 1961.

Gustafson, J. E., Winokur, G. & Reichlin, S. The effect of psychic and sexual stimulation on urinary and serum acid phosphatase and plasma non-esterified fatty acids. *Psychosomatic Medicine*, 1963, **25**, 101–105.

Hain, J. D. & Linton, P. H. Physiologic response to visual sex stimuli. *Journal of Sex Research*, 1969, **5**, 292–302.

Hammond, W. *A bibliography of aesthetics and the philosophy of the fine arts from 1900 to 1932*. New York: Longmans, Green, 1933.

Heath, R. G. Pleasure and brain activity in man: Deep and surface electroencephalograms during orgasm. *Journal of Nervous and Mental Disease*, 1972, **154**, 3–18.

Hyde, I. Effects of music upon electrocardiograms and blood pressure. *Journal of Experimental Psychology*, 1924, **7**, 213–224.

James, W. What is emotion? *Mind*, 1884, **9**, 188–204.

Johnson, W. R. (Ed.) *Science and medicine of exercise and sports.* New York: Harper, 1960.

Jokl, E. & Simon, E. *International research in sports and physical education.* Springfield, Ill.: Thomas, 1964.

Jovanovic, U. J. The recording of physiologic evidence of genital arousal in human males and females. *Archives of Sexual Behavior*, 1971, 3, 309–320.

Kasamatsu, A. & Hirai, T. An electroencephalographic study of Zen meditation (ZaZen). *Folia Psychiatrica et Neurologica Japonica*, 1966, 20, 315–336.

Kinsey, A., Pomeroy, W., Martin, C. & Gebhard, P. *Sexual behavior in the human female.* Philadelphia: Saunders, 1953.

Klausner, S. Z. (Ed.) *Why man takes chances.* Garden City, N. J.: Doubleday, 1968.

Koegler, R. R. & Kline, L. Y. Psychotherapy research: An approach utilizing autonomic response measurement. *American Journal of Psychology*, 1965, 19, 268–279.

Kreitler, H. & Kreitler, S. *Psychology of the arts.* Durham, N. C.: Duke University Press, 1972.

Külpe, O. *Grundriss der Psychologie*, Leipzig: Englemann, 1893.

Lange, C. *Om Leudsbeveegelser.* (original not available; see translation in Dunlap, K. [ed.] *The emotions.* Baltimore: Williams & Wilkins, 1922.)

Langevin, R. & Day, H. I. Physiological correlates of humor. In J. H. Goldstein & P. E. McGhee (Eds.), *The psychology of humor.* New York: Academic Press, 1972.

Lanier, L. H. An experimental study of 'affective conflict.' *Journal of Psychology*, 1941, 11, 199–217.

Levi, L. The urinary output of adrenalin and noradrenalin during pleasant and unpleasant emotional states. *Psychosomatic Medicine*, 1965, 27, 80–85.

Levi, L. Sympatho-adrenomedullary activity, diuresis, and emotional reactions during visual stimulation in human females and males. *Psychosomatic Medicine*, 1969, 31, 251–268.

Loisselle, R. H. and Mollenauer, S. Galvanic skin responses to sexual stimuli in a female population. *Journal of Genetic Psychology*, 1965, 73, 273–278.

Lunchen, G. *The cross-cultural analysis of sports and games.* Champaign, Ill.: Stipes, 1970.

Luthe, W. Autogenic training: Method, research and application in medicine. *American Journal of Psychotherapy*, 1963, 17, 174–195.

Martin, B. Expression and inhibition of sex motive arousal in college males. *Journal of Abnormal and Social Psychology*, 1964, 68, 307–312.

Martin, L. J. Psychology of aesthetics: Experimental prospecting in the field of the comic. *American Journal of Psychology*, 1905, 16, 35–116.

Maslow, A. H. *Motivation and personality.* New York: Harper, 1954.

Masters, W. H. and Johnson, V. *Human sexual response.* Boston: Little Brown, 1966.

McConaghy, N. Penile volume change to moving pictures of male and female nudes in heterosexual and homosexual males. *Behavior Research and Therapy*, 1967, 5, 43–48.

Morgan, C. T. *Physiological psychology* (3rd ed.). New York: McGraw-Hill, 1965.

Mosovich, A. & Tallaferro, A. Studies on EEG and sex function orgasm. *Diseases of the Nervous System*, 1954, 15, 218–220.

Mosso, A. *Sulla Curcolazione del sangue nel cervello dell' homo.* Rome, 1880.

Myrsten, A.-L., Hollstedt, C. & Holmberg, L. *Alcohol-induced changes in mood and activation in males and females as related to catecholamine excretion and blood-alcohol level.* Psychological Laboratories, University of Stockholm, No. 375, 1972.

Naranjo, C. & Ornstein, R. *On the psychology of meditation.* New York: Viking Press, 1971.

Ortman, O. The sensory bases of music appreciation. *Journal of Comparative Psychology*, 1922, 2, 227–256.

232

Pangborn, R. M. & Berggren, B. Human parotid secretion in response to pleasant and unpleasant odorants. *Psychophysiology*, 1973, **10**, 231–237.

Perl, R. E. A review of experiments on humor. *Psychological Bulletin*, 1933, **30**, 752–763.

Pilgrim, F. J. Human food attitudes and consumption. In C. F. Code (Ed.) *Handbook of physiology: Alimentary canal*, Vol. 1, Washington, D. C.: American Physiology Society, 1967.

President's Council on Physical Fitness and Sports. *Newsletter*, May, 1973.

Rachman, S. The role of muscular relaxation in desensitization therapy. *Behavior Research and Therapy*, 1968, **6**, 159–165.

Reich, W. *The discovery of the orgone*. Vol. 1. *The function of the orgasm; sex-economic problems of biological energy*. New York: Orgone Institute Press, 1942.

Roessler, R. & Collins, F. Physiological responses to sexually arousing motion pictures. *Psychophysiology*, 1970, **6**, 620. (Abstract)

Romano, K. Psychophysiological responses to a sexual and an unpleasant motion picture. Unpublished bachelor's thesis. University of Manitoba, Canada, 1969.

Ruckmick, C. A. *The psychology of feeling and emotion*. New York: McGraw-Hill, 1936.

Schachter, S. & Wheeler, L. Epinephrine, chlorpromazine and amusement. *Journal of Abnormal and Social Psychology*, 1962, **65**, 121–128.

Sears, G. A. & Manning, G. W. Routine electrocardiography: Post-prandial T-wave changes. *Aerospace Medicine*, 1959, **30**, 143. (Abstract)

Shapiro, A., Cohen, H. D., Di Bianco, P. & Rosen, G. Vaginal blood flow changes during sleep and sexual arousal. *Psychophysiology*, 1968, **4**, 394. (Abstract)

Shapiro, D., Barber, T. X., DiCara, L. V., Kamiya, J., Miller, N. E. & Stoyva, J. (Eds.) *Biofeedback and self-control, 1972*. Chicago: Aldine, 1973.

Shock, N. W. & Coombs, C. H. Changes in skin resistence and affective tone. *American Journal of Psychology*, 1937, **49**, 611–620.

Simpson, D. D., Dansereau, D. & Giles, G. *A preliminary evaluation of physiological and behavioral effects of self-directed relaxation*. Institute of Behavioral Research, Texas Christian University, No. 71–72, 1971.

Spencer, H. On the physiology of laughter. In *Essays on education*. London: Every man's Library, 1916.

Stern, J. A. Towards a definition of psychophysiology. *Psychophysiology*, 1964, **1**, 90–91.

Sternbach, R. Assessing differential autonomic patterns in emotions. *Journal of Psychosomatic Research*, 1962, **6**, 87–91.

Sternbach, R. A. *Pain: A psychophysiological analysis*. New York: Academic Press, 1968.

Stoyva, J., Barber, T. X., DiCara, L. V., Kamiya, J., Miller, N. E. & Shapiro, D. (Eds.) *Biofeedback and self-control, 1971*. Chicago: Aldine-Atherton, 1972.

Tart, C. T. *Altered states of consciousness*. New York: Wiley, 1969.

Tart, C. T. Personal Communication, 1973.

Taylor, W. J. R., Kerwin, A. J. & Franks, W. R. Post-prandial T-wave lowering in apparantly healthy young aviators—1959. *Journal of Aviation Medicine*, 1958, **29**, 251. (Abstract)

Timmons, B. Kamiya, J. The psychology and physiology of meditation and related phenomena: A bibliography. Chap. 8, pp. 146–167, in T. Barber, L. V. DiCara, J. Kamiya. N. E. Miller D. Shapiro & J. Stoyva (Eds) *Biofeedback and self-control*, Chicago: Aldine-Atherton, 1970.

Titchener, E. B. A textbook of psychology, New York: McMillan, 1901.

Treadwell, Y. Bibliography of empirical studies of wit and humor. *Psychological Reports*, 1967, **20**, 1079–1083.

Trigg, R. *Pain and emotion*. Oxford: Clarendon Press, 1970.

Wallace, R. Physiological effects of transcendental meditation. *Science*, 1970, **167**, 1751–1754.

Wallace, R. & Benson, H. The physiology of meditation. *Scientific American*, 1972, **226**, 84–90.

Wallgren, H. & Barry, H. III. *Action of alcohol.* Amsterdam: Elsevier, 1970.

Wenger, M. A., Averill, J. R. & Smith, D. D. B. Autonomic activity during sexual arousal. *Psychophysiology*, 1968, **4**, 468–478.

Wolff, H. A., Smith, C. E. & Murray, H. A. The psychology of humor. I. A study of responses to race-disparagement jokes. *Journal of Abnormal and Social Psychology*, 1934, **28**, 341–365.

Young, P. T. Palatability: The hedonic response to foodstuffs. In C. F. Code (Ed.) *Handbook of physiology: Alimentary canal*, Vol. 1, Washington, D. C.: American Physiology Society, 1967.

Zuckerman, M. Physiological measures of sexual arousal in the human. *Psychological Bulletin*, 1971, **75**, 297–329.

Chapter 10

The Psychosocial Environment and Precursors of Disease

MARGARET J. CHRISTIE

St. Mary's Hospital Medical School and
Bedford College, University of London, NW1 4NS

10.1. INTRODUCTION

This chapter is concerned with 'stress', with individual differences in the psychophysiological response to some aspects of the psychosocial environment, and with possible links between such individual differences and the development of disease. In this discussion of 'stress' it will, it is hoped, become apparent that there are links between areas of clinical medicine, psychophysiology, and experimental research within psychology. Such links arise from a view of stress as the state which exists when controlling mechanisms are strained in maintenance of the internal environment of vital areas such as brain or blood. Examples of exploratory work with this model, used in the investigation of potassium control, suggest that there may be individual differences in the efficiency of control. There may also be individual differences in the protection afforded by relaxing activities: such differences may lie in the speed with which recovery of homeostatic equilibrium is achieved in 'easement'. Individual differences in the maintenance of optimal potassium concentrations may be reflected in individual differences in mood, in information processing, and in development of stress induced myocardial breakdown.

10.1.1. A concept of stress

The concept of 'stress' which is used here has physiological origins in Cannon (1929) and Selye (1950): stress can be viewed as a response state of the organism, associated with strain on mechanisms which maintain the constancy of the internal environment. Thus, it will be argued, any psychophysiological methods which may be used to monitor the functioning of such controlling mechanisms have value for detecting the development of strain, and the subsequent existence of stress.

Relative constancy of the internal environment is essential for information from the external environment to be efficiently received, transmitted, and acted upon: Barcroft (1934) noted that 'working of the mind' required a medium of great constancy, and Tschirgi (1960) wrote that, 'minute changes in chemical or physical parameters of (the neuron's) microenvironment will alter the threshold of excitability ... and introduce noise in the communication sense, and there are unique homeostatic mechanisms designed to buffer the central nervous system against such changes and thereby to achieve a maximum signal to noise ratio'.

Given, then, that body cells require a relatively constant internal environment, there is a complexity of negative feedback systems maintaining homeostasis. One aspect of such maintenance is the *anticipation* of demand for additional materials from cells, activity of which may be temporarily increased. This is exemplified by Cannon's description of preparation for 'fight or flight', which includes the mobilization of stored glycogen to provide a temporary increase in blood glucose concentration.

Thus, when the human organism perceives *threat* there is a widespread physiological response which prepares for intense physical activity. This stereotyped, phylogenetically old adaptation pattern may, however, be distinctly maladaptive for contemporary man, for whom threat is more often symbolic, requiring cognitive activity not physical fight or flight. If mobilized metabolic resources are not required there is a temporary surfeit in circulation, and possible strain on mechanisms which should maintain the optimal conditions of the internal environment. An example of such a surfeit is the increase in plasma free fatty acids (FFA), which results from the mobilization of stored lipids in sympathetic arousal (Back & Bogdonoff, 1965). The increased levels of FFA in a non-active subject who is repeatedly aroused may be a factor in the development of coronary atherosclerosis: one important feature of this is the presence of lipid deposits on the walls of arteries. The significance of such 'furring up' is described in Section 6. Thus, the psychophysiological response to threat, though adaptive in stone-age man, may in contemporary conditions jeopardize that constancy of the internal environment which it is 'programmed' to maintain. In such circumstances the strain on the system of controlling mechanisms imposed by this maladaptive preparation for physical activity may be designated as stress, as defined on page 235.

Cannon's work emphasized the short-term sympatho-medullary response, whereas Selye (1950) highlighted the pituitary–adrenocortical response to relatively prolonged threats to homeostasis. So, for example, Cannon's description of glycogenolysis implicated adrenaline and glucagon in the mobilization of glucose, whereas Selye was concerned, in his earlier writing at least, with the increased use of protein under the influence of cortisol, for the emergency production of heat and energy. Selye also coined the term 'stressor'; this has value for defining stimulation originating from the external environment, which because of its frequency, intensity, or symbolic nature, so arouses neuroendocrine responses that the optimal state of the internal environment may be threatened.

Selye's later work has focused less on the glucocorticoids' role in maintaining life in stress, and more on mineralocorticoid effects. His concern has been primarily with relations between the potassium ion (K^+) and myocardial function in stress (Selye, 1970): this is examined in Section 6 where suggestions are made about the potential value of psychophysiology for 'psychocardiology' (Raab, 1971).

Consideration of the potassium ion is relevant to the notion that minute changes in the chemical microenvironemnt will alter neuronal thresholds of excitability (Tschirgi, 1960), and that unique homeostatic mechanisms exist to buffer vital body fluid compartments against such changes in their chemical composition. Such vital areas may be designated as *controlled* areas, and the relevant homeostatic mechanisms as *controlling* mechanisms. The next section describes examination of some controlling mechanisms which are associated with maintenance of appropriate potassium concentrations in extracellular fluids. It is suggested that if the state of stress is that physiological condition where controlling mechanisms are strained, such a state may be detected by examining the controlling mechanisms, as well as by looking for change in the vital controlled area.

10.2. K^+ AND THE STRESS RESPONSE

Selye's 1950 publication summarized the evidence at that time available on K^+ shifts in stress, and presented a figure (p. 279) showing the change in potassium concentration, $[K^+]$, of the blood from normal to increased values in the alarm-reaction (A–R) stage. The presence of this hyperkalaemia at the A–R stage reflects the discharge of K^+ from cells, and work since the 1950s has added greater detail to Selye's original description. Kernan's (1965) monograph on cell K^+, for example, details the shift of K^+ from intracellular fluid (ICF) to extracellular fluid (ECF) during glycogenolysis, as for example in Cannon's 'fight and flight' preparation. Any transient increase in ECF concentrations of K^+ probably leads to the ion being distributed between plasma and interstitial fluid (Woodbury, 1965). If, however, plasma $[K^+]$ is not adequately controlled, the transient hyperkalaemia may stimulate increased mineralocorticoid activity: Dluhy, Axelrod, Underwood & Wiliams (1972) have shown that in normal man increments of serum $[K^+]$ from 0·2 to 1·0 mEq/l can significantly increase blood aldosterone levels. Williams & Dluhy (1972) reviewed aldosterone output and concluded that in normal circumstances both the renin–angiotensin system and serum $[K^+]$ regulate aldosterone secretion through negative feedback loops. They viewed these two mechanisms as being of equal importance in normal circumstances, although adrenocorticotrophic hormone (ACTH) was a factor operative in more exceptional conditions.

If the concentration of K^+ in blood rises sufficiently to increase aldosterone production this increases the likelihood of K^+ being lost from the body. Thus, when under the influence of mineralocorticoids sodium (Na^+) is reabsorbed in the kidney, K^+ may be exchanged for this cation, and excreted in urine. This renal mechanism for maintaining suitable levels of ECF K^+ would seem, however, to be a drastic and irrevocable means of handling a transient hyperkalaemia. If such an increase in ECF K^+ is the result of shifts from cells of K^+, under the influence of temporary increases in sympatho-medullary activity, a more adaptive response would be the temporary withdrawal from blood of excess K^+, and its handling by non-renal controlling mechanisms. This 'handling' would prevent the stimulation by increased blood $[K^+]$ of aldosterone production and prevent a maladaptive loss of K^+ until the ion could be reincorporated within the cell. It is, then, possible to suggest that when non-renal controlling mechanisms are coping, shifts of K^+ from cell to ECF in sympathetic arousal do not necessarily result in hyperkalaemia. Thus only when extra-renal mechanisms are strained is the controlled blood compartment affected, and only in this case of increased blood $[K^+]$ is there stress as defined in the present chapter.

10.2.1. Methodology

If the state of stress if defined as the physiological condition in which controlling mechanisms are strained and there is a change in the controlled variable, then the human organism may be said to be in the state of stress when a transient hyperkalaemia follows the shift of K^+ from ICF to ECF in sympathetic arousal. Thus, monitoring of blood K^+ might detect the existence of stress. There are, however, disadvantages in such methodology: the procedure of venipuncture is a stressor capable of introducing error variance, and it is virtually impossible to make repeated measurements without disturbing a subject (Graham, 1971). Further, Graham (1971), in his consideration of contributions which could be made by psychophysiology to internal medicine, hoped ' . . . to see a clear delineation of the sequence of steps, neurologic, endocrine and other which occur in the development of disease processes.' One approach to such an endeavour might well be via investigation of individual differences in the capacity of controlling mechanisms to defend a controlled area. Thus with reference to K^+ it can be argued that blood levels need to be adequately controlled, that weakness of extra-renal control allows transient hyperkalaemia in sympathetic arousal, and that ensuing increase in aldosterone activity can result in a maladaptive loss of K^+ in urine. Such losses, if repeated, might reasonably be viewed as a step in the development of disease processes: for example, evidence shows the vital role of adequate body K^+ in maintaining healthy myocardial tissue (Raab, 1971; Selye, 1970) On two counts, therefore, it is of advantage to investigate extra-renal controlling mechanisms rather than blood levels of K^+: the first advantage is methodological and avoids the stressor potential of venipuncture. The second lies in the possibility of examining individual differences in strain on controlling mechanisms, that is, individual differences in the capacity of extra-renal mechanisms to maintain the relative constancy of blood K^+ values. There are thus advantages in examining the *development* of, rather than the *state* of, stress.

Having made such a statement, a question arising is inevitably: what methodology is available to the psychophysiologist for examining extra-renal control of K^+? The following section describes exploratory examination of saliva, following Bovard's suggestion (1959) that this fluid has value for psychologists engaged in stress research.

10.3. SALIVA

Bovard (1959) noted changes in salivary sodium/potassium ratio (Na/K) in stress; this could reflect mineralocorticoid (e.g., aldosterone) activity, and the subsequent reabsorption of Na^+ in exchange for K^+. Williams (1961, 1966) reported the use of saliva for detection of such an effect in climbers at altitude. Very little is known of normal changes in salivary Na/K in normal life situations, though Fowles & Venables (personal communication, 1968) observed a significant inverse correlation between corrected Na/K in stimulated saliva and neuroticism (N) scores of the Eysenck Personality Inventory (EPI) in a normal academic population.

10.3.1. Salivary physiology

Jenkins (1966) provides a brief introduction to salivary physiology, and Volume 2, Section 6 of the *American Physiological Society Handbook* (Code, 1967) contains a most useful collection of contributed chapters on various aspects (Schneyer & Schneyer, 1967; Emmelin, 1967; Blair-West, Coghlan, Denton & Wright, 1967). Saliva is produced by the three major pairs of parotid, submaxillary, and submandibular glands and several minor sources. Of these major glands the first two are within Thaysen's category of 'Group I' eccrine glands; these have a characteristic handling of Na^+ and K^+, by a limited maximal reabsorption capacity such that, at increasing rates of flow, there are increasing concentrations of Na^+. In the case of salivary K^+ there is an inverse relation between concentration and flow, but only at low flow rates.

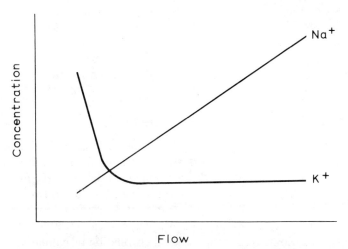

FIGURE 10.1. Schematic presentation of relations between salivary flow and concentrations of sodium and potassium

This limited maximal reabsorption capacity poses problems for interpretation of salivary Na^+ and K^+ values. For K^+ it may be possible to use samples only when flow rates are within the asymptotic portion of Figure 10.1 but for Na^+ some correction is advisable; Williams (1961) advocates computing an individual regression equation for each subject, but a group correction method is described by Fowles and Venables (1968).

Samples may be collected in 'resting' or 'stimulated' conditions; in the latter case a variety of stimuli have been employed including wax (Williams, 1961), rubber bands (Shannon, 1958), citric acid (Fowles & Venables, 1968), and acid drops (Ferguson, Fort, Elliott & Potts, 1973). 'Resting' saliva is probably not strictly so described, as collection methods inevitably tend to provide some stimulation: an operational definition, however, is given by Burgen (1967). Collection of whole saliva by spitting is a much-used technique (Wenger, 1966), the Lashley disc (Terry & Shannon, 1964) allows selection of parotid saliva, and dental rolls (washed before use if necessary) can be positioned over Stenson's duct to collect a sample which is probably of largely parotid origin. From such wool, saliva can then be eluted and analysed, as described briefly in Venables & Christie (1973).

10.3.2. Salivary analysis

Two methods for estimating K^+ and Na^+ in saliva are feasible for the psychologist, namely by use of ion-selective electrodes, or by flame photometry. The former method (used, for example, by Fowles & Venables, 1968) is not covered here; descriptions of ion-selective electrodes are available in Moody & Thomas (1971), Durst (1971), and Dahms, Rock & Seligson (1968).

Flame photometry provides a relatively simple means of estimating K^+ in body fluids. The least sophisticated equipment is probably a single cell instrument (Varley, 1967) using air and bottled gas; the concentration of the ion can be determined by burning the test solution in the gas/air mixture, the resulting light being passed through suitable filters to make it monochromatic (i.e., having the characteristic emission spectrum of the ion) and on to a photocell, when the current generated can then be taken as proportional to the ionic concentration of the test solution.

10.3.3. Preliminary explorations with salivary K^+

Preliminary studies with the dental roll method for collection of resting saliva were undertaken in the bed-rest conditions described by Christie & Venables (1971a) for recording 'basal' skin potential level (BSPL). In these conditions of collection salivary flow rates of $\geq 2 \cdot 0$ g/30 min were associated with asymptotic portion of the concentration/flow relation. Mean uncorrected K^+ concentrations were $37 \cdot 1$ and $33 \cdot 2$ mEq/l at noon and 6.00 p.m. respectively in summer conditions. In a winter study a correlation of palmar surface $[K^+]$ with uncorrected salivary $[K^+]$ (salivary flow rates being $\geq 2 \cdot 0$ g/30 min) was $\rho = 0 \cdot 76$, $P < 0 \cdot 05$, $N = 8$; in the winter mean salivary $[K^+]$ was $50 \cdot 2$ mEq/l, though flow rates were similar to those of summer. 'Basal' skin potential levels tended to be lower in winter: this can be interpreted as evidence for greater concentrations of K^+ in skin (Christie & Venables, 1971b) as well as in saliva. Correlations between BSPL and uncorrected K^+ were $-0 \cdot 85$ in a winter study, but use only of data from subjects with flow rates of $\geq 2 \cdot 0$ g/30 min resulted in a correlation of $-0 \cdot 6$ which did not reach significance. So, there are problems associated with the use of *resting* saliva, if flow rates tend to be low, but on the other hand, collection of *stimulated* samples may disturb the subject (Wenger, 1966), and may introduce further problems of interpretation. Examination of $[K^+]$ of resting saliva was reported by Venables & Christie (1974) in association with other indices of ECF $[K^+]$: it was suggested that the results indicated its value for psychologists. Similarly, De Marchi has reported the value of examining resting salivary electrolyte concentrations in his studies of menstrual cycle psychophysiology (personal communication). Thus, there may be such problems with resting saliva, but it does appear to have the value suggested by Bovard (1959).

Another approach to the extra-renal control of K^+ may be via the skin, as detailed in Section 4, which describes the use of an electrodermal measure as a putative index of ECF K^+ status.

10.4. THE SKIN AND EXTRA-RENAL CONTROL

Yoshimura (1964), Rothman (1954), and Cannon (1929) have all described the 'reservoir' function of the skin, and its ability to store water and electrolytes in defence of the intravascular compartment. It has been argued (Christie, 1972) that a number of findings from electrodermatology may be interpreted in terms of the skin's role as an extra-renal mechanism controlling the K^+ concentration of blood. The present section describes these findings, and suggests their significance for examining individual differences in defence of intravascular $[K^+]$.

10.4.1. Palmar skin potential level

During the 1960s the development of high impedence amplifiers made possible the recording of palmar skin *potential*, whereas in previous work the technically less demanding measurement of skin *resistance* had been the method of choice. In this decade Venables & Sayer (1963) reported their investigation of optimal methodology for recording palmar skin potential *level*, advocating the use of a matched pair of silver/silver chloride (Ag/AgCl) chamber electrodes, and 0·5 per cent KCl in 2 per cent agar jelly as the external electrolyte at the two electrode/epidermal interfaces. Human SPL is usually negative at a palmar surface electrode with reference to an 'inactive' electrode on an ipsilateral, abraded, forearm surface (Venables & Christie, 1973), though there were *positive* values recorded by Venables & Sayer (1963) when using external KCl concentrations markedly *below* 0·5 per cent.

The negativity of SPL decreases with decreasing arousal, a condition in which palmar eccrine sweat gland activity is reduced, if ambient temperatures are moderate (Neumann, 1968). The absolute value of SPL is, however, lowered when the concentration of the external electrolyte is reduced (Venables & Sayer, 1963; Rothman, 1954; Edelberg, 1963).

Examination of physiological mechanisms underlying the generation of SPL has suggested that although eccrine sweat glands are implicated, non-sudorific factors may be of significance: Venables & Martin (1967) blocked palmar eccrine sweat glands with hyoscyamine, measuring SPL before and after eccrine sweating had been eliminated. After such treatment SPL was reduced by only 25 per cent of its pre-treatment value (in contrast to a marked reduction in skin conductance level), thus leaving a major portion of measured SPL to be accounted for by non-sudorific mechanisms.

A condition of eccrine sweat glands similar to that of pharmacological inactivation is reached when relaxed subjects are maintained in an unarousing environment (Christie & Venables, 1971a); inactivity of palmar eccrine sweat glands can be assumed after a period of rest if no phasic electrodermal activity (i.e., skin potential or skin conductance responses: SPRs or SCRs) is observed. During such rest tonic levels of skin conductance (SCL) show gradual reduction, but SPL can exhibit a phenomenon described by Lykken, Rose, Luther & Maley (1966), namely, the reaching of a low value below which there is no

242

further decrease with decreases in arousal. These authors noted individual differences in the value of this, which they were unwilling to attribute to differences in arousal.

Suggestions had been made, however, concerning possible relations between individual differences in measured SPL and body fluid cations (Venables, 1963; Venables & Sayer, 1963; Martin & Venables, 1966), and work was undertaken to examine relations between the concentration of K^+ in the external electrolyte and individual differences in both body fluid K^+ concentration and the low, 'basal' SPL.

10.4.2. Basal Palmar Skin Potential Level

Investigation of the 'basal' SPL recorded from relaxed subjects maintained in an unarousing environment (Christie & Venables, 1971a, b, c; 1972) suggested that individual differences in BSPL, when measured with physiologically appropriate KCl ($[K^+] \leq 67$ mEq/l) could be interpreted in terms of a simple Nernst model:

$$BSPL = constant \times \log_{10} \frac{[K^+]_{external}}{[K^+]_{internal}}$$

where $[K^+]$ = potassium concentration (or in this context, perhaps, more strictly 'activity'). Thus lowered negativity of BSPL is associated with lowered values of $[K^+]_{external}$ (i.e., electrode electrolyte) or raised values of $[K^+]_{internal}$. Very low BSPL negativity approaches zero, after which *positive* values are recorded at the palm with reference to an abraded forearm site. This phenomenon can perhaps be more readily appreciated in Figure 10.2 which shows the effects on measured BSPL of lowering the external electrolyte concentration, i.e. $[K^+]_{external}$ below 67 mEq/l. The Nernst model predicts that at zero BSPL, when $[K^+]_{external} = [K^+]_{internal}$ the concentration in the epidermis would be in the region of 16 mEq/l. An attempt was made to compare this theoretical figure with tissue fluid values: palmar surface film was collected with suitable precautions (see method in Bell, Christie & Venables, 1974) from subjects in the 'basal' state of low arousal, and in temperate surroundings. Given such conditions, and the consequent quiescence of palmar eccrine sweat glands, it was assumed that palmar surface film reflected, not the composition of eccrine sweat, but of the intercellular fluid in clefts of the horny layer which opened on to the palmar surface, as shown in Figure 10.3. The K^+ of such intercellular fluid is not known with any certainty (Greisemer, 1959), but its origin is said to be the plasma of looped capillary nets in the corium (Kuno, 1956). As the fluid moves upward to the intercellular spaces of the horny layer its $[K^+]$ is probably augmented by sweat residues and keratinization products (Rothman, 1954). The $[K^+]$ of surface film collected from the palm varied between 16·20 and 20·80 mEq/l, with lower values recorded during hot summer weather (when, however, the weight of surface film was lowest).

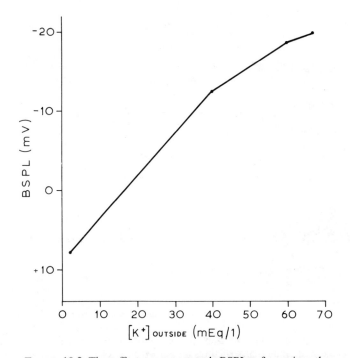

FIGURE 10.2. The effect on measured BSPL of varying the external potassium concentration. (From M. J. Christie & P. H. Venables, *Japanese Journal of Physiology*, 1971, **21**, 659–668, with permission.)

Such values seem to agree reasonably with the theoretical $[K^+]$ derived from the Nernst model and Figure 10.2. If the Nernst model is applicable, one should be able to record low BSPL when there is high epidermal $[K^+]$; but it could be the case that epidermal $[K^+]$ has no general significance, and is a purely local phenomenon. It thus becomes of interest to relate BSPL values to plasma $[K^+]$. This was undertaken by examining relations between BSPL and the electrocardiogram (ECG) T-wave, as described below.

10.4.3. BSPL and the electrocardiogram T-wave

Electrocardiographic literature occasionally mentions the ECG change which accompany changes in cation status; of particular interest in the present context are reports of positive relations between T-wave amplitude and ECF $[K^+]$ (Turner, 1967; Wood, 1968), and Mashima, Fu & Fukishima's (1965) report of increases in T-wave amplitude after ingestion of KCL.

Papadimitriou, Roy & Varkarakis (1970), in the context of monitoring patient state during renal dialysis, described the value of using T-wave amplitude as index of plasma $[K^+]$. They reported a positive correlation ($r = 0.68$, $P < 0.01$) between T-amplitude and plasma $[K^+]$, suggesting that a close approximation to plasma values can be derived from $K = 3t/2$, where $K = [K^+]$ of plasma in

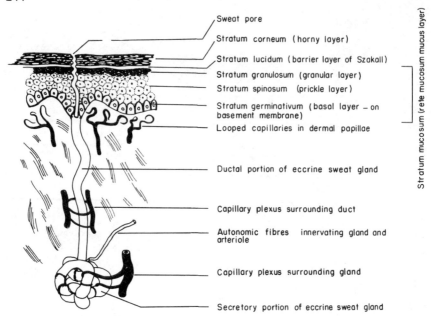

Sweat pore

Stratum corneum (horny layer)

Stratum lucidum (barrier layer of Szakall)

Stratum granulosum (granular layer)

Stratum spinosum (prickle layer)

Stratum germinativum (basal layer – on basement membrane)

Looped capillaries in dermal papillae

Ductal portion of eccrine sweat gland

Capillary plexus surrounding duct

Autonomic fibres innervating gland and arteriole

Capillary plexus surrounding gland

Secretory portion of eccrine sweat gland

Stratum mucosum (rete mucosum mucus layer)

FIGURE 10.3 Schematic presentation of a section of palmar skin showing an eccrine sweat gland and epidermal structures concerned in electrodermal activity. (From P. H. Venables & M. J. Christie. In W. F. Prokasy & D. S. Raskin (Eds.), *Electrodermal Activity in Psychological Research*, 1973. By permission of Academic Press Inc.)

in mEq/l, and t = amplitude of the T-wave in limb lead II of the ECG recorded at 1 mV/cm. Examples of T-wave characteristics through a range of plasma $[K^+]$ values can be found in Kernan (1965), and Laks & Elek (1967) provided a description of relations between events at a cellular level, ECF/ICF $[K^+]$ gradient, and inscription of the T-wave.

The report by Venables (1963) of an inverse correlation between the total *area* of ECG waveforms and negativity of a resting measure of SPL had included suggestions that body fluid electrolytes might be implicated. It was possible that, T-wave area being large in relation to other ECG waveforms, the SPL/ECG-area relation might be reflecting a common influence of ECF $[K^+]$. ECG waveform amplitudes were examined in conjunction with recording of BSPL, on the assumption that if the Nernst model held, and if epidermal conditions reflected more general ECF $[K^+]$, there should be an inverse relation between T-amplitude and BSPL, $[K^+]_{external}$ being held constant at 67 mEq/l.

Although the T-wave is reported to be the most labile of the ECG complexes, and known to be influenced by the short-term effects of many factors (Marriott, 1960), the conditions of BSPL recording (Christie & Venables, 1971a) appeared to provide an adequate control of at least some unwanted variance.

Summarizing the findings from a preliminary study (Christie & Venables, 1971c) of both bed-rest and chair-rest conditions, there were significant

$(r = -0.70, P < 0.001 ; r = -0.61, P < 0.01)$ inverse relations between T-amplitude and BSPL, though no relation with P or QRS $(-0.07$ and $-0.14)$. There was a consistent positive relation (significant around the 0·05 level) between heart period (HP) and T-amplitude, but also between HP and summed amplitudes of all the ECG waveforms. These measurements were made on 10 cycles of ECG about the point of BSPL, and comparisons of these data with that obtained from 30 cycle lengths indicated that the longer interval was not needed.

Thus there was a significant relation between BSPL and T-wave amplitude, in the direction predicted by the Nernst model, and this could be interpreted as indicating a relation between $[K^+]_{internal}$ at the palm and the more general status of ECF $[K^+]$.

10.4.4. BSPL and the state of stress

During investigation of BSPL phenomena atypically low values were occasionally noted. These were invariably associated with some psychosocial stressor such as an immediately previous academic examination, or an over-demanding working day. Following the Nernst model such low BSPL values indicated unusually high values of epidermal K^+ concentrations, such as might be expected if the skin were holding a temporary excess of K^+ after its shift from ICF in sympathetic arousal.

Further, a diurnal variation in BSPL is evident (Christie, 1972) with a nadir in the early afternoon. At this time there was an associated zenith in skin conductance levels, in heart rate, and in oral temperature, indicating a zenith in general activation. It has been reported (Fröberg, Karlsson, Levi & Lidberg, 1972) that there are increases in excreted adrenaline in the early afternoon, so the possibility exists that K^+ would shift from ICF to ECF under its influence. There have been no successful attempts to demonstrate diurnal variation in blood K^+ (Pollard, 1964; Seaman, Engel & Swank, 1965), though there *are* reported circadian rhythms in urine (Lobban, 1965) and saliva (de Traverse & Coquelet, 1952) which suggest increases in K^+ in the early afternoon. Thus, the nadir in BSPL could be interpreted in terms of the skin's function as an extra-renal mechanism which handles K^+ in defence of the blood.

A further observation was that atypically low BSPL values were occasionally recorded on Mondays. This raised questions about the possible significance of such observations, and led to a period of research in which there was less emphasis on academic electrodermatology and more interest in examining *changes* in variables such as salivary $[K^+]$, BSPL, and T-wave amplitude between the Friday and Monday of a working week. A summary of this period of research follows in Section 5, in which there is a broadening of scope to include some account of work on mood assessment by means of the Nowlis Mood Adjective Check List (MACL), and on individual differences in 'personality' assessed by the extraversion and neuroticism scales of the EPI.

10.5. THE WORKING WEEK—STRESSORS AND EASEMENTS

The Psychosocial Environment and Psychosomatic Disease (Levi, 1971) details the effects on the working population of stressors arising from today's urban, industrialized environment. Levi (1971) defines such psychosocial stressors as stimuli originating in social relationships or arrangements of the environment which may influence the psychological state of the organism through the mediation of higher mental processes. Fröberg *et al.* (1971) comment in the same volume that '. . .the constellations of stressors inherent in everyday life are very complex'; they report their work on stress responses in telephone operators, clerks working on salaried and piece-work schedules, office staff subjected to changes from conventional 'cell' conditions to open-plan landscaping, supermarket cash girls in rush periods and in normal conditions, and in shift-workers. Raab (1968) has described the stress response to intermittently ringing telephone bells, and Taggart (1971) has reviewed the effects of car driving.

It can, then, be assumed that for most workers there is stressor potential in their typical 5-day week. Stress responses may be cumulative, and by Friday the individual who has been exposed to significant stressor influence may well be in a different psychophysiological state from that in which he began the week on the previous Monday. There may, however, be individual differences in the extent of this cumulative stress response: there are 'protective interacting variables', and 'predisposing and protective factors may differ in effect in different individuals' (Kagan & Levi, 1971). One such protective factor may well be the putative 'easements' (Handlon, 1962) of working life such as lunch breaks and weekends. There may well be individual differences in the psychophysiological response to these, as to stressors, but virtually nothing is known about the former, in contrast to growing research interest in the latter. Some examination of the effects on psychological and physiological state of a substantial midday meal has now been undertaken, but the present section focuses primarily on examination of Friday and Monday state, beginning with some account of work on mood assessment by means of the MACL.

10.5.1. Monday morning mood

Two different areas of research stimulated interest in assessing mood in conjunction with K^+ investigation. The first was the work on electrolyte/mood relations within clinical psychiatry, the second was studies of individual proneness to Monday absenteeism (Froggatt, 1970a, b, c).

Coppen (1967) reviewed the biochemistry of affective disorders, including descriptions of K^+ in depression (Shaw & Coppen, 1966). Maas (1972) and Bunney, Murphy & Goodwin (1972) have also described relations between cation status and mood, but there is virtually no account of electrolyte/mood relations in normal subjects. Skoglund (1967) has hypothesised relations between plasma $[K^+]$, neuronal excitability, and developmental changes in rat and kitten, but what would be of great interest would be studies of ECF [K$^+$], neuronal excitability and behavioural reactivity in humans. The nearest approach is perhaps McDaniel's (1971) examination of plasma [K$^+$], EEG and information processing in patients with renal failure who were being treated by intermittent haemodialysis. He interprets his findings as indicating an underlying relationship between elevated plasma [K$^+$], a relative shift to lower frequency EEG activity, and difficulty in information processing. McDaniel cites the statement of Fishman & Raskin (1967) that the uraemic brain encephalopathy can be related to disordered membrane functioning, but notes that visual-motor integration does not appear to be appreciably affected. He concludes by stating that complex psychological functions may be mediated by metabolically activated exchange of sodium and potassium. Cell membrane potentials and the ion pump theory of neuronal activity are well-known neurophysiological events. If disruptions in cellular metabolism, specifically Na$^+$/K$^+$ transfer, affect behaviour directly, the cellular basis of psychological functioning becomes more credible.'

Given, then, a relation between ECF [K$^+$] and mood it can be asked whether a cumulative stress response in normal subjects exposed to a stressful week capable of producing significant changes in ECF [K$^+$], would be associated with any significant change in mood.

Secondly, one might ask whether the 'blue Monday' mood documented by Froggatt (1970, a, b, c) reflects in any way K$^+$ status on Monday mornings, and whether this itself reflects in any way easement or stressor effects of the weekend, and/or of the previous working week.

An initial, exploratory study was undertaken, using the Nowlis MACL, as described below. In an attempt to get insight into possible individual differences in Monday morning mood the EPI also used, to provide scores of extraversion (E) and neuroticism (N).

10.5.2. Friday and Monday mood and EPI scores

The Nowlis Mood Adjective Check List (MACL) has, in the three decades of its use and development, indicated its value for examining relatively small changes in 12 dimensions of mood (Nowlis, 1966). Nowlis sees mood as 'the effect on a person of his own configurations of activity ...' and describes these configurations in terms of general functioning such as 'level of activation'. Further details of the MACL and its development are available in Nowlis & Green (1965), and Green (1965). The study (Christie & Venables, 1973) compared Friday and Monday mood, in 80 male subjects working in 'service' occupations such as teaching, the Civil Service, etc. In addition to the MACL at the beginning and end of a Monday and an adjacent Friday, subjects also completed an Eysenck Personality Inventory (EPI) and a questionnaire concerned with their experience of stress in their jobs, and the extent to which they liked their occupations. When the subject-group had been broken down into sub-groups of personality type by a series of binary cuts, it became apparent that the group with extraversion score above the mean in association with neuroticism scores below the mean (stable extraverts) and the group having extraversion scores below the mean in association with neuroticism scores above the mean (unstable introverts) had distinctive mood characteristics. Stable extraverts showed, for example, much smaller changes in mood between morning and evening than did unstable introverts. Further, the latter group was characterized by highest arousal in association with lowest reported social affection and pleasantness on Monday mornings, and the former by highest arousal and highest euphoria on Friday evenings. Examination of K^+ changes between Friday and Monday was undertaken in the exploratory study (Venables & Christie, 1974) described below.

10.5.3. Friday and Monday K^+ and the change in neuroticism

Eighteen male subjects between the ages of 20 and 30 were examined on a Friday, and again at the same time on the following Monday. All subjects reported having a week divided into five working days with a Saturday/Sunday weekend. 'Resting' saliva was collected, ECG and BSPL recorded, mood assessed with the MACL, and subjects completed EPIs at *both* testing periods. E scores were virtually identical on Friday and Monday, but there was a significant reduction in N scores on Monday. These data showed that subjects could be broken down into two groups: nine subjects, in all of whom there was a reduction in N score (mean $= -2.5$ points) and a group of nine in which there was no change, or a minimal increase (mean $= +0.9$ points). When the groups' physiological data were examined by means of analyses of variance, significant interaction effects were found to be associated with BSPL ($P = 0.046$) and salivary $[K^+]$ (corrected by the method of Fowles & Venables, 1968), such that a reduction in neuroticism was associated with an increase in ECF $[K^+]$, i.e., with an increase in salivary $[K^+]$ and a reduction in BSPL, and vice versa. There was no significant interaction effect shown in the T-wave data, though there was a main effect of day in that T-amplitudes were lower on Monday ($P = 0.04$). However, QRS amplitude showed a similar reduction ($P = 0.03$) on Monday, and interpretation of these main effects is probably more appropriate in terms of an associated reduction in heart period. The main effect of day was not significant for this variable, though the direction of change was downwards on Monday: this is similar to the significant increase in Monday heart rate reported by (Malstrom, 1973). The data were also examined for any evidence of individual differences in the relation between BSPL change and T-amplitude change. Thus it was argued that if BSPL changed while T-amplitude remained relatively constant this indicated the controlling function of the skin defending plasma $[K^+]$. There was a significant inverse correlation ($r = -0.5$) between BSPL change and T-amplitude change, a significant positive correlation of 0.50 between T-amplitude change and neuroticism, and significant negative correlation ($r = -0.55$) between T-amplitude change and a score of 'stable extraversion'. This latter score was obtained by suitably combining each subject's N and E scores. Stable extraversion was significantly associated with stable T-amplitudes in the Friday/ Monday comparison (Venables & Christie 1974) and thus with stable plasma $[K^+]$. A question now arising is the relation, in *normal* human subjects between stability of plasma $[K^+]$, stability of $[K^+]$ in the neuronal microenvironment (Tschirgi, 1960) and stability of mood. The mood data were, however, less clear-cut, and there were no significant interaction effects. It is, however, possible to regard changes in N score as reflecting generalized changes in mood state, and reasonable to suggest the value of investigating cumulative stress in normal subjects by examining cation shifts and mood changes. Further, such investigations may have relevance for the study of short-term absenteeism, as described below.

10.5.4. Individual differences in 'recovery'

At the beginning of Section 5 it was suggested that there may be individual differences in the psychophysiological *recovery* during easement as there are in *response* to stressors. Expansions of this statement have been made recently (Christie & Venables, 1974); relevant aspects of this are summarized below.

There are very little data on recovery from stress: some are available in Johansson & Frankenhaeuser (1973); Bull & Nethercott (1972); Freeman (1939). There appear to be, however (apart from Farmer & Chambers, 1925), no data available on recovery over periods such as the 2-day weekend, from the cumulative effects of a stressful working week. If, however, 'rapid recovery' restores homeostatic equilibrium in 2 days, may not 'slow recovery' require longer? And if longer time is required, may not slow recoverers be psychophysiologically unready to face another stressful working week on Monday morning? Returning to the Monday morning mood data (Christie & Venables, 1973) unstable introverts were, on Monday mornings, in a state of high arousal in association with low social affection and pleasantness. Referring to Froggatt's comprehensive review of short-term absenteeism (Froggatt, 1970a, b, c) there are individual differences in the liability or proneness to Monday absence, about which there is a dearth of information. If, however, one takes a definition of mood from Nowlis's co-worker Green (1965) as the 'predisposition to respond', then the predispositions of the unstable introverts might, in less congenial working environments than the service occupations of the reported study (Christie & Venables, 1973), manifest themselves as Monday absence.

10.6. THE DEVELOPMENT OF STRESS DISEASE

Wadsworth (1973) has described current theories of sickness causation, and their move away from simple single-cause to multi-factorial models. Wadsworth also presented Figure 10.4, from Wadsworth, Butterfield & Blaney (1971), which exemplifies '...the older kind of disease pattern which the Western urbanized world is leaving behind...' contrasted with the present

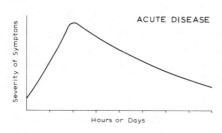 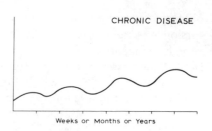

FIGURE 10.4. Patterns of development of acute and chronic disease. (From M. E. J. Wadsworth, W. J. H. Butterfield and R. Blaney, *Health and Sickness: The Choice of Treatment*, 1973, with permission of Associated Book Publishers Ltd.)

predominant pattern of the typical course of a chronic illness. This latter pattern is, Wadsworth argued, characterized by a period of self-medication preceding a patient's eventual appearance in his doctor's surgery, and this pre-consultation period has, for social scientists, become an important area of investigation. One line of investigation described by Wadsworth (1973) concerns the homeostatic model of Sheldon *et al.* (1970), and his suggestion that the continual onslaught of stressors may sequentially modify the capacity of homeostatic feedback mechanisms to maintain a constant internal environment.

If the maintenance of a constant $[K^+]$ in vital body fluid compartments is jeopardized there is, it has been suggested, the risk of effects on cell excitability, which might be reflected in behavioural change. There is, however, evidence that depletion of K^+ has effects on cell function in heart muscle: these have been reviewed by Selye (1970) and Raab (1968, 1969, 1971), the latter having coined the term 'psychocardiology' to describe the psychophysiology of degenerative heart disease. Raab's model is summarized in a useful figure (Raab, 1969); as this field of research may be relatively unfamiliar to the general reader (while degenerative heart disease is a most pressing problem urgently requiring transdisciplinary investigation) Raab's model will be described in some detail. Two recent publications provide overviews: a popular introduction is available in Carruthers (1974), and a volume of contributed papers in Eliot (1974).

Raab (1969) has argued that Western cardiological research and thinking has been mesmerized by the vascular, 'plumbing' aspect of cardiac pathology. This mechanistic view that degenerative heart disease is caused exclusively by reduction or interruption of the oxygen supply to heart muscle, and that such damage to heart muscle is the consequence of altherosclerotic 'furring up' of coronary arteries, has, he argues, blinded orthodox cardiology to the significance of neuroendocrine factors. Raab (1969) emphasizes the need for close conceptual rapport between cardiologists and psychologists familiar with neuroendocrine physiology.

His model (1969) centres on cation shifts from heart muscle cells: in normal cardiac function with the spreading action currents of systole, K^+ moves from ICF to ECF, and during its return against the gradient in diastole, metabolic energy is required. Na^+ moves in opposite directions in both phases and the speed of transmembranous active transport is accelerated under the influence of adrenergic catecholamines. Adrenocortical hormones reported to have significance are those with combined mineralo- and glucocorticoid activity, e.g. cortisol.

Reduction of alimentary $[K^+]$ results in reduction of serum $[K^+]$; associated myocardial dysfunction has been reported in both rat and human, but early myocardial changes can be reversed by appropriate intake of K salts.

If there is significant anoxia myocardial K^+ depletion may result from reductions in cellular energy, which is essential for active return to the cell of systolically extruded K^+. In normal conditions coronary arteries can dilate to maintain adequate oxygen supplies, when cellular demands increase, as for example, when oxygen consumption increases during accelerated cation transport under the influence of catecholamines. If there is artherosclerosis, however, this adaptive dilation may not be possible. Thus, sympathetic arousal may threaten myocardial K^+, and be particularly damaging when cortisol affects the tissue, when there is inadequate vascular dilatability, and when vagal and sympatho-inhibitory counter-regulation is inefficient (Raab, 1969).

Given Raab's case for transdisciplinary study of cardiac pathology, it becomes apparent that psychophysiology has much to contribute: there is, for example, considerable evidence concerning individual differences in catecholamine responses in stress (Frankenhaeuser, 1971, 1975). There is also growing sophistication in analysis of heart rate change (Hayes, 1974; Lobstein, 1974) and a relevance of this to consideration to vagal counter-regulation of sympathetic arousal. Approaches within cardiology to individual differences in development of myocardial disease have been dominated by Friedman & Rosenman's description (e.g., 1971) of Type A and B behaviour patterns. Mai (1968) describes theirs as 'perhaps the most comprehensive and certainly the most provocative' work on personality factors in relation to development of coronary heart disease. Type A is typically driving and ambitious with a well-developed sense of time and urgency, always meeting deadlines. Type A shows also sympathetic overactivity, raised serum cholesterol, reduced clotting time, and higher incidence of myocardial infarction. One criticism voiced by Mai (1968) is that proposed prospective studies require prior identification of Type A individuals, but such identification is dependent on the re-latively crude and somewhat esoteric methods of Friedman & Rosenman; Mai concluded by commenting that the evidence remains equivocal.

An example of Raab's own work on individual differences is a study of the effects of minor sensory and mental annoyances (1968). These consisted of 20 min of interrupted ringing of a telephone bell combined with a flickering bright light: during the latter half of this 20-min period two mental arithmetic problems had to be solved. These stressors provoked significant elevations of plasma cortisol level together with evidence of cardiac sympathetic stimulation (cardiac and blood pressure acceleration). The degree of intra-subject adrenergic cardiovascular reaction was virtually unchanged after several years. Thirty-four subjects were rated by means of a questionnaire (Raab & Krywanek, 1965) for emotional excitability and attitude toward everyday annoyances. A binary cut divided these Ss in 2×17 sub-groups of high/low emotional excitability. The high emotional group was characterized by significantly greater deviations in stress from baseline values, and Raab (1968) contrasts what he designates 'Type A' personality (being more excitable, having more intense cardiovascular reactions and a prolonged rise of plasma cortisol) with 'Type B', (a placid individual reacting with weak cardiac acceleration, fall of systolic blood pressure, and a delayed, moderate rise of cortisol) Raab (1968) concludes with the suggestion that the development of objective criteria for early detection of a predisposing over-reactivity to a modest stress situation such as his sensory and mental annoyance would have value for investigation of degenerative heart disease. Within this context of individual differences in response to, and also in *recovery* from, stressors psychophysiology has a contribution to make.

Our own interest in examining 'recovery' has now moved from the molar analyses of Friday/Monday changes to the molecular level of a laboratory stressor. This is a Sidman avoidance situation using aversive noise, following the design of Stern (1966) and Russell & Stern (1967). In such a situation, with yoked 'executive' and control, it is possible to examine resting values, stressor induced response, and post-stressor recovery, to compare these parameters in both subjects, and to look at characteristics of resting state, response and recovery in relation to 'personality' differences. Initial results are available in Christie & Venables (1974), which reports the effects on SPL of 10 min of noise-avoidance.

Lastly, a contribution from psychophysiology to investigation of the development of myocardial dysfunction is suggested by Mai's (1968) review: from his writing it becomes apparent that investigation of relations between 'personality' and angina have proved the most rewarding. In view of suggestions made by Raab (1969) that the pain of angina is associated with loss of ICF K^+ from the myocardium, investigation of relations between angina and adequacy of extra-renal controlling mechanisms for plasma $[K^+]$ might well be a profitable undertaking. The putative relation between 'stable extraversion' and constancy of plasma $[K^+]$ (Venables & Christie, 1974) provides one approach to such an undertaking.

In summary, then, research in psychophysiology may contribute to the understanding of stages in the development of stress-induced disease; psycho-cardiology exemplifies a multidisciplinary area to which psychophysiology may make a major contribution. One approach to this may be via investigation of individual differences in the *control* of K^+ in plasma, and of individual differences in *recovery* from stressor effects.

10.7. ACKNOWLEDGMENT

This chapter was written during tenure of a grant from the Social Science Research Council, and while the author was in the Department of Psychology, Birkbeck College, University of London.

10.8. REFERENCES

Back, K. W. & Bogdonoff, M. D. Plasma lipid responses to leadership, conformity and deviation. In P. H. Leiderman & D. Shapiro (Eds.), *Psychobiological approaches to social behaviour*. London: Tavistock, 1965.

Barcroft, J. *Features in the architecture of physiological function*. London: C.U.P., 1934.

Bell, B., Christie, M. J. & Venables, P. H. Menstrual cycle variation in potassium. *Journal of Interdisciplinary Cycle Research*, 1974. (In press).

Blair-West, J. R., Coghlan, J. P., Denton, D. A. & Wright, R. D. Effects of endocrines on salivary glands. Chapter 38, In C. F. Code (ed.), *Handbook of physiology: Alimentary canal*. Baltimore: Williams and Wilkins, 1967.

Bovard, C. W. The effects of social stimuli on the response to stress. *Psychological Review*, 1959, **66**, 267–277.

Bull, R. H. C. & Nethercott, R. E. Physiological recovery and personality. *British Journal of Social and Clinical Psychology*, 1972, **11**, 297.

Bunney, W. E., Goodwin, F. K. & Murphy, D. L. The 'switch process' in manic-depressive illness. III. Theoretical implications. *Archives of General Psychiatry*, 1972, **27**, 312–317.

Burgen, A. S. V. Secretory processes in salivary glands. Chapter In Code, C. F. (Ed.), *Handbook of physiology: Alimentary canal*. Baltimore: Williams and Wilkins, 1967.

Cannon, W. B. *Bodily changes in pain, hunger, fear and rage*. Boston: Branford, 1929.

Carruthers, M. *The Western Way of Death*. London: Davis-Poynter, 1974.

Christie, M. J. 'Basal' palmar skin potential and body fluid potassium. Section of Measurement in Medicine, Royal Society of Medicine, October, 1972.

Christie, M. J. & Venables, P. H. Characteristics of palmar skin potential and conductance in relaxed human subjects. *Psychophysiology*, 1971, **8**, 523–532(a).

Christie, M. J. & Venables, P. H. Sodium and potassium electrolytes and 'basal' skin potential levels in male and female subjects. *Japanese Journal of Physiology*, 1971, **21**, 659–668(b).

Christie, M. J. & Venables, P. H. Basal palmar skin potential and the electrocardiogram T-wave. *Psychophysiology*, 1971, **8**, 779–786(c).

Christie, M. J. & Venables, P. H. Site, state, and subject characteristics of resting skin potentials. *Psychophysiology*, 1972, **9**, 645–649.

Christie, M. J. & Venables, P. H. Mood changes in relation to age, EPI scores, time and day. *British Journal of Social and Clinical Psychology*, 1973, **12**, 61–72.

Christie, M. J. & Venables, P. H. Change in palmar skin potential level during relaxation after stress. *Journal of Psychosomatic Research*, 1974, **18**, 301–306.

Code, C. F. (Ed.). *Handbook of physiology: alimentary canal*. Baltimore: Williams and Wilkins, 1967.

Coppen, A. The biochemistry of affective disorders. *British Journal of Psychiatry*, 1967, **113**, 1237–1264.

Dahms, H., Rock R. & Seligson, D. Ionic activities of sodium, potassium and chloride in human serum. *Clinical Chemistry*, 1968, **14**, 859–870.

Davis, R. C. & Berry, F. Gastrointestinal reactions to a noise-avoidance task. *Psychological Reports*, 1963, **12**, 135–137.

De Traverse, P. M. & Coquelet, M.L. Variations nycthemerales du rapport sodium/ potassium dans la saline et l'urine. *Biologie Comptes Rendus*, 1952, **146**, 1099–1102.

Dluhy, R. G., Axelrod, L., Underwood, R. H. & Williams, G. H. Studies of the control of plasma aldosterone concentration in normal man. II. Effect of dietary potassium and acute potassium infusion. *Journal of Clinical Investigation*, 1972, **51**, 1950–1957.

Durst, R. A. Ion-selective electrodes in science, medicine and technology. *American Scientist*, 1971, **59**, 353–361.

Edelberg, R. Electrophysiologic characteristics and interpretation of skin potentials. *USAF School of Aerospace Medicine Technical Documentary Report No. SAM-TDR-63–95*, 1963.

Eliot, R. S. (Ed.), *Stress and the Heart*. New York: Futura, 1974.

Emmelin, N. Nervous control of salivary glands. Chapter 37, In Code, C. F. (Ed.), *Handbook of physiology; Alimentary canal*. Baltimore: Williams and Wilkins, 1967.

Farmer, E. & Chambers, E. G. Concerning the use of psychogalvanic reflex in psychological experiments. *British Journal of Psychology*, 1925, **15**, 237–254.

Fedor, J. H. & Russell, R. W. Gastrointestinal reactions to response-contingent stimulation. *Psychological Reports*, 1965, **16**, 95–113.

Ferguson, D. B., Fort, A., Elliott, A. L. & Potts, A. J. Circadian rhythms in human parotid saliva flow rate and composition. *Archives of Oral Biology*, 1973, **18**, 1155–1173.

Fishman, R. & Raskin, N. Experimental uremic encephalopathy. *Archives of Neurology*, 1967, **17**, 10–21.

Fowles, D. C. & Venables, P. H. Endocrine factors in palmar skin potential. *Psychonomic Science*, 1968, **10**, 387–388.

Frankenhaeuser, M. Experimental approaches to the study of human behaviour as related to neuroendocrine functions. In L. Levi (Ed.), *Society, Stress and Disease*. Volume 1. London: Oxford University Press, 1971.

Frankenhaeuser, M. Sympathetic-adrenomedullary activity, behaviour and the psychosocial environment. Chapter 4, In P. H. Venables & M. J. Christie (Eds.), *Research in Psychophysiology*. London: Wiley, 1975. (In preparation)

Freeman, G. L. Toward a psychiatric plimsoll mark: physiological recovery quotients in experimentally induced frustration. *Journal of Psychology*, 1939, **8**, 247–252.

Friedman, M. & Rosenman, R. H. Type A behavior pattern: its association with coronary heart disease. *Annals of Clinical Research*, 1971, **3**, 300–302.

Fröberg, J., Karlsson, C.-G., Levi, L. & Lidberg, L. Physiological and biochemical stress reactions induced by psychosocial stimuli. In L. Levi (Ed.), *Society, Stress and Disease*, Volume 1. London: Oxford University Press, 1971.

Fröberg, J. Karlsson, C.-G., Levi, L. & Lidberg, L. Circadian variations in performance, psychological ratings, catecholamine excretion and diuresis during prolonged sleep deprivation. *International Journal of Psychobiology*, 1972, **2**, 23–36.

Froggatt, P. Short-term absence from industry. I Literature, definitions, data, and the effect of age and length of service. *British Journal of Industrial Medicine*, 1970, **27**, 199–210(a).

Froggatt, P. Short-term absence from Industry. II. Temporal variation and inter-assocation with other recorded factors. *British Journal of Industrial Medicine*, 1970, **27**, 211–224(b).

Froggatt, P. H. Short-term absence from industry. III. The inference of proneness and a search for causes. *British Journal of Industrial Medicine*, 1970, **27**, 297–312(c).

Graham, D. T. Psychophysiology and medicine. *Psychophysiology*, 1971, **8**, 121–131.

Green, R. F. On the measurement of mood. *Technical Report No. 10*. Project No. NR 171–342 Office of Naval Research, 1965.

Greisemer, R. D. Protection against the transfer to matter through the skin. In S. Rothman (Ed.), *The human integument*. Washington: A.A.A.S., 1959.

Handlon, J. H. Hormonal activity and individual responses to stresses and easements in everyday living. Chapter 8. In R. Roessler & N. S. Greenfield (Eds.), *Physiological correlates of psychological disorder*. Madison: University of Wisconsin Press, 1962.

Hayes, R. Measuring heart rate responses in psychophysiology. Paper presented to the Foundation Meeting of the Psychophysiological Section of the British Psychological Society, London, 1973.

Jenkins, G. N. *The physiology of the mouth*. Chapter 9. Oxford: Blackwell, 1966.

Johansson, G. & Frankenhaeuser, M. Temporal factors in sympatho-adrenomedullary activity following acute behavioural activation. *Biological Psychology*, 1973, **1**, 53–73.

Kagan, A. & Levi, L. Adaptation of the psychosocial environment to man's abilities and needs. In L. Levi (Ed.), *Society, Stress and Disease*, Volume 1. London: Oxford University Press, 1971.

Kernan, R. P. *Cell K*. London: Butterworths, 1965.

Kuno, Y. *Human perspiration*. Springfield, Illinois: Charles C. Thomas, 1956.

Laks, M. M. & Elek, S. R. The effect of potassium on the electrocardiogram. *Diseases of the Chest*, 1967, **51**, 573–586.

Levi, L. (Ed.), The psychosocial environment and psychosomatic diseases. *Society, stress and disease*. London: Oxford University Press, 1971.

Lobban, M. C. Time, light and diurnal rhythms. In O. G. Edholm & A. L. Bacharach (Eds.), *The physiology of human survival*. London: Academic Press, 1965.

Lobstein, T. J. Heart rate and skin conductance activity in schizophrenia. Unpublished Ph.D. thesis, University of London, 1974.

Lykken, D. T., Rose, R., Luther, B. & Maley, M. Correcting physiological measures for individual differences in range. *Psychological Bulletin*, 1966, **66**, 481–484.

Maas, J. W. Adrenocortical steroid hormones, electrolytes, and the disposition of cate-cholamines with particular reference to depressive states. *Journal of Psychiatric Research*, 1972, **9**, 227–241.

Mai, F. M. M. Personality and stress in coronary disease. *Journal of Psychosomatic Research*, 1968, **12**, 275–287.

Malstrom, E. D. Basal heart rate variations by day of week. *Psychophysiology*, 1973, **10**, 218–220.

Marriott, H. J. L. Coronary mimicry: normal variants and physiologic, pharmacologic, and pathologic influences that simulate coronary patterns in the electrocardiogram. *Annals of Internal Medicine*, 1960, **54**, 411–427.

Martin, I. & Venables, P. H. Mechanisms of palmar skin resistance and potential. *Psychological Bulletin*, 1966, **65**, 347–357.

Mashima, S., Fu, L. & Fukushima, K. The effect of oral potassium chloride on the normal and abnormal electrocardiogram. *Japanese Heart Journal*, 1965, **6**, 463–473.

McDaniel, J. W. Metabolic and CNS Correlates of cognitive dysfunction with renal failure. *Psychophysiology*, 1971, **8**, 704–713.

Martin, I. & Venables, P. H. Mechanisms of palmar skin resistance and skin potential. *Psychological Bulletin*, 1966, **65**, 347–357.

Moody, G. J. & Thomas, J. D. R. *Selective ion sensitive electrodes*. Watford: Merrow, 1971.

Neumann, E. Thermal changes in palmar skin resistance patterns. *Psychophysiology*, 1968, **5**, 103–111.

Nowlis, V. Research with the Mood Adjective Check List. In S. S. Tomkins & C. E. Izard (Eds.), Affect, cognition and personality. London: Tavistock, 1966.

Nowlis, V. & Green, R. F. Factor analytic studies of the mood adjective checklist. (*Technical Report No. 11. Project No. NR 171–342*. Office of Naval Research).

Papadimitriou, M., Roy, R. R. & Varkarakis, M. Electrocardiographic changes and plasma potassium levels in patients on regular dialysis. *British Medical Journal*, 1970, **2**, 268–269.

Pollard, A. C. The quantitative changes which occur throughout the day in some commonly determined plasma constituents. *Technicon 3rd symposium on Automation in Analytical Chemistry*, London, 1964.

Raab, W. Correlated cardiovascular, adrenergic and adrenocortical responses to sensory and mental annoyances in man. *Psychosomatic Medicine*, 1968, **30**, 809–818.

Raab, W. Myocardial electrolyte derangement: Crucial feature of pluricausal, so-called coronary, heart disease. *Annals of the New York Academy of Sciences*, 1969, **147**, Art. 17, 627–686.

Raab, W. Cardiotoxic biochemical effects of emotional-environmental stressors-fundamentals of psychocardiology. In L. Levi (Ed.), *Society, stress and disease*. London: Oxford University Press, 1971.

Raab, W. & Krzywanek, H. J. Cardiovascular sympathetic tone and stress response related to personality patterns and exercise habits. *American Journal of Cardiology*, 1965, **16**, 42–53.

Rothman, S. *Physiology and biochemistry of the skin*. Chicago: University of Chicago Press, 1954.

Rothman, S. (Ed.). *The human integument*. Washington: A.A.A.S., 1959.

Russell, R. W. & Stern, R. M. Gastric motility: The electrogastrogram. Chapter 7, In P. H. Venables & I. Martin (Eds.), *A manual of psychophysiological methods*. Amsterdam: North-Holland Publishing Co., 1967.

Schneyer, L. H. & Schneyer, C. A. Inorganic composition of saliva. Chapter 33, In C. F. Code (Ed.), *Handbook of physiology: alimentary canal*. Baltimore: Williams and Wilkins, 1967.

Seaman, F. F., Engel, R. & Swank, R. L. Circadian periodicity in some physico-chemical parameters of circulating blood. *Nature*, 1965, **207**, 833–835.

Selye, H. *The physiology and pathology of exposure to stress*. Montreal: Acta Inc., 1950.

Selye, H. The evolution of the stress concept. *American Journal of Cardiology*, 1970, **26**, 269–299.

Shannon, I. L. Sodium and potassium levels of human whole stimulated saliva collected under two forms of stimulation from subjects in a select age grouping. *Journal of Dental Research*, 1958, **37**, 391–400.

Shaw, D. M. & Coppen, A. Potassium and water distribution in depression. *British Journal of Psychiatry*, 1966, **112**, 269–276.

Sheldon, A., Baker, F. & McLaughlin, C. P. *Towards a general theory of disease and medical care*. Cambridge; Massachusetts: M.I.T. Press, 1970.

Skoglund, S. Plasma ion concentration as a basis for an hypothesis regarding neuronal excitability changes during development. *Acta Societatis Medicorum Upsaliensis*, 1967, **72**, 76–84.

Stern, R. M. A re-examination of the effects of response–contingent aversive tones on gastro-intestinal activity. *Psychophysiology*, 1966, **2**, 217–223.

Taggart, P. Driving and heart response. *Community Health*, 1971, **2**, 185–188.

Teichner, W. Interaction of behavioural and physiological stress reactions. *Psychological Review*, 1968, **75**, 271–291.

Terry, J. M. & Shannon, I. L. Modification of a self-positioning device for the collection of parotid fluid. *Tech. Doc. Rep. No. SAM. TDR*-1964, 64–71.

Tschirgi, R. D. Chemical environment of the central nervous system. Chapter 78. In J. Field (Ed.), *Handbook of physiology*, Volume III. Section I *Neurophysiology*, Baltimore: Williams and Wilkins, 1960.

Turner, R. W. D. *Electrocardiography*. Edinburgh: Livingstone, 1967.

Varley, H. *Practical clinical biochemistry*. London: Heinemann, 1967.

Venables, P. H. Amplitude of the electrocardiogram and level of skin potential *Perceptual and Motor Skills*, 1963, **54**.

Venables, P. H. & Christie, M. J. Mechanisms, instrumentation, recording and quantification. Chapter 1. In W. F. Prokasy & D. C. Raskin (Eds.), *Electrodermal activity in psychological research*. New York: Academic Press, 1973.

257

Venables, P. H. & Christie, M. J. Neuroticism, physiological state and mood: An exploratory study of Friday/Monday changes. *Biological Psychology*, 1974, **1**, 201–211.

Venables, P. H. & Martin, I. The relation of palmar sweat gland activity to level of skin potential and conductance. *Psychophysiology*, 1967, **3**, 302–311.

Venables, P. H. & Sayer, E. On the measurement of the level of skin potential. *British Journal of Psychology*, 1963, **54**, 251–260.

Wadsworth, M. Health and sickness: The choice of treatment. Paper presented to the 17th Annual Conference of the Society for Psychosomatic Research, 1973.

Wadsworth, M., Butterfield, W. J. H. & Blaney, R. *Health and sickness: The choice of treatment.* London: Tavistock, 1971.

Wenger, M. A. Studies of autonomic balance: A summary. *Psychophysiology*, 1966, **2**, 173–186.

Williams, E. S. Salivary electrolyte composition at high altitude. *Clinical Science*, 1961, **21**, 37–42.

Williams, E. S. Electrolyte regulation during the adaptation of humans to life at high altitude. *Proceedings of the Royal Society*, B., 1966, **165**, 266–280.

Williams, G. H. & Dluhy, R. G. Aldosterone biosynthesis: Inter-relationships of regulatory factors. *American Journal of Medicine*, 1972, **53**, 595–605.

Wood, P. *Diseases of the heart and circulation.* London: Eyre and Spottiswode, 1968.

Woodbury, D. M. Physiology of body fluids. In T. C. Ruch & H. D. Patton (Eds.), *Physiology and biophysics.* Philadelphia: Saunders, 1965.

Yoshimura, H. Organ systems in adaptation: The skin. In D. B. Dill (Ed.), *Adaptation to the environment.* A.P.S. Handbook of Physiology, Section 4. Baltimore: Williams and Wilkins, 1964.

Chapter 11

The Affective Disorders

MALCOLM LADER and PETER NOBLE

Institute of Psychiatry,
University of London

11.1. INTRODUCTION

Psychiatric classification is so rudimentary that several systems co-exist. The division of psychiatric patients into the psychotic, the neurotic and the personality-disorders represents one basic system. Another, which cuts right across these categories, recognizes a group of disorders which have as a common element a disordered emotional state. This group of 'affective disorders' comprises anxiety states, depressive illnesses and manic conditions.

There is a close relationship between anxiety and depression seen in the clinical context. For example, a patient with severe anxiety may become depressed as a reaction to the social and personal handicaps consequent upon the anxiety state. Depressed patients may show extreme anxiety and agitation. As well as both affects occurring together they may succeed each other in time. For example, a patient may present in the clinic with 'free-floating' anxiety which soon becomes attached to certain situations, i.e., the patient develops phobic anxiety. Later an overt depressive illness may develop which responds to antidepressive treatment, the last symptom to remit being anxiety.

In both anxiety states and depressed patients the clinical picture is coloured by an abnormal emotion. In anxiety states and in reactive depressions such as grief reactions the emotion is more intense, pervasive or persistent than normal but it is qualitatively identical to the corresponding emotions experienced at some time or another by normal people. With depression of the type variously categorized as 'endogenous', 'psychotic', 'biological', or 'vital', the affect appears to be unlike that experienced by normal subjects as its quality seems so abnormal to the patient. The entire affective life of the patient is coloured grey by the depression so that no hope for the future remains. This clinical impression is an important one to bear in mind as it influences the experimental approach to using psychophysiological methods in such patients.

It has been shown useful to maintain a clinical distinction between anxious and depressed patients as the clinical features, treatment and prognosis differ in some crucial respects (Gurney, Roth, Garside, Kerr & Schapira, 1972; Kerr, Roth, Schapira & Gurney, 1972; Mendels, Weinstein & Cochrane, 1972; Roth, Gurney, Garside & Kerr, 1972; Schapira, Roth, Kerr & Gurney, 1972). Accordingly, we have organized this chapter to deal first with the psychophysiological researches carried out in patients with anxiety states and then to outline similar studies in depressed patients. Where particularly relevant, work with normal subjects has been included. We conclude with a discussion of a selected number of basic difficulties in applying this area of research to clinical problems.

11.2. ANXIETY

11.2.1. Introduction

Physiological changes accompanying anxiety and fear are usually so marked as to be easily apparent to both the subject and the observer. The subjective changes include palpitations, flushes, dry mouth, clammy palms, intestinal discomfort, shakiness and unsteadiness, and muscular tension. The objective assessment of these changes contributes to the clinical evaluation of anxiety. Psychophysiological measures used in this context include surface electromyography, skin conductance, a variety of cardiovascular measures, the electroencephalogram and certain endocrine indices.

11.2.2. Electromyography

Anxiety is frequently associated with increased muscle tension and for this reason would be expected to produce high EMG levels. Some authors have reported high EMG levels in anxious patients (Malmo & Shagass, 1949; Malmo, Shagass & Davis, 1951), but others have found no consistent alteration (Sainsbury & Gibson, 1954; Martin, 1956).

In one study, an attempt was made to correlate increased EMG activity with specific symptom patterns (Sainsbury & Gibson, 1954). Patients were sub-divided into those with headache and those with aching in the limbs. The first group had significantly higher frontalis EMG's while the second group had higher forearm EMGs. Some of the contradiction in earlier studies may be due to this 'symptom-specificity'.

On balance, most studies suggest that there is in fact a relationship between anxiety and raised EMG levels but this is not particularly marked and is too unreliable to be useful as an index of clinical anxiety.

11.2.3. Skin conductance

Sweaty palms are a common accompaniment of anxiety. An increase in sweating leads to an increase in skin conductance. Fluctuations in conductance, apparently occurring independently of any identifiable external influence ('spontaneous fluctuations'), increase in frequency as the level of anxiety rises.

The results of skin conductance studies on patients categorized as 'anxiety state' or 'anxiety neurosis' are relatively uniform. When compared to controls these patients show an increase in skin conductance and in the number of spontaneous fluctuations. The individual GSRs are small and show delayed habituation. The literature on this subject has been reviewed elsewhere in detail (Lader & Wing, 1966).

Studies comparing broader patient categories such as 'neurotic' or 'psychotic', or anxious patients suffering from a variety of psychiatric disorders have generally yielded conflicting results. These categories are heterogeneous and some of the studies have been poorly controlled. Hoch, Kubis & Rouke (1944) found greater reactivity in the skin conductance tracings of neurotics and cited similar findings in their survey of the literature. In contradiction, Altschule (1953) concluded from his review of the literature that the GSRs of 'neurotics' were variously described. Other studies have shown no differences in skin conductance levels or flunctuations between normals and neurotics (Eysenck, 1956; Sherman & Jost, 1945).

11.2.4. Cardiovascular variables

Pronounced cardiovascular changes occur during states of high arousal such as anxiety or fear. A rapid pulse, 'palpitating' heart and pallor of the skin contribute to the symptomatology and to the clinical picture of severe anxiety. The cardiovascular variables delineated below enable quantitative measurement of this well documented clinical picture. Thus finger plethysmography reflects the peripheral vasoconstriction which causes skin pallor;

arterial blood pressure depends on the balance between cardiac output and peripheral resistance; and increased forearm bloodflow during anxiety stems from increased muscle bloodflow.

11.2.4.1. Arterial pressure

Altschule (1953) reviewed the literature then available and concluded that there was no evidence that chronic anxiety, personality disorder or conflict were associated with a sustained rise in arterial pressure. Neurotic patients were generally reported as having normal or slightly increased arterial pressures and some subjects diagnosed as circulatory asthenia showed a labile hypertension on exercise.

11.2.4.2. Pulse rate

A transient increase in pulse rate in response to fear-provoking situations is common and frequently observed clinically.

Altschule (1953) noted that most studies reported a normal, or only slightly accelerated pulse rate in patients suffering from 'neurosis' or 'neurocirculatory asthenia'. White & Gildea (1937), Wenger (1947) and Wishner (1953) all reported higher pulse rates in patients suffering from anxiety states than in normal controls. However, other findings are contradictory. No difference in pulse rate between anxiety states and controls was found in one study (Malmo & Shagass, 1949) and, in another, no difference was detected in pulse rate between a psychoneurotic group of patients and normal controls (Jurko, Jost & Hill, 1952). The mean waking pulse rate in anxious patients and controls was similar but a greater drop in the pulse rate of the anxious patients with the onset of sleep was observed (Ackner, 1956a). Lader & Wing (1966) reported significantly higher pulse rates in 20 anxious subjects compared with normal controls. Kelly & Walter (1968) computed correlations between pulse rate and psychometric measures for 60 controls and 203 patients suffering from a wide range of psychiatric states. The correlation coefficient between pulse rate and anxiety self rating was $+0.24$, which was statistically significant but of a low order.

Although not all work is in agreement and the results of some studies are inconsistent, anxious patients appear to have higher pulse rates than normals although there is often considerable overlap between the two groups. The correlation between anxiety and pulse rate is positive, but not sufficiently high to enable the pulse rate to be used as a reliable indicator of anxiety.

11.2.4.3. Finger plethysmography

The blood flow in the finger is predominantly to the skin. Changes in finger plethysmography monitor skin vasoconstriction and vasodilatation.

Burch, Cohn & Neumann (1942) studied the spontaneous fluctuations in finger volume of a group of normal subjects: phlegmatic and emotionally stable subjects showed small and relatively constant deflections while excitable subjects showed a wide variation in the size of the deflection. A later study showed that 'relaxation' was associated with vasodilatation and large pulse waves and 'anxiety' with vasoconstriction and small pulse waves (Neumann, Lhamon & Cohn, 1944). In other studies finger plethysmography was correlated with an 'emotional stability–lability' factor derived from the Bell Adjustment Inventory (Van der Merwe & Theron, 1947; Theron, 1948). The more 'tense' subjects had smaller pulse volumes and the more 'emotionally labile' subjects showed a greater rate of change of finger volume during the performance of various tasks. The same technique was used to compare 'anxiety neurotics', 'hysterics' and controls (Van der Merwe, 1948). There was considerable overlap between the groups but the mean pulse volumes of the anxiety neurotics tended to be small and those of the 'hysterics' large when compared with the control group.

Ackner (1956a) reviewed previous work on the relationship between anxiety and the level of peripheral vasomotor activity. Although mean levels often differentiated between groups of anxious subjects and controls the degree of overlap made individual assessment difficult. Ackner (1956b) also demonstrated that anxious subjects displayed a marked vasodilatation during barbiturate induced sleep.

11.2.4.4. Forearm plethysmograph

The increase in muscle blood that occurs during stress may be recorded by forearm plethysmography. Using this technique forearm blood flow levels of 20 patients suffering from long-standing anxiety were compared with those of 40 mixed psychoneurotic and 40 normal controls (Kelly, 1966). The mean basal flow for the normal controls was 2·19 ml/100 ml arm volume per minute, for the mixed psychoneurotics 2·31, and for the anxiety group 4·78. The difference in basal forearm flow between the anxiety group and the other two groups was highly significant ($P<0·001$). However, it is of interest that there was no significant difference in forearm blood flow between the controls and mixed psychoneurotics, although the latter scored significantly higher on anxiety ratings. Kelly & Walter (1968) provide further information on the relationship between blood flow and anxiety. In a series of 263 subjects the overall correlation between forearm blood flow and anxiety self rating was 0·24 which was no higher than that for pulse rate.

Two studies on small numbers of patients failed to show a significant difference between anxious and non anxious subjects (Harper, Gurney, Savage & Roth, 1965; Bloch & Davies, 1969). These results are not surprising. The low, but statistically significant, correlation between forearm blood flow and anxiety is such that one would only expect statistically significant differences in forearm blood flow to emerge when large numbers of patients, showing marked differences in anxiety, are studied.

11.2.5. Electroencephalogram

There have been relatively few studies of the EEG in anxious patients but the results have been quite consistent. In an early study involving 100 psychoneurotics and 100 normal control subjects, alpha activity was less abundant in the patients, especially the chronic anxiety states (Strauss, 1945). The alpha activity which is present is faster in anxiety states (mean value of 11·2 Hz) than in normals (mean of 10 Hz) (Brazier, Finesinger & Cobb, 1945). The EEG's of anxious patients thus show less alpha and more beta activity than normal (Lindsley, 1950; Kennard, Rabinovitch & Fister, 1955). This reflects these patients' inability to relax so that they continue to have an activated EEG pattern under conditions where calm normals show much alpha activity (Ellingson, 1954).

The results of 'driving' the EEG by photic stimulation are in accord with the findings in the resting EEG. Thus, anxious patients show more response to stimulation at 15 Hz (Shagass, 1955).

Various aspects of the contingent negative variation (CNV) have been examined in anxious patients. The mean CNV during acquisition trials was significantly smaller in 40 highly anxious patients than 40 control subjects. When a distracting noise was added, the CNV in the normals initially diminished but then was steadily restored; in the patients, however, it remained small. A complicating factor was that the patients were receiving sedatives but, even so, the authors' conclusions, that anxious patients are over-distractible, seem justified (McCallum & Walter, 1968).

Although the CNV presents many technical problems and many factors influence it (Tecce, 1972), it would appear to provide a useful and versatile technique for exploring both physiological and psychological characteristics of brain function in anxious patients.

11.2.6. Hormonal function

Complex techniques in specialized laboratories are required for accurate estimates of various hormones in blood, urine and cerebro-spinal fluid. The main hormonal groups in the psychophysiological context are the adrenocortical hormones, the catecholamines and the thyroid hormones.

Cortisol is the main adrenocortical hormone in man and can be estimated in plasma or as 17-oxogenic steroid metabolites in the urine (Jenkins, 1968). The adrenal cortex is under the control of the hypothalamus and anterior pituitary and there are several tests of the integrity of this axis. Both biological and chemical methods exist for the estimation of adrenaline and noradrenaline in the plasma, the latter techniques being more convenient but less specific. Small quantities of catecholamines are excreted unchanged in the urine where their estimation provides a rough index of catecholamine production (Levi, 1972). Thyroid function can be estimated by analysing the thyroid hormones circulating in the blood and by assessing the rate of uptake of radioactive iodine by the thyroid gland.

11.2.6.1. Normals

Many studies have been carried out which evaluate changes in adrenocortical function as related to alterations in affect in normal subjects. Admission to hospital, i.e. a change in environment, raises cortisol levels, and venepuncture, or at least the anticipation of it, itself increases plasma cortisol levels, and these factors must be taken into account. Real-life stressful situations such as college examinations, surgical operations, paratroop training and piloting aircraft produce marked increases both in plasma cortisol and urinary cortisol metabolites. However, the increases in steroid levels reflect more the subject's emotional involvement in the situation rather than the physical danger or stress itself. For example, soldiers in training were exposed to five simulated (but real to the subjects) situations: (i) an aircraft emergency during flight; (ii) the disruption of a military exercise by misdirected incoming shells; (iii) a forest fire; (iv) radioactive fallout; and (v) the soldier was made to feel responsible for a situation in which a comrade seemed seriously injured. Situation (v) had the greatest effect on steroid levels (Berkun, Bialek, Kern & Yagi, 1962).

Hypnotic induction of anxiety in normal subjects is attended by rises in plasma cortisol levels although induction of the trance itself may be accompanied by a drop in these levels (Persky, Korchin, Basowitz, Board, Sabshin, Hamburg & Grinter, 1959). Personality anxiety as assessed by the Taylor Manifest Anxiety Scale is also related to plasma cortisol levels: the mean plasma cortisol level was 13·0 μg/ml in a group of 19 subjects scoring in upper 15 percentile of the scale as compared with 9·9 in 31 subjects in the lower 15 percentile (Fiorica & Muehl, 1962).

That adrenaline is released from the adrenal medulla in states of effort and emotional arousal is well-known. Urinary excretion of catecholamines increases in sportsmen, aviators, paratroop trainess and subjects undergoing similar activities. There is some tendency for the secretion of adrenaline to parallel the subject's level of emotion whereas noradrenaline reflects the physical effort involved.

Motion pictures have provided the stimulation situation in one series of studies (Levi, 1972). Adrenaline excretion in the urine increased with viewing emotionally arousing films whether their content was anxiety-provoking, sad, or amusing, the *degree* of the emotional arousal being the important factor.

Several studies have examined the effects of catecholamines given by injection or infusion (Breggin, 1964). Adrenaline and noradrenaline produced the expected physiological effects such as changes in blood-pressure but 'the subjective feeling of anxiety was almost negligible in relation to the subjective viscerosomatic reactions.' However, occasional episodes of 'real' anxiety did occur (Hawkins, Monroe, Sandifer & Vernon, 1960). In emotionally labile subjects, excess symptoms but few cardiovascular changes have been noted; in rigid personalities, no symptoms but marked physiological changes occurred (Basowitz, Korchin, Oken, Goldstein & Gussack, 1956).

In general, then, infusion experiments suggest that true affects cannot be reproduced in this way, the subject feeling 'as if' he were anxious. However, anxious patients are more likely to have genuine panic attacks induced and this may reflect a learned association between somatic symptoms and anxiety attacks. Lactate infusions also produce adrenaline-like effects. Nevertheless, although the increased arousal induced by the adrenaline or lactate may be non-specific, it can act as the substrate upon which an emotion can be grafted, the quality of the emotion depending on the cognitive clues provided for the subject (Schachter, 1966).

Thyroid function is a less sensitive indicator of emotional change than adrenocortical or adrenomedullary indices but some increases with stressful situations such as examinations and a 75-h vigil have been reported.

11.2.6.2. Anxious patients

An early finding which has been amply replicated was that patients with high levels of anxiety have plasma cortisol levels at least 50 per cent higher than normal. Patients during calm periods showed no such rise, patients in panic attacks particularly high levels. Stressful interviews increase plasma cortisol levels but anxiety, anger and depression may all be the predominant accompanying affect (Persky, Hamburg, Basowitz, Grinter, Sabshin, Korchin, Herz, Board & Heath, 1958). An especially marked effect was noted when the anxiety was of a 'disintegrative' character, e.g. fear of loss of sanity or of control.

Psychoneurotic patients have been noted as over-responsive to adrenocorticotrophin injections and as having high plasma cortisol turnover rates.

A detailed study compared 10 male and 10 female inpatients, judged clinically to show intense emotions such as anxiety, depression, anger and elation, with 10 male and 10 female patients with low affect levels and with a group of affectively stable normal subjects. Plasma cortisol levels were raised above normal levels in both the high and low affect groups (Curtis, Fogel, McEvoy-Zorate, 1966). It was suggested that plasma cortisol levels reach an asymptotic level (at about 20 $\mu g/ml$) because the transport proteins in the blood (mainly transcortin, a high-affinity cortisol-binding protein) become saturated and any excess free cortisol is rapidly metabolized. This study emphasizes the importance of assessing fully the physiological systems involved and not naively assuming that the variable under study has an indefinite range.

There have been surprisingly few studies of adrenomedullary function in anxious patients. Regan & Reilly (1958) classified patients diagnostically, and according to intensity of emotional arousal. Catecholamine levels in the plasma were within the normal range but there was some tendency for levels to be higher in patients with high emotional ratings, especially paranoid patients.

Various groups of subjects with overt affects of anger, anxiety etc. were examined with respect to their urinary catecholamine excretion (Silverman, Cohen, Shmavonian & Kirschner, 1961). Excretion of adrenaline was highest among the primarily anxious, lowest among the primarily angry; the reverse pattern was noted for noradrenaline. The mean values (in μg/l) for normal subjects ($N = 54$) were 1·6 for adrenaline and 2·5 for noradrenaline; corresponding values for neurotic patients ($N = 33$) were 2·0 and 2·8, and for psychotic patients ($N = 30$), 3·8 and 6·3. The psychotic patients' values were significantly higher than those for the other two groups but there was no difference between the neurotic group and the normals.

Thyroid function has not been systematically evaluated in anxious patients although, of course, increased thyroid function as in thyrotoxicosis presents many features similar to that of anxiety states.

11.3. DEPRESSION

11.3.1. Introduction

Severe depressive illness is accompanied by pronounced physical and behavioural changes. The autonomic accompaniments of depression have been less studied than those of anxiety. Biological studies of depression are difficult because depression cannot be induced experimentally, as can anxiety, and because depression rarely occurs without some anxiety, which may itself be responsible for some of the physiological changes observed.

11.3.2. Vascular responses to methacholine

An excessive and prolonged drop in blood pressure in depressed patients following the intramuscular administration of methacholine has been described (Funkenstein, 1954). This response was reported in 90 per cent of involutional and manic depressive patients. On the basis of these findings it was claimed that the methacholine test distinguished between endogenous depression and other psychiatric categories. The fall in blood pressure was attributed to a postulated excessive secretion of noradrenaline in endogenous depression.

The clarity of this physiological demarcation of endogenous depression is in itself surprising as many workers would find it difficult to demonstrate clinically this conditions with such accuracy. Subsequent workers (e.g., Feinberg, 1956; Rose, 1962) were generally unable to replicate these findings. Davies & Palmai (1964) assessed the blood pressure response of 22 female depressed patients to methacholine. There was some evidence that the more severely depressed patients showed a more marked drop in blood pressure.

There is an association between a positive methacholine test and increasing age (Hamilton, 1960). In several of the studies using methacholine the depressed patients were appreciably older than the controls which would produce a spurious difference in the methacholine response. The evidence is so contradictory that no reliance may be placed on this investigation. Certainly Funkenstein's original claim to demarcate between endogenous and reactive depression is without basis.

11.3.3. Sedation and sleep thresholds

The intravenous injection of a barbiturate, such as pentothal, produces drowsiness, slurring of speech, and eventually sleep. The amount of barbiturate necessary to produce sleep as determined by the onset of verbal unresponsiveness is known as the sleep threshold. The onset of sleep is associated with an increase in frontal EEG activity. The sedation threshold is the amount of barbiturate necessary to produce a specified increase in this activity.

Shagass and his co-workers reported on large numbers of patients (Shagass & Jones, 1958). The sedation threshold was low in psychotic depression and high in neurotic depression and anxiety. It was concluded that the test enabled an objective distinction to be made between psychotic and neurotic depression. Early findings were in accordance with Shagass' claims. However, subsequent workers have found it difficult to obtain a reliable end point—with either clinical or EEG assessment of the onset of sleep—and have failed to confirm any clear-cut distinction between psychotic and neurotic depression (Ackner & Pampiglione, 1959; Martin & Davies, 1962; Friedman Granick, Freeman-Stewart, 1965).

A link has been suggested between reduced sedation threshold, reduced arousal and memory loss (Caird, Laverty & Inglis, 1963). Hemsi, Whitehead & Post (1968) found a lower sleep threshold in 13 brain-damaged patients than in 13 elderly depressives. Rather surprisingly, they found no increase in the sleep thresholds of the depressed patients after recovery with ECT. Verbal unresponsiveness and inhibition of the GSR have been used as criteria for judging the sedation threshold of depressed patients (Perez-Reyes, 1968; Perez-Reyes & Cochrane, 1967). Eighty-two psychotic and 108 neurotic depressed patients were compared with 69 normal controls; the mean sedation threshold was low in the psychotic group and high in the neurotic. Again the experimental work is contradictory and difficult to summarize. Sedation threshold does not distinguish clearly between psychotic and neurotic depression and even the more limited hypothesis that sedation threshold is reduced in depressive illness cannot be taken as proven.

Wakefulness or arousal is maintained by excitatory impulses from the ascending reticular system. Barbiturates induce sleep by blocking these impulses. Those who have reported a low sedation threshold in endogenous depression (e.g., Perez-Reyes, 1968) tend to look upon severe depression as being predominantly a central inhibitory state. This is an attractive but over-simple hypothesis. Behaviourally, depressed patients are often slow and 'inhibited' but there is no direct evidence of inhibition of the central nervous system. Moreover, depressive illness, even of the 'endogenous' type, is often associated with raised anxiety and even severe agitation. Anxiety and agitation are indicators of high arousal and by the same analogy might lead to the postulation of central excitation. Central excitation and inhibition are potentially useful unitary concepts but there are dangers both in equating a complex syndrome such as depression with central inhibition and also in assuming that central inhibition may be adequately measured by the response to a single drug.

A startling omission is that none of the many workers studying sedation threshold have taken the trouble to measure plasma barbiturate levels in their subjects. High muscle blood flow facilitates the uptake of barbiturates from the circulation (Balasubramanian, Mawer & Simons, 1970). Thus barbiturate plasma levels after a standard dose are likely to be inversely related to the muscle blood flow which has already been shown to reflect anxiety levels. It is thus possible that sedation and sleep thresholds are little more than indirect measures of the state of the peripheral vascular systems.

11.3.4. Salivation

Dryness of the mouth is a common somatic complaint in depressed patients and reduced salivary secretion in depression was first reported over 30 years ago (Strongin & Hinsie, 1938). More recently, a simple technique for measuring total salivary flow using absorbent dental rolls has been described (Peck, 1959). Since then a number of studies have appeared which are usually interpreted as evidence of diminished salivation in depression. However, not all studies are comparable because of differences in the selection of patients and some results are frankly contradictory.

An investigation of a diagnostically heterogenous group of psychiatric inpatients revealed that those with depressed mood salivated less than others, although the reduction in salivation was unrelated to the severity of the depression (Peck, 1959). Several authors using the same technique have demonstrated that the salivary flow of depressed, hospitalized patients is less than that of normal, non-hospitalized controls (Davies & Gurland, 1961; Gottlieb & Paulson, 1961; Busfield & Wechsler, 1961; Davies & Palmai, 1964; Palmai & Blackwell, 1965; Palmai, Blackwell, Maxwell & Morgenstern, 1967). It has also been found that salivary secretion in non-depressed inpatients was less than that of non-hospitalized controls (Busfield & Wechsler, 1961). Thus some of the reduction in salivary flow ascribed to depression may be due to hospitalization and associated changes in diet and activity. Attempts to relate the impairment of salivation to the severity of depressive symptoms have produced discordant results. Davies & Palmai (1964) describe a progressive diminution in salivation with increasing severity, whereas others found no relationship at all (Peck, 1959; Busfield & Wechsler, 1961).

If depression is associated with diminished salivary flow, the salivation of depressed patients should increase with clinical improvement. However, the results of longitudinal studies are inconsistent. In one study the salivation of depressed patients remained unchanged in spite of clinical improvement (Gottlieb & Paulson, 1961), and a similar finding has been reported in patients over the age of 60 (Hemsi, Whitehead & Post, 1968). An increase in the salivation of depressed patients to control level before discharge from hospital has been claimed (Davies & Palmai, 1964; Palmai & Blackwell, 1965; Palmai, Blackwell,

Maxwell & Morgenstern, 1967). However the achievement of normal salivary flow rates in these patients is unexpected, as studies on the outcome of depressive illness indicate that about a third of the patients are unimproved after treatment (for example, Carney, Roth & Garside, 1965; Medical Research Council Report, 1965). In one paper, 22 consecutively admitted female patients are described as 'recovered' and 'free' from depressive symptoms on retesting (Davies & Palmain, 1964). Such complete recovery in a group of depressed patients selected in this way is uncommon and suggests that the subjects were unusual in their response to treatment.

An alternative approach is to attempt to distinguish different patterns of salivary secretion within groups of depressed patients. Thus, patients categorized as 'agitiert' (agitated) or 'ängstlich aggressiv-depressiv' (anxious, depressive, agressive) had lower salivary secretion than those who were 'gehemmt, apathisch, depressiv' (inhibited, apathetic, depressive), who in turn secreted less saliva than control subjects (Loew, 1965). In another study, the salivary secretion of 34 depressed patients was measured before and after a course of ECT (Noble & Lader, 1971a). Prior to ECT the most retarded patients secreted least saliva. Overall the patients' mean salivary secretion did not change subsequent to ECT. But a more detailed analysis showed that the salivation of the most retarded subjects was low prior to ECT and increased subsequently, whereas that of the least retarded subjects was high prior to ECT and diminished subsequently. Brown (1970) also reported low salivation in retarded depression.

The relationship between retardation and salivary flow may well explain the discrepant results from earlier longitudinal studies. A group of predominantly retarded depressives would be likely to show an increase in salivary flow after clinical improvement, while a sample containing an appreciable number of non-retarded patients would show no mean change.

11.3.5. Electromyography

Claims have been made that the EMG levels in depressed patients are markedly raised, particularly in conjunction with retardation (Whatmore & Ellis, 1959). Subsequently, the EMG levels in severe recurrent depressive illness were studied (Whatmore & Ellis, 1962). EMG levels were elevated both during the depressive episodes and prior to relapse but dropped temporarily in response to treatment.

There are several reasons for expecting depressed patients to show an increase in muscle tone and EMG levels. Depression is almost always accompanied by anxiety which is itself associated with an increase in muscle tone. An agitated depressed patient who continually paces the floor wringing his hands must have an increase in the activity of the muscles responsible for these actions. In general, experimental work confirms these expectations, but the findings are not clear cut and several results are either inconsequential or contradictory (Noble & Lader, 1971b).

11.3.6. Skin conductance

Although skin conductance has been extensively used as an index of arousal, studies of the skin conductance changes in depression are relatively few.

Richter (1928) investigated the skin conductance of psychiatric patients and found that those who felt 'definitely depressed' had low conductance levels. Using a plastic paint technique to measure palmar sweat gland activity in 18 depressed female inpatients it was found that sweating was reduced during the depression and increased significantly with recovery (Bagg & Crookes, 1966). Twenty depressed patients and 20 controls were rated on a depressive scale derived from the MMPI (Greenfield, Katz, Alexander & Roessler, 1963). Subjects with higher depressive scores showed a reduction in galvanic skin response to auditory stimuli. Goldstein (1965) reported that depressives were more responsive than normal controls on a number of physiological variables that included skin conductance. In a series of 73 psychiatric patients, nine patients designated 'depressive' had a low skin conductance, small amplitude galvanic skin responses (GSR's) and a diminished responsivity to stress (Gilberstadt & Maley, 1965).

The GSR's to auditory stimuli were recorded from 35 depressed patients who were subdivided into 17 agitated, 13 retarded and five 'uncomplicated' depressives (Lader & Wing, 1969). A clear cut difference was found between the agitated and retarded groups, the agitated patients having a higher skin conductance level and more spontaneous fluctuations. This relationship between retardation, agitation, and skin conductance has been confirmed more recently (Noble & Lader, 1971c).

11.3.7. Cardiovascular variables

The cardiovascular accompaniments of depressive illness have been little studied. An increased pulse rate in agitated depression has been reported (Lader & Wing, 1969; Kelly & Walter, 1969).

A significant increase in the forearm blood flow of depressed patients subsequent to recovery after a course of ECT has been demonstrated (Noble & Lader, 1971d). The initial blood flows (2·1 ml/100 ml/min) were disproportionately low considering the high anxiety levels of the subjects. Retarded depressed patients evidenced a particularly poor vasodilatory response to the stress of mental arithmetic. Kelly & Walter (1969) suggested that depressive illness did not influence forearm blood flow, since 'non-agitated depressives' had a mean blood flow of 2·1 ml/100 ml arm volume/min), similar to that of normal subjects (2·2) but lower than that of both 'agitated depressives' (3·2) and patients with anxiety state (4·4). However, their data show that the non-agitated depressives had an anxiety level (self-rating 3·8) close to that of the anxiety state group (4·1), although the high anxiety rating of these non-agitated depressives was not associated with an elevated blood flow. The agitated depressives had higher anxiety levels (5·0) and significantly lower blood flows than the anxiety state groups. Thus the blood flow levels of both the agitated and non-agitated depressives were substantially lower than their high anxiety levels would lead one to predict. It is thus likely that depressive illness, particularly in conjuction with retardation, is associated with a diminution in the vasodilatory effect of anxiety.

11.3.8. Electroencephalogram

Initial studies of the EEG in depressive patients were concerned with identifying 'abnormalities' such as slow-wave or paroxysmal activity. As these features could be found in a small proportion of normal subjects and in appreciable numbers of schizophrenics, psychopaths and patients with organic brain pathology, their significance remains unclear. The EEG shows more abnormalities in the elderly making it imperative to match patients and controls for the variable of age (Greenblatt, 1944; Hurst, Mundy-Castle & Beerstacher, 1954; Maggs & Turton, 1956).

Broad-waveband analyses were carried out on the EEGs of 20 severely depressed patients and 20 normal subjects matched for age and sex (Julier & Lader, unpublished data). The patients had smaller amounts of slow-wave activity (2·3–4·0 Hz) and greater amounts of fast-wave activity (13·5–26·0 Hz). However, most patients were receiving hypnotic drugs and as similar EEG changes have been found following such drugs (Bond & Lader, 1972), the difference might be attributable at least in part to this factor. The activity in the 7·5–13·5 Hz waveband was also higher in the patients and this may represent a real inter-group difference as hypnotics tend to *decrease* this waveband.

Sleep is frequently disturbed in depressed patients who tend to have fitful, unsatisfying sleep and to wake early (Hinton, 1963). EEG studies confirm the brevity and broken nature of sleep in depressives and that they take longer to fall asleep than normals (Gresham, Agnew & Williams, 1965; Mendels & Hawkins, 1967). Some controversy exists regarding the pattern of sleep. One study suggested that depressed patients, when asleep, spend a greater proportion of the time in deep sleep (Oswald, Berger, Jaramillo, Keddie, Olley & Pluntelt, 1962); other investigators reported the opposite (Diaz-Guerrero, Gottlieb & Knott, 1946; Gresham *et al.*, 1965; Hawkins & Mendels, 1966).

EEG responses in depressed patients have been the focus of much attention. The duration of alpha blocking in response to photic stimulation is longer in patients and habituation of the response is delayed (Wilson & Wilson, 1961). Depressed patients show more EEG reactivity during sleep than normals and than themselves when recovered (Zung, Wilson & Dodson, 1964).

Somatosensory evoked responses increase with increased shock intensity. The rate of increase appeared greater in psychotic depressed patients (Shagass & Schwartz, 1964) but this finding of larger responses in patients at high stimulus levels could not be replicated (Shagass, 1968). More recently, visual evoked responses have been elicited with flashes at four different intensities. Most normal subjects show an increase in amplitude with increasing stimulation intensity, i.e. they 'augment'. Patients with so-called 'bipolar' depressive illnesses (mania being present at some stage) also augmented whereas patients with 'unipolar' illnesses (no history of mania) showed smaller responses with stronger stimulation i.e., they 'reduced' (Borge, Buchsbaum, Goodwin, Murphy & Silverman 1971; Buchsbaum, Goodwin, Murphy & Borge, 1971). This is an intriguing finding but the clinical difficulties in categorizing patients in this way should not be underestimated.

Evoked responses have also been used to study 'cortical recovery cycles'. This is a concept akin to that of neuronal recovery cycles and involves the presentation of two stimuli over a range of interstimulus intervals. There are undoubtedly many technical as well as theoretical problems but this approach has been regarded as particularly appropriate to study depressive patients. In general, the results have been dauntingly complex with somatosensory stimulation with several components of the evoked response being analysed at a large number of interstimulus intervals (For a full review see Shagass, 1972). Some abnormalities were described, especially with respect to responses elicited at inter-stimulus intervals less than 20 msec but these findings applied to most groups of psychiatric patients (Shagass, 1968). Nevertheless, other studies using visual stimulation have also suggested that psychiatric patients in general, and psychotic depressives in particular, show impaired recovery of the second response (Speck, Dim & Mercer, 1966; Vasconetto, Floris & Morocutti, 1971). This approach, despite its technical complexities, does have the virtue of analysing brain responses in psychiatric patients within a theoretical framework which is derived from clinical observation of severely depressed patients.

11.3.9. Hormonal function

Affective changes occur in patients with adrenocortical abnormalities: lowered adrenal function is often attended by apathy, mild depression, irritability and tiredness; patients with adrenocortical hyperfunction or receiving steroids therapeutically may evidence depression, anxiety, paranoid states, acute confusional excitement or euphoria.

Quite high within-patient correlations have been found between urinary steroid excretion and the intensity of depressive affect. However, the intensity of anxiety was also important. Two groups of patients were distinguished, one characterized by high depression rating but low and stable steroid excretion levels, the other also by high depression ratings but with high and fluctuating steroid levels. The former group had elaborate psychological defences, often with marked denial of their illness, the latter patients were aware of and engaged in a struggle with their illnesses (Bunney, Mason & Hamburg, 1965). Behavioural deterioration and rise in urinary steroids occurred together suggesting that the steroid levels were a concomitant of but not a cause of the psychological changes (Bunney, Mason, Roatch & Hamburg, 1965).

Admission to hospital itself produced rises in urinary steroid excretion of about 20 per cent. The decreases on clinical recovery were quite small, of the order of 10 per cent (Sachar, 1967). However, other similar studies have not confirmed these findings (Gibbons, Gibson, Maxwell & Willcox, 1960).

Patients with manic-depressive cycles have attracted much attention as some endocrinological contrasts between the phases might be expected. In general, steroid levels mirror the intensity of the affect and the patient's involvement in his illness rather than the type of affect.

Plasma cortisol level studies have generally confirmed the findings with urinary steroids. For example, very high cortisol levels were associated with 'very intense distress (especially of a depressive affect in the presence of retarded behavior)' and with the development of extensive personality disintegration, especially depressive psychoses (Board, Persky & Hamburg, 1956). It has been confirmed that retarded depressives have higher plasma cortisol levels (mean 25·3 μg/ml) than non-retarded depressives (mean value 18·3). Intense suffering and inability to cry were also associated with high cortisol levels (Board, Wadeson & Persky, 1957).

Plasma cortisol levels show a diurnal variation, being highest in the morning. Plasma cortisol levels in depressives are most elevated in the early morning and, as some steroids increase brain excitability, it has been suggested that early morning wakening in such patients might be related to this (McClure, 1966).

Cortisol secretion rate and plasma corticotrophin levels are raised in depressed patients (Gibbons, 1966), and this may be due to an insensitivity of the hypothalamus to cortisol (Carroll, Martin & Davies, 1968) which results in over-production of corticotrophin. Cortisol levels in the cerebrospinal fluid of depressives are within the normal range (Coppen, Brooksbank, Noguera & Wilson, 1971).

Catecholamine excretion has been reported as low in depressive patinets in contrast to manic patients where it is very high (Bergsman, 1959). This may reflect the physical overactivity of the manic patients.

Thyroid function is not disordered in depressives although plasma thyroid hormone levels do tend to rise a little during episodes of acute emotional distress. Retarded patients have somewhat higher levels than non-retarded patients (Board, Wadeson & Persky, 1957). Levels of thyroid-stimulating hormone have been reported as abnormally high in depressives (Dewhurst, El Kabir, Hams & Mandelbrote, 1969), and it may be that the hypothalamus is insensitive to thyroid hormone in the same way as it appears insensitive to cortisol.

It would appear that raised hormone levels in patients with anxiety and/or depression are not specific to either emotion. Mason (1959) concluded 'the pituitary-adrenal cortical system is remarkably sensitive to psychological influences in man and monkey, and that ACTH release occurs, not in association with a specific emotional state, but rather with a wide variety of emotional disturbances which may have the relatively undifferentiated element of distress or arousal'. One can echo these sentiments for adrenaline and noradrenaline, and for the less sensitive measure, thyroid function.

11.4. CONCLUSION

The review of psychophysiological studies of clinical anxiety and depression which we have presented has concentrated on the empirical approach. Groups of patients with certain clinical features are compared with 'normal' subjects, or the patient is re-tested when improved or cured. The problems of control have exercised researchers in this field and aspects such as age, sex, diurnal and seasonal variations, dealt with by other contributors to this volume, are equally important in the clinical context. Some factors are especially noteworthy. The doctor–patient relationship is different from the experimenter–subject relationship and from the experimenter–patient relationship. Moreover, a paranoid patient will have different attitudes to the experimenter from a depressive patient who regards the experimental procedures, despite their innocuousness, as just retribution for his real or imagined peccadilloes. Control for such factors is impossible but note can be taken of the attitudes of the patients or more formal psychometric assessment undertaken.

Another important factor is the degree of laboratory sophistication. This can operate in either direction: a newly-admitted patient will probably know much less about laboratory procedures than, say, a nurse acting as control; however, a patient who has been through a series of diagnostic procedures may be much more blasé about laboratory testing than a control subject obtained from the general population. Admission to hospital itself appears to influence certain physiological measures so that mixed patient groups should be first analysed as sub-groups of in-patients and out-patients.

A wide range of other factors should be kept in mind—diet, exercise, sexual activity, leisure opportunities—and all make full control impossible. However, if any of these factors is so important that it would obscure differences between patients and controls it would probably have been detected within the patient population.

A further difficulty stems from the fact that all the psychotropic drugs in current vogue have marked autonomic and metabolic effects which may persist for a prolonged time after the medication is stopped. An experimenter who takes this into account in designing his methods usually faces a dilemma. If he is stringent in his requirement that the patients studied be drug free he will obtain few, or none, or thoroughly atypical subjects. If he relaxes his criteria his subjects become more numerous and representative, but the risk of error due to spurious drug effects increases. Most studies describe small numbers of patients, selected by an undiscernable process from an undescribed and generally unknown population. Workers who study a series of patients—such as 'consecutive admissions'—have an advantage. But even here it must be cautioned that many non-medical factors determine admission to a particular hospital. The clientele of one institution may differ markedly from that of another. The answer lies in a collaborative approach between the research worker and the clinician to create a management policy which is compatible with the needs of the patient and with research. This would facilitate the study of representative samples of illness categories. Ideally the patients should also come from a defined population, which is assessed demographically and monitored by a case register system.

The non-specificity of the psychophysiological correlates of clinical states cannot be stressed too strongly. In other words, there are no pathognomonic (exclusively characteristic) physiological signs of any particular clinical entity. In part, this must reflect the unsatisfactory nature of psychiatric classification. One cardinal feature of a taxonomic classification is the mutual exclusivity of the categories. This is manifestly not so in psychiatry. The alternative is to categorize each patient along a series of continua such as the extroversion–introversion, stable–neurotic and normal–psychotic ones of Eysenck. Here again concepts of the 'structure' of mental illnesses intrude on empirical observations. And the relationships between psychophysiological measures and global dimensions of this sort seem, if anything, to be even more confused than those derived from clinical categories.

The non-specificity extends to the type of emotion present and to clinical states. The differences claimed in physiological patterns accompanying various emotions are unimpressive. The intensity rather than the type of emotion is the main determinant of level of physiological activity. To approach this problem emotional traits and symptoms should be established, which with multivariate analyses, might result in clearer relationships with physiological measures being discerned. What is crucial is the reliability of such measures. There is no hope of establishing any concurrent validity if the reliability is low. It is notorious that inter-psychiatrist reliability for diagnosis is low and often only moderately higher for symptoms and signs. However, most research psychiatrists would be presumed to be fairly consistent in the ratings of a group of patients and especially of patients on successive occasions otherwise few controlled clinical trials would show significant results. Thus, within-patient correlations should be the most sensitive method for establishing clinical–physiological relationships.

Observable phenomena in the patient, especially those easily and accurately quantifiable, are potentially more useful for study than global disease concepts or syndromes. For example, we have found it useful to rate depressed patients for retardation and agitation. This is not to gainsay the difficulties and inaccuracies of such ratings but they are preferable to rating of mood as expressed by a psychiatrically ill patient. Of course, other methods of categorizing patients might be even more heuristic, e.g. dividing depressives into unipolar and bipolar cases (Perris, 1973).

In conclusion, hope for the future lies in the time-honoured techniques of close clinical observation, and the construction of hypotheses testable by using rigorous psychophysiological techniques. The major questions regarding the fundamental physiological abnormalities in anxiety and depression are slowly being answered. Meanwhile, the methods provide useful quantitative measures to complement clinical assessment of illness severity and to monitor behavioural, pharmacological and other treatments.

11.5. REFERENCES

Ackner, B. Emotions and the peripheral vasomotor system. A review of previous work. *Journal of Psychosomatic Research*, 1956, **1**, 3–20(a).

Ackner, B. The relationship between anxiety and the level of peripheral vasomotor activity. *Journal of Psychosomatic Research*, 1956, **1**, 21–48(b).

Ackner, B. & Pampiglione, G. An evaluation of the sedation threshold test. *Journal of Psychosomatic Research*, 1959, **3**, 271–281.

Altschule, M. D. *Bodily physiology in mental and emotional disorders.* Grune and Stratton: New York, 1953.

Bagg, C. E. & Crookes, T. G. Palmar digital sweating in women suffering from depression. *British Journal of Psychiatry*, 1966, **112**, 1251–1255.

Balasubramaniam, K., Mawer, G. E. & Simons, P. J. The influence of dose on the distribution and elimination of amylobarbitone in healthy subjects. *British Journal of Pharmacology*, 1970, **40**, 578P–579P.

Basowitz, H., Korchin, S. J., Oken, D., Goldstein, M. S. & Gussack, H. Anxiety and performance changes with a minimal dose of epinephrine. *Archives of Neurology and Psychiatry*, 1956, **76**, 98–108.

Bergsman, A. The urinary excretion of adrenaline and noradrenaline in some mental diseases: a clinical and experimental study. *Acta Psychiatrica et Neurologica Scandinavia*, 1959 (Suppl. 133).

Berkun, M. M., Bialek, H. M., Kern, R. P. & Yagi, K. Experimental studies of psychological stress in man. *Psychological Monographs*, 1962, **76**, No. 15, Whole No. 534.

Bloch, S. & Davies, B. Forearm blood-flow in anxious and non anxious patients. *Australian and New Zealand Journal of Psychiatry*, 1969, **3**, 86–88.

Board, F., Persky, H. & Hamburg, D. A. Psychological stress and endocrine functions. Blood levels of adrenocortical and thyroid hormones in acutely disturbed patients. *Psychosomatic Medicine*, 1956, **18**, 324–333.

Board, F., Wadeson, R. & Persky, H. Depressive affect and endocrine functions. Blood levels of adrenal cortex and thyroid hormones in patients suffering from depressive reactions. *Archives of Neurology and Psychiatry*, 1957, **78**, 612–620.

Bond, A. J. & Lader, M. H. Residual effects of hypnotics. *Psychopharmacologia*, 1972, **25**, 117–132.

Borge, G. F., Buchsbaum, M., Goodwin, F., Murphy, D. & Silverman, J. Neuropsychological correlates of affective disorders. *Archives of General Psychiatry*, 1971, **24**, 501–504.

Brazier, Mary A. B., Finesinger, J. E. & Cobb, S. A contrast between the electroencephalograms of 100 psychoneurotic patients and those of 500 normal adults. *American Journal of Psychiatry*, 1945, **101**, 443–448.

Breggin, P. R. The psychophysiology of anxiety with a review of the literature concerning adrenaline. *Journal of Nervous and Mental Diseases*, 1964, **139**, 558–568.

Brown, C. C. The parotid puzzle: a review of the literature on human salivation and its application to psychophysiology. *Psychophysiology*, 1970, **7**, 66–85.

Buchsbaum, M., Goodwin, F., Murphy, D. & Borge, G. AER in affective disorders. *American Journal of Psychiatry*, 1971, **128**, 19–25.

Bunney, W. E., Mason, J. W. & Hamburg, D. A. Correlations between behavioural variables and urinary 17-hydroxy-corticosteroids in depressed patients. *Psychosomatic Medicine*, 1965, **27**, 299–308.

Bunney, W. E., Mason, J. W., Roatch, J. F. & Hamburg, D. A. A psychoendocrine study of severe psychotic depressive crises. *American Journal of Psychiatry*, 1965, **122**, 72–80.

Burch, G. E., Cohn, A. E. & Neumann, C., A quantitative study of spontaneous variation in volume of the finger tip, toe tip and posterosuperior position of the pinna in resting normal white adults. *American Journal of Physiology*, 1942, **136**, 433–447.

Busfield, B. L. & Wechsler, H. Studies of salivation in depression. *Archives of General Psychiatry*, 1961, **4**, 10–15.

Caird, W. K., Laverty, S. G. & Inglis, J. Sedation and sleep thresholds in elderly patients with memory disorder. *Gerontology Clinics*, 1963, **5**, 59–60.

Carney, M. W. P., Roth, M. & Garside, R. F. The diagnosis of depressive syndromes and the prediction of ECT response. *British Journal of Psychiatry*, 1965, **111**, 659–674.

Carroll, B. J., Martin, F. I. R. & Davies, B. Resistance to suppression by dexamethasone of plasma 11–O.H.C.S. levels in severe depressive illness. *British Medical Journal*, 1968, **3**, 285–287.

Coppen, A., Brooksbank, B. W. L., Noguera, R. & Wilson, D. A. Cortisol in the cerebrospinal fluid of patients suffering from affective disorders. *Journal of Neurology, Neurosurgery and Psychiatry*, 1971, **34**, 432–435.

Curtis, G. C., Fogel, M. C., McEvoy, D. & Zarate, C. The effect of sustained affect on the diurnal rhythm of adrenal cortical activity. *Psychosomatic Medicine*, 1966, **28**, 696–713.

Davies, B. M. & Gurland, J. B. Salivary secretion in depressive illness, *Journal of Psychosomatic Research*, 1961, **5**, 269–271.

Davies, B. M. & Palmai, G. Salivary and blood pressure responses to methacholine in depressive illness. *British Journal of Psychiatry*, 1964, **110**, 594–598.

Dewhurst, K. E., El Kabir, D. J., Harris, G. W. & Mamdelbrote, B. M. Observations on the blood concentration of thyrotropic hormone (T.S.H.) in schizophrenia and affective states. *British Journal of Psychiatry*, 1969, **115**, 1003–1011.

Diaz-Guerrero, R., Gottlieb, J. S. & Knott, J. R. The sleep of patients with manic-depressive psychosis, depressive type. An electroencephalographic study. *Psychosomatic Medicine*, 1946, **8**, 399–404.

Ellingson, R. J. The incidence of EEG abnormality among patients with mental disorders of apparently nonorganic origin: a critical review. *American Journal of Psychiatry*, 1954, **111**, 263–275.

Eysenck, S. B. G. An experimental study of psychogalvanic reflex responses of normal neurotic and psychotic subjects. *Journal of Psychosomatic Research*, 1956, **1**, 258–272.

Feinberg, I. Current status of the Funkenstein test. *Archives of Neurology and Psychiatry*, 1956, **80**, 488–499.

Fiorica, V. & Muehl, S. Relationship between plasma levels of 17-hydroxycorticosteroids (17-OH-CS) and a psychological measure of manifest anxiety. *Psychosomatic Medicine*, 1962, **24**, 596–599.

Friedman, A. S., Granick, S., Freeman, L. & Stewart, M. Cross-validation of the low (EEG) sedation threshold of psychotic depressives. Paper presented at Annual Meeting of American Psychological Assocation Chicago, September 1965.

Funkenstein, D. H. Physiologic studies of depression, In P. W. Hoch & J. Zubin (Eds), *Depression*. New York: Grune & Stratton, 1954. Chapters 10, 11.

Gibbons, J. L. The secretion rate of corticosterone in depressive illness. *Journal of Psychosomatic Research*, 1966, **10**, 263–266.

Gibbons, J. L., Gibson, J. G., Maxwell, A. E. & Willcox, D. R. C. An endocrine study of depressive illness. *Journal of Psychosomatic Research*, 1960, **5**, 32–41.

Gilberstadt, H. & Maley, M. GSR, clinical state and psychiatric diagnosis. *Journal of Clinical Psychology*, 1965, **21**, 233–238.

Goldstein, Iris B. The relationship of muscle tension and autonomic activity to psychiatric disorders. *Psychosomatic Medicine*, 1965, **27**, 39–52.

Gottlieb, G., & Paulson, G. Salivation in depressed patients. *Archives of general Psychiatry*, 1961, **5**, 468–471.

Greenblatt, M. Age and electroencephalographic abnormality in neuropsychiatric patients. A study of 1593 cases. *American Journal of Psychiatry*, 1944, **101**, 82–90.

Greenfield, N. S., Katz, D., Alexander, A. A. & Roessler, R. The relationship between physiological and psychological responsivity, depression and galvanic skin response. *Journal of Nervous and Mental Disease*, 1963, **136**, 535–539.

Gresham, S. C., Agnew, H. W. & Williams, R. L. The sleep of depressed patients. An EEG and eye movement study. *Archives of general Psychiatry*, 1965, **13**, 503–507.

Gurney, C., Roth, M., Garside, R. F., Kerr, T. A. & Schapira, K. Studies in the classification of affective disorders. The relationship between anxiety states and depressive illness. II. *British Journal of Psychiatry*, 1972, **121**, 162–166.

Hamilton, M. Quantitative assessment of the mecholyl test. *Acta Neurologica Psychiatrica Scandinavica*, 1960, **35**, 156–162.

Harper, M., Gurney, C., Savage, D. R. & Roth, M. Forearm blood flow in normal subjects and patients with phobic anxiety states. *British Journal of Psychiatry*, 1965, **111**, 723–731.

Hawkins, E. R., Monroe, J. D., Sandifer, M. G. & Vernon, C. R. Psychological and physiological responses to continuous epinephrine infusion. *Psychiatric Research Report American Psychiatric Association*, 1960, **12**, 40–52.

Hawkins, D. R. & Mendels, J. Sleep disturbance in depressive syndromes. *American Journal of Psychiatry*, 1966, **123**, 682–690.

Hemsi, I. K., Whitehead, A. & Post, F. Cognitive functioning and cerebral arousal in elderly depressives and dements. *Journal of Psychosomatic Research*, 1968, **12**, 145–56.

Hinton, J. M. A comparison of the effects of six barbiturates and a placebo on insomnia and motility in psychiatric patients. *British Journal of Pharmacology*, 1963, **20**, 319–325.

Hoch, P., Kubis, J. F. & Rouke, F. L. Psychometric investigations in psychosis and other abnormal mental states. *Psychosomatic Medicine*, 1944, **6**, 237–243.

Hurst, L. A., Mundy-Castle, A. C. & Beerstacher, D. M. The electroencephalogram in manic-depressive psychosis. *Journal of Mental Science*, 1954, **100**, 220–240.

Jenkins, J. S. *An introduction to biochemical aspects of the adrenal cortex*. London: Edward Arnold, 1968.

Jurko, M., Jost, H. & Hill, T. S. Pathology of the energy system. *Journal of Psychology*, 1952, **33**, 183–198.

Kelly, D. H. W. Measurement of anxiety by forearm blood flow. *British Journal of Psychiatry*, 1966, **112**, 789–798.

Kelly, D. H. W. & Walter, C. J. S. The relationship between clinical depression and anxiety assessed by forearm blood flow and other measurements. *British Journal of Psychiatry*, 1968, **114**, 611–627.

Kelly, D. H. W. & Walter, C. J. S. A clinical and physiological relationship between anxiety and depression. *British Journal of Psychiatry*, 1969, **115**, 401–406.

Kennard, M. A., Rabinovitch, M. S. & Fister, W. P. The use of frequency analysis in the interpretation of the EEGs of patients with psychological disorders. *Electroencephalography and Clinical Neurophysiology*, 1955, **7**, 29–38.

Kerr, T. A., Roth, M., Schapira, K. & Gurney, C. The assessment and prediction of outcome in affective disorders. *British Journal of Psychiatry*, 1972, **121**, 167–174.

Lader, M. H. & Wing, L. *Physiological measures, sedative drugs and morbid anxiety*. Maudsley Monograph No. 14. London: Oxford University Press, 1966.

Lader, M. H. & Wing, L. Physiological measures in agitated and retarded depressed patients. *Journal of Psychiatric Research*, 1969, **7**, 89–100.

Levi, L. Psychological and physiological reactions to and psychomotor performance during prolonged and complex stressor exposure. *Acta Medica Scandinavica*, 1972, suppl. *528*, 119–142.

Lindsley, D. B. Emotions and the electroencephalogram. In M. L. Reymert (Ed.), *Feelings and emotions*. New York: Mc-Graw-Hill, 1950. pp. 238–246.

Loew, D. Syndrom, Diagnose und Speichelsekretion bei depressiven Patienten. *Psychopharmacologia*, 1965, **7**, 339–348.

McCallum, W. C. & Walter, W. G. The effects of attention and distraction on the contingent negative variation in normal and neurotic subjects. *Electroencephalography and Clinical Neurophysiology*, 1968, **25**, 319–329.

McClure, D. J. The effects of antidepressant medication on the diurnal plasma cortisol levels in depressed patients. *Journal of Psychosomatic Research*, 1966, **10**, 197–202.

Maggs, R. & Turton, E. C. Some EEG findings in old age and their relationship to affective disorder. *Journal of Mental Science*, 1956, **102**, 812–818.

Malmo, R. B. & Shagass, C. Physiologic studies of reaction to stress in anxiety and early schizophrenia. *Psychosomatic Medicine*, 1949, **11**, 9–24.

Malmo, R. B., Shagass, C. & Davis, J. F. Electromyographic studies of muscular tension in psychiatric patients under stress. *Journal of Clinical Experimental Psycho-pathology*, 1951, **12**, 45–66.

Martin, I. Levels of muscle activity in psychiatric patients. *Acta Psychologica*, 1956, **12**, 326–341.

Martin, I. & Davies, B. M. Sleep thresholds in depression. *Journal of Mental Science*, 1962, **108**, 466–473.

Martin, I. & Davies, B. M. The effect of Na amytal in autonomic and muscle activity of patients with depressive illness. *British Journal of Psychiatry*, 1963, **111**, 168–75.

Mason, J. W. Psychological influences on the pituitary-adrenal cortical system. *Recent Progress in Hormone Research*, 1959, **15**, 345–378.

Medical Research Council Report Clinical trial of the treatment of depressive illness. *British Medical Journal*, 1965, **1**, 881–886.

Mendels, J. & Hawkins, D. R. Sleep and depression. A follow-up study. *Archives of General Psychiatry*, 1967, **16**, 536–542.

Mendels, J., Weinstein, N. & Cochrane, C. The relationship between depression and anxiety. *Archives of General Psychiatry*, 1972, **27**, 649–653.

Neumann, C., Lhamon, W. T. & Cohn, A. E. Study of emotional factors responsible for changes in the pattern of rhythmic volume fluctations of the finger tip. *Journal of Clinical Investigation*, 1944, **23**, 1–9.

Noble, P. J. & Lader, M. H. Salivation and depressive illness: a psychometric and physiological study. *Psychological Medicine*, 1971, **1**, 372–376(a).

Noble, P. J. & Lader, M. H. An electromyographic study of depressed patients. *Journal of Psychosomatic Research*, 1971, **15**, 233–239(b).

Noble, P. J. & Lader, M. H. The symptomatic correlates of the skin conductance changes in depression. *Journal of Psychiatric Research*, 1971, **9**, 61–69(c).

Noble, P. J. & Lader, M. H. Depression and forearm blood flow. *British Journal of Psychiatry*, 1971, **119**, 261–66(d).

Oswald, I., Berger, R. J., Jaramillo, R. A., Keddie, K. M. G., Olley, P. C. & Plunkett, G. B. Melancholia and barbiturates: a controlled EEG, body and eye movement study of sleep. *British Journal of Psychiatry*, 1962, **109**, 66–78.

Palmai, G. & Blackwell, B. Diurnal pattern of salivary flow in normal and depressed patients. *British Journal of Psychiatry*, 1965, **111**, 334–38.

Palmai, G., Blackwell, B., Maxwell, A. E. & Morgenstern F. Pattern of salivery flow in depressive illness and during treatment. *British Journal of Psychiatry*, 1967, **113**, 1297–1308.

Peck, R. E. The SHP test: an aid in the detection and measurement of depression. *Archives of General Psychiatry*, 1959, **1**, 35–40.

Perez-Reyes, M. Differences in sedative susceptibility between types of depression, clinical and neurophysiological. *Archives of General Psychiatry*, 1968, **19**, 64–71.

Perez-Reyes, M. & Cochrane, C. Differences in sodium thiopental susceptibility of depressed patients as evidenced by the GSR inhibition threshold. *Journal of Psychiatric Research*, 1967, **5**, 335–47.

Perris, C. A new approach to the classification of affective disorders. In R. Garcia (Ed.), *Aspects of depression*. Barcelona, World Psychiatric Association, 1973.

Persky, H., Hamburg, D. A., Basowitz, H., Grinker, R. R. Sabshin, M. Korchin, S. J. Herz, M. Board, F. A. and Heath, H. A. Relation of emotional responses and changes in plasma hydrocortisone level after stressful interview. *Archives of Neurology and Psychiatry*, 1958, **79**, 434–447.

Persky, H., Korchin, S. J., Bosowitz, H., Board, F. A., Sabshin, M., Hamburg, D. A. & Grinker, R. R. Effects of two psychological stresses on adrenocortical function studies in anxious and normal subjects. *Archives of Neurology and Psychiatry*, 1959, **81**, 219–232.

Regan, P. F. & Reilly, J. Circulating epinephrine and norepinephrine in changing emotional states. *Journal of Nervous and Mental Disease*, 1958, **127**, 12–16.

Richter, C. P. The electrical skin resistance. *Archives of Neurology and Psychiatry*, 1928, **19**, 488–508.

Rose, J. T. Autonomic function in depression: a modified methaeholine test. *Journal of Mental Science*, 1962, **108**, 624–641.

Roth, M., Gurney, C., Garside, R. F. & Kerr, T. A. Studies in the classification of affective disorders. The relationship between anxiety states and depressive illness. 1. *British Journal of Psychiatry*, 1972, **121**, 147–161.

Sachar, E. J. Corticosteroids in depressive illness. I. A reevaluation of control issues and the literature. *Archives of General Psychiatry*, 1967, **17**, 544–553.

Sainsbury, P. & Gibson, J. G. Symptoms of anxiety and tension and the accompanying physiological changes in the muscular system. *Journal of Neurology, Neurosurgery and Psychiatry*, 1954, **17**, 214–216.

Schachter, S. The interaction of cognitive and physiological determinants of emotional state. In C. D. Spielberger (Ed.), *Anxiety and Behavior*. New York: Academic Press, 1966, pp. 193–224.

Schapira, K., Roth, M., Kerr, T. A. & Gurney, Clair. The prognosis of affective disorders: the differentiation of anxiety states from depressive illnesses. *British Journal of Psychiatry*, 1972, **121**, 175–181.

Shagass, C. Differentiation between anxiety and depression by the photically activated electroencephalogram. *American Journal of Psychiatry*, 1955, **112**, 41–46.

Shagass, C. Averged somatosensory evoked responses in various psychiatric disorders, In J. Wortis (Ed.), *Recent advances in biological psychiatry*. New York: Plenum Press, 1968. pp. 205–219. Vol. X.

Shagass, C. *Evoked brain potentials in psychiatry*. New York: Plenum Press, 1972.

Shagass, C. & Jones, A. L. A neurophysiological test for psychiatric depression: results in 750 patients. *American Journal of Psychiatry*, 1958, **114**, 1002–1009.

Shagess, C. & Schwartz, M. Evoked potential studies in psychiatric patients. *Annals of New York Academy of Sciences*, 1964, **112**, 526–42.

Sherman, M. & Jost, H. Quantification of psychophysiological measures. *Psychosomatic Medicine*, 1945, **7**, 215–219.

Silverman, A. J., Cohen, S. I., Shmavonian, B. M. & Kirschner, N. Catecholamines in psychophysiologic studies. *Recent Advances in Biological Psychiatry*, 1961, **3**, 104–117.

Speck, L. B., Dim, B. & Mercer, M. Visual evoked responses of psychiatric patients. *Archives of General Psychiatry*, 1966, **15**, 59–63.

Strauss, H. Clinical and electroencephalographic studies: the electroencephalogram in psychoneurotics. *Journal of Nervous and Mental Diseases*, 1945, **101**, 19–27.

Strongin, E. I. & Hinsie, L. E. Parotid gland secretions in manic depressive patients. *American Journal of Psychiatry*, 1938, **94**, 1459–1466.

Tecce, J. J. Contingent negative variation (CNV) and psychological processes in man. *Psychological Bulletin*, 1972, **77**, 73–108.

Theron, P. A. Peripheral vasomotor reactions as indices of basic emotional tension and lability. *Psychosomatic Medicine*, 1948, **10**, 335–46.

Van der Marwe, A. B. The diagnostic value of peripheral vasomotor reactions in psychoneurosis. *Psychosomatic Medicine*, 1948, **10**, 347–354.

Van der Merwe, A. B. & Theron, P. A. A new method of measuring emotional stability. *Journal of General Psychology*, 1947, **37**, 109–124.

Vasconetto, C., Floris, V. & Morocutti, C. Visual evoked responses in normal and psychiatric subjects. *Electroencephalography and clinical Neurophysiology*, 1971, **31**, 77–83.

Wenger, M. A. Preliminary study of the significance of measures of autonomic balance. *Psychosomatic Medicine*, 1947, **9**, 301–9.

Whatmore, G. B. & Ellis, R. M. Some neurophysiologic aspects of depressed states. An electromyographic study. *Archives of General Psychiatry*, 1959, **1**, 70–80.

Whatmore, G. B. & Ellis, R. M. Further neurophysiologic aspects of depressed states: an electromyographic study. *Archives of General Psychiatry*, 1962, **6**, 243–253.

White, B. V. & Gilden E. F. 'Cold pressor test' in tension and anxiety. A cardiochronographic study. *Archives of Neurology and Psychiatry*, 1937, **38**, 964–84.

Wilson, W. P. & Wilson, N. J. Observations on the duration of photically elicited arousal responses in depressive psychoses. *Journal of Nervous and Mental Diseases*, 1961, **133**, 438–440.

Wishner, J. Neurosis and tension: an exploratory study of the relationship of physiological and Rorschach measures, *Journal of abnormal and social Psychology*, 1953, **48**, 253–260.

Zung, W. W. K., Wilson, W. P. & Dodson, W. E. Effect of depressive disorders on sleep EEG responses. *Archives of General Psychiatry*, 1964, **10**, 439–445.

Chapter 12

Psychophysiological Studies of Schizophrenic Pathology

P. H. VENABLES

Department of Psychology,
University of York

12.1. GENERAL CONSIDERATIONS

Schizophrenic pathology was chosen as part of the title of this chapter as a label to cover aspects of behaviour subsumed under the general rubric of schizophrenia with no commitment to any notion that there exists a unitary disease entity—schizophrenia. Nevertheless, in attempting to review work under this general title it must be recognized that there is tacit assumption in the approach made by many workers that there is a basic disease, and this may or may not be subdivided. It is, therefore, convenient in our present state of knowledge to retain the general term schizophrenia to encompass a set of behaviours, even if there are indications that as our knowledge develops the sub-divisions within this general disease construct may widen so greatly as to suggest that it would be more appropriate to consider the sub-divisions as separate entities.

12.1.1. Sub-divisions of schizophrenia

As in so many instances where two cognate aspects of a subject come together, different amounts of expertise are brought to bear from the separate disciplines. Thus, in some studies we may have expert psychophysiology paired with a fairly naive approach to the clinical aspects of the subject, and in other cases a sophisticated realization of the problems of working with patient groups coupled with psychophysiology which verges on what appears to be a disregard for the basic principles of electrophysiology. However, there is undoubtedly a growing acceptance of the necessity for any work using patients labelled as schizophrenic as an experimental group to employ carefully defined subdivisions of the experimental population. In some cases the sub-categorization starts from earlier psychiatric classification such as the quadripartite division of Kraepelin (1913). There does, however, seem to be almost universal acceptance of the idea that this is more sensibly reduced to the dichotomy paranoid and non-paranoid (Shakow, 1962; Silverman, 1967). There is a consequence of the use of this dichotomy in the suggestion which perhaps goes back as far as Kraepelin (1913) that paranoid patients (or at least some of them) should not be included under the rubric of schizophrenia (Foulds & Owen, 1963). Certainly, psychophysiological data, in an experiment by Venables & Wing (1962) suggested that patients labelled as paranoid schizophrenics and who expressed their delusions in a coherent fashion, behaved in an entirely different way from non-paranoid patients and those called paranoid but whose delusions were not expressed coherently and in whom there were other signs of deterioration of personality.

In other instances the division of patients into process and reactive groups appears to have been useful (Herron, 1962; Higgins & Peterson, 1966). This division although deriving from a different background has a virtual identity with that described as 'poor' versus 'good' pre-morbid (Phillips, 1953) and empirical studies using scales to measure each dimension has shown them to be correlated ($r = +0.62$) (Johannsen, Friedman, Leitschuch & Ammons, 1963). Basically the idea underlying the division would seem to be the old one of organic on the one hand and psychogenic on the other. In the case of the 'process', 'poor pre-morbid' patient there is no necessity for an identifiable external event to be present to trigger off the disease process, the seeds of the disease lie in the unfortunate endowment of the patient. On the other hand, in the case of the 'reactive' patient whose status prior to disease onset was 'good', external precursors of the disease can be identified. Probably no-one, among those who use a process-reactive dichotomy would now hold to an idea of an alternative organic or psychogenic basis for some patients within the group of schizophrenias. A 'stress-diathesis' approach is far more acceptable and consequently the process-reactive dichotomy becomes a dimension of level of threshold at which external events react with a predisposed system to produce pathology. A further division of patients into acute and chronic is often made. Formerly, before the introduction of tranquillizers a division at 2 years hospitalization based on the function relating probability of discharge to stay in hospital (Brown, 1960) was potentially useful. Since the introduction of tranquillizers however, with the greater ability of clinicians to discharge patients after a short stay in hospital an acute–chronic dichotomy based on hospitalization becomes relatively meaningless. There is also a confounding between the ideas of acute versus chronic and process versus reactive, in so far as a process patient in whom pathology has an insidious onset cannot be said to present an acute phase in the same manner as a reactive patient. Further discussion of this point is taken-up in Section 12.1.4.

So far sub-classifications which exist prior to the execution of an experimental study have been discussed. Other sub-divisions arise because of the manner in which the experimental data forces interpretation. For example, the division along the dimensions of 'activity–withdrawal' (Venables, 1957), arose from the way patients performed in a reaction time study (Tizard & Venables, 1957), and later was shown to have validity in psychophysiological investigation (Venables, 1960; Venables & Wing, 1962). In another example, the sub-division of the patient population has arisen directly from a psychophysiological investigation; thus Gruzelier & Venables (1972) found that a large group of undifferentiated schizophrenic patients could be divided into more or less equal sized sub-groups depending on the extent to which they did or did not shown skin conductance orienting responses to simple non-signal auditory stimuli.

While there has thus been an improvement since the early days in the degree to which experimental variance may be sub-divided and hence better understood, and there has been a parallel development in psychophysiological techniques, so that the degree of error variance in measurement has been reduced, a major experimental problem which has arisen in the past two decades has been the almost universal use of major tranquillizing drugs in the treatment of schizophrenic patients. In considering the consequences of medication it is, however, important to view them only as one of the sources of difficulty which prevent direct study of fundamental pathology (cf. Sections 12.1.3 and 12.1.4.)

12.1.2. The problems imposed by patient medication

The investigator is faced with a series of problems which appear to be only capable of solution by compromise. The ideal experiment using schizophrenic patients takes an unequivocally diagnosed population, divided into clearly defined sub-groups, desirably matched on other relevant variables with suitably selected controls, and tests them at balanced, allocated times of day, etc. The medication problem, among others tends to impose departures from this ideal position. While reports undoubtedly still appear in the literature where patients who are not on drugs form part of the experimental population, doubts must be felt about the extent to which either clinical or experimental ethics have been satisfied. It is recognized that not all medication is effective all of the time with all patients and that in many instances undesirable side effects accompany ineffective treatment, nevertheless, the removal of patients for experimental purposes from a regime which has potential benefits, is not undertaken lightly. It is generally acknowledged that complete excretion of phenothiazines may take at least one month (e.g., Forrest, Forrest & Mason, 1961). During this time the patient may become a nursing problem. If he is put back on medication, the representativeness of the original sample which was taken off drugs is destroyed, if he remains off medication then his responses to testing are at least in part contaminated by his reaction to drug withdrawal. A possibility, which is at least feasible, is to accept the fact that the patient is on drugs and bear in mind what is already known, from experiments which have been carried out, about the effect of the drug on the variable of interest. Thus, the patient is acknowledged to be, for instance, a schizophrenic receiving a known dose of chlorpromazine and the results interpreted in light of this knowledge. The patient on drugs still exhibits symptoms, or he would not be a patient, and the relation of overt symptomatology to conservatively interpreted psychophysiological data is of value.

Three ways of working with patients on drugs seem feasible; the first, which does not seem to have been tried, is to persuade the clinician to put all the patients in the experimental population on equal dosages of a particular drug (matched for body weight). This might be a more defensible procedure than withdrawing medication. The second technique is to use an index method such as the 'Phenothiazine Dosage Index' of Spohn, Thetford & Cancro (1971) where drug dosage (made equivalent over different types of drugs) may be entered as a factor for statistical control. The third technique, in a way equivalent to the second, is to show statistically that dosages and types of drugs do not distinguish the patient sub-populations divided on the variable on interest. There are, however, dangers from hidden interaction in these techniques. If, for instance, the effect of phenothiazine medication is to raise the value of some variable in paranoid patients and the effect of the same dosage is to lower the value of the variable in non-paranoid patients, then the measured difference between paranoids and non-paranoids on the same dosage of the drug will be due to differential pharmacological action rather than to a 'real' difference between paranoids and non-paranoids. Only by taking patients on different dosages as subjects would the interaction be shown up. None of these three methods remove the effect of the drug dosage, they rather are means by which patients-on-drugs may be studied in a more standardized way. One technique sometimes used is to examine samples of patients, almost always to be found in a large hospital, who are unmedicated because medication has not been effective. Here again, the sample is undoubtedly unrepresentative (Chapman, 1963). It should, however, be noted that important theoretical work has been done (e.g., Itil, Keskiner & Fink, 1966; Saletu, Saletu & Itil,

1973) comparing the responses of 'therapy resistant' and 'therapy responsive' patients. These patients are operationally defined as falling in one category or the other to the extent to which medication does or does not produce clinical improvement. The definition does not directly take into account the extent to which the medication has or has not an effect because it is or is not metabolized and therefore is or is not present in blood to have a therapeutic effect (Curry, 1971).

A final strategy in dealing with the problem of medication is to arrange that patients newly contacting medical agencies be tested before therapy begins. One psychiatrist known to the author reports that he has managed to examine three unmedicated acute schizophrenic patients in the past 2 years by adopting this policy. In most cases, patients contacting the psychiatrist have already been given tranquillizers by their general practitioners. In any case, the representative nature of the population gathered in this way must be in doubt. Whatever technique is adopted is a compromise. However, comparison of data so obtained with data (perhaps imperfectly collected) from the earlier, pre-tranquillizer era, may enable some approximation to a picture to be built up.

12.1.3. 'High-risk' studies

The problem of working with adult schizophrenic patients, whether medicated or not, is not confined to psychophysiological research. Mednick & McNeil (1968) have strongly suggested that in the adult patient the condition of schizophrenia is heavily overlaid with the consequences of the illness including 'bachelorhood, misery, loneliness, educational and social disadvantages, and institutionalization'. It is thus virtually impossible to study the schizophrenic process *per se* independently of these other variables in somebody who is already a patient. With this point of view in mind the interference of medication in research is no more of a stumbling-block than others included in the list of consequences above. For these reasons, Mednick & McNeil (1968) advocate the use of 'high-risk' methodology, where the subject is studied before he shows schizophrenic pathology and before the consequents of the illness have had the opportunity to interact with the illness itself to produce an unseparable amalgam of interrelated factors. It is important at this stage to bring out a difficulty in this type of research, particularly in so far as psychophysiological measurement is at the core of the problem. The difficulty is to some extent one of definition. If the subject already, as a prepubertal child, shows *overt* psychopathological behaviour, then, to the extent that the behaviour is psychotic he is not a 'true schizophrenic' because the classic disease may be said to manifest itself only from puberty onwards. If, however, the subject manifests no 'covert' (i.e., measured for instance by psychophysiological techniques) behaviour, there is nothing to study. If he does show 'covert' abnormality, to what extent is he already reacting to that abnormality, and to what extent is his behaviour becoming a mixture of primary symptoms and reaction to those symptoms? At least it is possible to say that the interaction is less than that in the case of the manifest patient in whom the results of the disease are that people react to him in a particular way. If his pathology is 'covert' in the sense that an abnormal skin conductance response suggests that he reacts to external circumstances in a particular way then at least the interaction between the patient and his environment may be partially asymmetric.

12.1.4. Primary and secondary aspects of the disease

The undesirable consequences of the disease have been outlined in the previous section. It is important to recognize that not only does the primary disease process result in consequences which become factors bringing about the present social condition of the adult patient, but also that the present condition of the patient is also the result of his attempts to build 'crutches' in the form of defences which enable him to gain even partial mastery over his developing primary illness. The operation of these defences is learned to the extent that they are effective in preventing what would otherwise be an intolerable degree of disturbance. These defences are, however, part of the pathology—'in them, however, may be seen the elements of the disease process as it is manifest to the outside observer' (Venables, 1967). Analysing, in this way, the possibilities of interaction within the schizophrenic process, we may see at least for pragmatic purposes, the following separate stages which may be studied. Firstly, the pre-patient who, showing no, or minimal, overt signs of the disease may nevertheless show covert indications capable of being studied psychophysiologically. Secondly, there is the patient with the first early overtly recognizable signs of the disease. At this stage, the process patient having already experienced the insidious onset of disturbance may already have developed some defence systems. Thirdly, there is the reactive patient, in whom the onset of the disease follows some identifiable external stress, and may show different aspects of the disease in so far as in his case the disease is grafted on top of a more mature set of behaviours. Fourthly, there is the chronologically defined 'chronic' patient in whom the primary disease process may have abated and in whom both the overt and covert symptoms are largely aspects of secondary and learned processes.

Shakow (1971) also advocates recognition of the secondary aspects as subsidiary to the primary disease process. In addition to the secondary aspects of the disease as such, he counsels the need to include recognition of the patient's reaction to the testing situation. He suggests that there is a 'need to be sensitive in studies with schizophrenics to distinguish between defects that are blanketing and those that are basic. Both kinds of defect are important, but they must be kept sharply separated since they have quite different theoretical implications'.

12.1.5. Descriptive or theoretically oriented research

The title of this section does of course present an artificial dichotomy for what is essentially a continuum. Nevertheless, at one end of the continuum there would appear to be studies, which although perfectly justifiable in the light of the dearth of data about the psychophysiology of schizophrenia, have apparently only an aim akin to that of differential diagnosis. An example on the borderline of psychophysiology would be sedation threshold measurements which allocate different psychopathological sub-groups to positions on a continuum which might be considered to be one of 'arousal'. At the other end of the range of studies are those which start out in a more hypothetico-deductive way to suggest that clinical or experimental psychological data would lead to the proposal that with a certain kind of pathology a certain psychophysiological response pattern might be expected. Clearly, both kinds of studies are required, but it is suggested that psychophysiological studies of schizophrenia are less likely to remain outside the mainstream of psychopathological investigation if ideas from one branch of investigation fully inseminate ideas from other branches. With the points in this section in mind, the remainder of the chapter will be concerned with a more definitive examination of some of the psychophysiological data available which throws light on the mechanism of the schizopherenic disease. There is not, nor is there ever likely to be, a definitive experiment in this field. Developing knowledge would appear to be achieved through successive iteration to a hoped-for convergence where the combined weight of many pieces of evidence dictates the direction to be taken.

12.1.6. Definitions of types of activity

Before embarking upon a review of empirical data it is probably worthwhile considering three types of activity, that, for clarity, require definition and discussion. These are levels of activity, phasic activity and spontaneous activity.

12.1.6.1. Levels of activity

Data under this heading are those representing tonic levels of activity or the changes in tonic activity resulting from alterations in amounts of stimulation or situational conditions. A distinction is thus drawn between changes in ongoing tonic levels and phasic activity resulting from discrete stimulation and usually having identifiable morphological features. A word should probably be said about the definition of 'basal' levels of activity. By implication basal activity is that level which is a datum from which other activity may be measured. Except in highly sophisticated and habituated normal subjects, search for such a basal level may be illusory. Placing the subject in a laboratory probably raises the levels of psychophysiological activity above true resting levels and may do so to a different extent in schizophrenics and in normals. On the other hand, if the subject goes to sleep, another set of considerations come into play and if, for instance, the measure being examined is spontaneous electrodermal activity there will be a 'paradoxical' increase in this activity as sleep proceeds (Johnson & Lubin, 1966). The only sensible course when examining work with schizophrenic subjects would appear to be to consider as closely as possible the conditions involved in obtaining 'resting' levels and interpret the findings in this light; almost certainly no theoretically perfect 'basal' level will have been achieved.

12.1.6.2. Phasic activity

Under this head fall data resulting from the presentation of discrete stimuli. In general the resulting responses are characterized by identifiable wave-forms having temporal and magnitude characteristics. They are thus to be distinguished from change in tonic levels of activity where what is being measured is a difference in two ongoing states having relatively (in relation to phasic changes) long-term continuity. The measures which characterize any phasic response are numerous, and perusual of the literature on normal subjects gives some indication of their range. Unfortunately, not all of the aspects of response are measured in the majority of studies of schizophrenics and consequently not all the possible information which might be derived from recordings is available. Recent work on electrodermal activity tends to make use of most of the possible data but that on phasic heart rate measures seems to lag behind the available expertise provided by such workers as Uno & Grings (1965), Graham & Clifton (1966), Lacey (1967), Connor & Lang (1969), Smith & Strawbridge (1968, 1969).

In the case of EEG derived measures there is in general a close parallel in the degree of methodological expertise employed by workers using abnormal subjects and those working in non-clinical laboratories. However, one AER component which has provided considerable possibilities for integration between psychological and psychophysiological thought, the late positive component P_3 (see Sutton, Chapter 14, this volume) appears only to have been the subject of one study on schizophrenics (Roth & Cannon, 1972).

12.1.6.3. Spontaneous activity

Spontaneous activity falls in an intermediate position in relation to the two forms of activity already discussed. While, in general being definable as activity which takes the *form* of phasic responses, but without the property of having been elicited by identifiable stimuli, in many ways the use of the measure of frequency of spontaneous activity is more akin to that of a tonic level measure than one of phasic activity. In Section 2 it is described for instance how the effect of phenothiazines is most often to change tonic levels of activity and frequencies of spontaneous activity while phasic, elicited activity was not effected. In a somewhat similar way, Depue & Fowles (1973) reviewing work on electrodermal activity in schizophrenia suggest the superiority of frequency of spontaneous fluctuations over skin conductance level as a measure of 'arousal'. In a parallel fashion, as reviewed in Section 12.2.3, variability of the integrated EEG, a measure which appears analagous to spontaneous activity in autonomic systems is far more a measure of tonic status than of responsivity.

12.2. THE INFLUENCE OF MAJOR TRANQUILLIZERS ON PSYCHOPHYSIOLOGICAL MEASURES

As discussed in the previous section, a major problem with psychophysiological research in schizophrenia is the almost universal medication with tranquillizing drugs. Although other forms of medication are employed, their regular usage is not so widespread and it is therefore of less importance to deal with them than with the effects of major tranquillizers.

Tecce & Cole (1972) have recently presented an important review of the literature, which makes extended reiteration of their material unnecessary. It is, however, worthwhile at this stage pointing out some areas of particular importance against which examination of psychophysiological measures of pathology may be placed. Throughout the chapter attention is focused on electrodermal, heart rate and cortical activity and therefore the effects of tranquillizers on these systems are the main point of interest.

12.2.1. Effects of electrodermal activity

One of the clearest demonstrations of the effect of phenothiazines on skin conductance measures is the study by Spohn, Thetford & Cancro (1971). Their work is of particular interest because in addition to showing the effect of removing medication from a group of schizophrenic patients, relations between drug dosage and skin conductance measures are also examined. The study commenced with a representative group of 32 long- and short-stay schizophrenics including paranoid and non-paranoid patients, of whom 29 were receiving phenothiazine medication; in the case of 20 of these, medication was withdrawn and replaced by placebo, and of these, 15 remained without medication for 3 months. While the patients were still on drugs it was shown that their SCLs were lowered proportionally to drug dosage. (Drug dosage was equated over different phenothiazines by means of the Phenothiazines Dosage Index (PDI), Spohn et al., 1971). When patients were taken off medication their SCL increased, and did so in comparison to those patients in whom medication was continued. SCL in the patients from whom medication was withdrawn was found to increase to a level higher than that of 16 normal controls who also took part in the study.

In the case of SCRs to specific stimuli, frequency of response was inversely proportional to drug dosage but when the effect of the relation between SCL and drug dosage was partialed out, the relation between SCR frequency and drug dosage was insigificant. When medication was withdrawn there was an increase in frequency of SCRs but the relation between SCL and SCR which was present under medication disappeared. No evidence was found of effect of medication on SCR amplitude.

In the case of non-specific skin conductance responses or spontaneous fluctuations, there was, however, an increase in the number of fluctuations on drug withdrawal.

The general conclusions from this study would, therefore, seem to be that phenothiazines appear to effect those aspects of electrodermal activity which might be considered to reflect *tonic* levels of arousal, that is, SCL and numbers of spontaneous fluctuations (see Depue & Fowles (1973) for a recent statement on this point). However, there would seem to be no effect of phenothiazine upon phasic activity, i.e. specific SCRs.

The study by Spohn *et al.* has been reviewed in some detail because it presents a particularly clear picture against which other studies can be compared. Goldstein, Acker, Crockett & Riddle (1966) working with a chronic schizophrenic population, randomly allocated members of the group to drug (thiordizane) or placebo status, and examined electrodermal activity during the presentation of movie films. Unfortunately, the SCL data are not presented in a manner which makes direct comparison with other studies possible, although the indication is one of reduced tonic reactivity under medication In a later study Goldstein, Rodnick, Jackson, Evans, Bates & Judd (1972) used a population of acute schizophrenic patients, allocated to drug or placebo status and showed a higher skin resistance level (i.e., reduced SCL) in the drugged patients.

Interestingly, in view of the caveat suggested in Section 12.1.2 of the possible interaction artefact in examining the effect of drugs on different sub-groups of patients, Goldstein *et al.* (1972) say that as far as electrodermal reactivity is concerned 'goods' on drugs become more reactive, 'goods' on placebo less reactive, while the reverse pattern was true for 'poors'. A similar pattern of findings is shown by Magaro (1973) who found that phenothiazine medication decreased SCR amplitude for patients rated as 'poor' (Phillips, 1953), and also for paranoid schizophrenics, but increased SCR amplitudes for patients rated as 'good'. If in these two studies only those patients on drugs had been examined and the drug dosages received by the groups had not been significantly different: then a statement might have been made that 'good' premorbid patients were more reactive than 'poor' premorbid patients. Interaction of this kind can clearly lead to false conclusions.

Pugh (1968), in a study of schizophrenic women medicated with chlorpromazine showed a significant reduction in spontaneous GSRs with medication. This was accompanied by a fall in SCL but due to a fall in SCL of comparable magnitude over the same period in control patients, this effect was not significant. As far as reactivity is concerned there was, in line with the Spohn *et al.* data, no change in the numbers of specific SCRs, although there was a reduction in SCR amplitude with chlorpromazine medication. Pugh's patients were of chronic status and not sub-divided.

Bernstein (1964, 1967) in studies of the electrodermal orienting response and tonic arousal level provides data to show that while tonic levels and the reactivity shown by changes in tonic level in response to stimulation are diminished by phenothiazines, there appear to be no significant drug effects on OR. He does not, however, examine the interaction between his 'remitted' and 'regressed' schizophrenic allocation and drug states which might suggest whether there is a parallel to the differential reactivity of 'goods' and 'poors' shown by Goldstein *et al.* (1972) and Magaro (1973). An indication of some similarity of effect, however, is shown in his 1967 data where there is a trend for there to be a smaller number of spontaneous fluctuations under phenothiazines in a group which might be similar to 'poors' (LO.MRS) but this effect was not shown in the HI.MRS group who might be similar to 'goods'. LO.MRS and HI.MRS refer to extreme scores on the Montrose Rating Scale (Rackow, Napoli, Klebanoff & Schillinger, 1953). However, as Bernstein notes in his study the drug status was that determined by clinical requirements and was not an experimental variable, hence confounding of drug status and sub-diagnosis is highly likely.

Further data are reviewed by Tecce & Cole (1972) and these together with the studies covered here suggest a major effect of lowering by phenothiazines of electrodermal activity indicative of tonic level of function i.e. SCL and spontaneous SCRs, while there is a minimal data showing an effect on elicited phasic activity. The data showing a possible differential effect with patients in the good/poor, reactive/process category clearly needs to be born in mind for future study. It is worthwhile noting at this point that no data appear to be available on the effect of phenothiazines on the latency or recovery time of the SCR. As the latter, particularly, appears to be of particular relevance with work on schizophrenics this is an unfortunate absence of information.

12.2.2. Effects on heart rate

As with electrodermal data, it is convenient to take the data of Spohn *et al.* (1971) as an initial example. Their HR data was collected at the same time as the electrodermal data and thus the experimental conditions described earlier are applicable. Data are available for 5 beats pre-stimulus and 5 beats post-stimulus. The very small number of post-stimulus beats sampled allows only limited conclusions to be drawn as it is to be expected from work on normal subjects (e.g., Smith & Strawbridge, 1968; 1969) that information may be obtained from the HR record up to 15 beats post-stimulus. For patients on phenothiazines, 'peak' heart rate scores, i.e., the fastest HR either pre- or post-stimulus was not related to dosage; however, 'low' HRs, i.e. the slowest rate pre- or post-stimulus was. Small variability in peak HRs suggests that no dosage effect was found with peak HRs because the operation of the Law of Initial Values (LIV) allowed no increases in HR from already high levels. A decline in both 'peak' and 'low' HRs was shown after drug withdrawal to a level which nevertheless remained higher than that of normal controls. A measure of 'cyclic variability' (i.e., peak-low HRs) was negatively correlated to drug dosage and remained so even when the effect of 'low' HR was removed by partial correlation. An increase in variability was shown on drug withdrawal. HR response, i.e. HR peak pre-stimulus–HR peak post-stimulus showed no effect of medication. In both normals and controls the response was one of deceleration, an appropriate response to stimuli composed of tachistoscopically exposed visual displays (Lacey, 1967). The general finding from this study is that phenothiazines raise tonic levels of HR and reduce non-specific variability, due possibly to the operation of the LIV. Specific HR orientation appears to be unaffected by medication. These results, therefore, provide a partial parallel to those from the electrodermal system in that it is the tonic levels of both variables which are affected by medication and not specific phasic activity.

Goldstein *et al.* (1966) interpreted their findings on a study of 40 chronic schizophrenic patients divided at random for allocation to drug or placebo status, as suggesting that phenothazines reduce HR acceleratory activity resulting from anxiety provoking stimuli. This result was also shown in a study by Goldstein & Acker (1967) where higher levels of basal HR under phenothiazine were also reported. These studies replicate findings by Acker (1965) showing higher HRs under phenothiazine than placebo and reduced tonic HR reactivity in a word-association test. Spiegel & Keith-Spiegel (1967) differentiating between types of medication showed an increase in tonic HR in a group of schizophrenics on chlorpromazine as compared to previous placebo level, while patients on carphenazine and trifluophenazine showed a decrease in tonic HR under similar circumstances.

The finding of increased tonic HR under chlorpromazine and possibly other phenothiazine medication seems well-established. The effect of phenothiazines on responsivity would appear from the data available to depend on the nature of the stimuli used. With anxiety provoking stimuli, such as films or words in a word-association task, there would seem to be a reduction of responsivity which appears to be in the accelerative direction in patients on phenothiazine medication. In the absence of studies using discrete stimuli and fairly standardized ways of reporting HR responses, the data are, however, equivocal. Where the stimuli brought about an HR deceleration, i.e. a defensive response was shown by neither normals nor schizophrenics, phenothiazine medication, as might be expected, brought about no change in responsivity (Spohn *et al.*, 1971).

12.2.3. Effects on cortical activity

The data in this area present a problem. In so far as electroencephalography in use with patient subjects is often more a clinically oriented tool rather than a source of data for theoretical studies, there is a tendency for the available data to be collected in ways that are not so easily aligned with those presented in the previous two sections. Furthermore, the patterns of data, arising from visual analysis of EEG recordings, from some form of automatic analysis (e.g., integration), or from more sophisticated computer-based techniques (e.g., the averaged evoked response) are not easily encompassed in a consistent manner.

Fink (1963, 1973) presents data arising from traditional clinical EEG analyses. He states that 'antipsychotic compounds which are associated with sedation' are characterized by decreased fast waves, a regularity of EEG rhythms ('synchronization') and increased slow waves or increased alpha activity. In the case of medication by chlorpromazine, Fink reports an increase in delta (0–3·5 Hz) and theta (3·5–7·5 Hz) activity, a variable effect on alpha (7·5–13 Hz) activity and a decrease in fast beta activity (22–33 Hz). He also reports (1963) in the case of schizophrenic patients medicated with phenothiazines, that in addition to an increase in slow wave activity there may also be a slowing of central alpha frequencies by 1 Hz or more. The work of Serafetinides (1972, 1973) presents an interesting extension of this area of study by showing that there are voltage laterality shifts in some schizophrenic patients treated with antipsychotic medication. 'Such shifts were consistent; the left side of the brain (dominant for speech) gaining voltage as a result of drug (especially chlorpromazine) administration or clinical improvement'. Improvement in clinical status in a disease particularly associated with deficiencies in speech and thought processes, in conjunction with voltage increase in the left hemisphere, where other studies tend to show voltage increase to be associated with effective medication is certainly worthy of further investigation. The method of measurement of the EEG used by Serafetinides is the planimetric method of Bruck (1962) for the determination of voltage. The integration method of Drohocki (1948) used by Goldstein and his colleagues may be though of as an automatic equivalent to Bruck's method.

Two measures are available from the Drohocki integrator, both are derived from unfiltered EEG and thus represent the activity in all frequency bands present at the time of integration. The integrator may be classified as a 'constant reset level' type (Shaw, 1967) and produces a series of pulses, the frequency of which can be considered as proportional to the cumulative energy of the EEG trace. If the mean energy content (MEC) of successive time intervals is obtained, then the variation of this mean energy content expressed as a coefficient of variation (CV) is a further parameter of measurement. Using this system, Sugarman, Goldstein, Murphree, Pfeiffer & Jenney (1964) examined the effect of long-term administration of chlorpromazine, perphenazine and placebo in a group of chronic schizophrenic patients. It was shown that the effect of phenothiazines was to increase the variability of the integrated EEG and that this increase was accompanied by an improvement in the patients' clinical status. A somewhat paradoxical finding was that of an association between a decrease in mean energy content of the EEG associated with clinical improvement after medication. This finding is peculiar in so far as low MEC has been shown to characterize chronic schizophrenic patients (Goldstein, Murphree, Sugarman, Pfeiffer & Jenney, 1963; Goldstein, Sugarman, Stolberg, Murphree & Pfeiffer, 1965). Further, if the results reported by Fink of an increase in low frequency activity of the EEG following phenothiazine administration are also taken into account an increase in energy content under medication might be expected. The effect of antipsychotic drugs on the averaged evoked response (AER) of schizophrenics appears to be reasonably consistent. It is generally found that phenothiazine induced AER changes occur predominantly in the late components, while the early primary part of the response is relatively unaffected (Ciganek, 1959; Shagass & Schwartz, 1965). Heninger & Speck (1966) showed an increase in latency of the visual evoked response in schizophrenics treated with trifluoperazine and chlorpromazine. This result was confirmed and extended by Saletu, Saletu, Itil & Marasa (1971), and Saletu, Saletu & Itil (1973), who showed an increase in latency and a decrease in amplitude of somatosensory, auditory and visual evoked responses during haloperidol, thiothixene and fluphenazine treatment after 2 months maintenance on placebo. These changes were shown markedly in those patients classed on the basis of clinical change as therapy responsive, but were minimal, or even in the contrary direction in those classed as therapy resistant. A contrary finding is presented by Jones, Blacker, Callaway & Layne (1965) who showed that there was an increase in the amplitude of the AER in those patients who improved with phenothiazine treatment.

This section on the effect of phenothiazine medication has been introduced before considering the data on psychophysiological characteristics of schizophrenic patients in order that the effects of these drugs should be borne in mind in the interpretation of available data. The general findings seem to indicate that the main effect of phenothiazine medication is to change tonic activity, to lower SCL, to raise tonic heart rate and possibly to change those indicants of cortical activity in a direction which suggests a lowering of tonic arousal. There appears to be no effect of tranquillizing medication upon the orienting aspects of autonomic activity, however, in so far as the heart rate accelerating response appears to be reduced, defensive activity appears reduced by medication. At this state in our knowledge it would not appear to be possible to accommodate changes in AERs in this summary statement.

12.3. PSYCHOPHYSIOLOGICAL CHARACTERISTICS OF SCHIZOPHRENIC PATIENTS

An approach to the psychophysiology of schizophrenia depends to a large extent upon the theoretical stance from which one starts. Given a point of view which states that there is some unitary basic defect which characterizes all schizophrenics it might be possible to ask such a question as: Are schizophrenics as a whole more or less aroused than normals? Starting from the position that schizophrenia is an umbrella term for different sub-groupings within the basic diagnostic category then a possible question which might be asked is: Have process patients different psychophysiological characteristics from reactive patients? On the other hand, an interactive point of view is possible which suggests that a patient's psychophysiological state at any one time is a function not only of his fundamental pathology but also the situational and stimulus condition under which he is tested. Nor will this function always be tidily linear as might be expected with a person with a 'strong nervous system' obeying the 'law of strength', rather, if following the Pavlovian (1941) notion that schizophrenics are characterized by 'weak nervous system' we might expect that under certain situational circumstances there would be a decrease in activity in certain psychophysiological indices as the impact of external factors increased. A version of this type of approach is that of Epstein (1967, 1970), Epstein & Coleman (1970), where it is suggested that the basic defect in schizophrenia is an inadequately modulated inhibitory system which gives rise to a tendency for the patient either to under-respond or over-respond. This approach leads to the supposition that schizophrenics might occupy extreme positions in either direction on continua of psychophysiological levels or reactivity if under-responding or over-responding is a relatively permanent characteristic of the patient. If these characteristics are relatively labile, however, the expectation is for a larger than normal variability in patient behaviour. This is not a new point of view, the high within and between subject variability of the schizophrenic has long been recognized and is fully reviewed by Shakow (1963) and Silverman (1967).

Even if the investigation recognizes that schizophrenics' data tend to oocupy the extremes of continua the question may still be asked, how far is it possible to identify with labels derived from clinical or experimental observations the patients who tend to occupy one or the other extreme position? Or, more pessimistically, is the ultimate analytic stance to be that the only constancy in schizophrenic behaviour is extreme variability? A final question which must be approached is to what extent do any of the theoretical positions outlined above depend on the particular psychophysiological or behavioural variable which is measured. Undoubtedly, sufficient is known about the physiological bases of the two most investigated variables, cardiovascular and electrodermal activity to suggest that they cannot be expected to co-vary together and that therefore a simple 'unitary arousal' type of approach is not likely to be productive.

12.3.1. Skin conductance

12.3.1.1. Tonic levels

Lang & Buss (1965) reviewing studies of 'basal skin resistance' in schizophrenic patients up to that time, point to the general apparent inconsistency of findings, a similar conclusion about the lack of unanimity of results using tonic levels of conductance is reached in a recent review by Depue & Fowles (1973), in which they advocate the use of the habituation rate of orienting response and frequency of spontaneous electrodermal responses as measures which 'appear to reflect arousal and yield results indicating that chronic schizophrenics are over-aroused'. If the techniques which are used for measuring skin conductance are not themselves productive of error variance (Lykken & Venables, 1971; Montagu, 1973; Venables & Christie, 1973) and the fundamental phenomenon of schizophrenia is not random lability then a lack of consistency of findings on levels of conductance should indicate either that there is insufficient control (or knowledge) of important subject, situational, stimulus or temporal variables or that skin conductance level is irrelevant as a measure in this area. While it is not impossible that the latter conclusion may regrettably be correct, sufficient optimism has been generated and sufficient investment made in the use of the measure over the past 80 years to suggest that it is lack of understanding of experimental variables that is the crux of the issue. The very fact that electrodermal activity produces inconsistent results while, for instance, cardiovascular activity is much more consistent (Broen, 1968) may reflect the fact that electrodermal activity is in a way a more complicated or more sensitive indicator than cardiovascular activity. One point of view which would support this is that whereas cardiovascular activity is clearly a vital system, constrained within fairly narrow limits by dual innervation from both branches of the ANS, a fact which is indicated by the general applicability of the 'Law of Initial Values' in this area, electrodermal activity, as measured, is an epiphenomenon of the activity of several systems. While it would be unthinkable to suggest that these systems did not have vital function and were just provided by kindly nature as a convenient 'one-way screen' for psychophysiologists the fact that a major source of variance is from singly innervated eccrine sweat glands does potentially allow for a greater range of variability than is the case with cardiovascular activity.

Central control of electrodermal activity is supra-segmental (Wang, 1957, 1958) and reflects activity at spinal, reticular, limbic and cortical levels; in addition there is some control by circulating steroid hormones (Venables & Christie, 1973). It is therefore suggested that studies which attempt to use electrodermal activity require that considerable attention be paid to a particularly wide range of factors which may influence the activity.

It is at this point worthwhile examining some further studies concerned with tonic levels of SC activity which have appeared since Lang & Buss's review in 1965. Bernstein (1967) presents results of a study on chronic schizophrenic patients divided into four groups depending on drug states (on or off phenothiazines), and on their position on the Montrose Rating Scale (MRS). Patients scoring low on the MRS were described as in the following terms 'wholly or partially disoriented, regressed disorganized, tangential, incoherent speech (autism in some), and physical untidiness'. Patients scoring high, on the other hand, were 'well oriented, in good contact with logical thought, coherent, with well-organized speech and were largely symptom free'. The scale has thus some affinities with the process-reactive, poor-premorbid–good premorbid dichotomies. In resting conditions, prior to visual stimulation, the high MRS patients who were not on drugs had a higher SC level than controls, the low MRS patients not on drugs did not differ from controls. Both schizophrenic samples not on drugs showed greater tonic reactivity to visual stimulation than normals or patients on drugs. In a study by Ax, Bamford, Beckett, Fretz & Gottlieb (1970) of skin conductance levels during conditioning, in a group of 28 chronic drug free schizophrenics, there was an overall tendency for the schizophrenics to have significantly higher levels of SC than normals. Zahn, Rosenthal & Lawlor (1968) in a study basically designed to investigate orienting responses, also showed a higher level of SC in 52 chronic schizophrenic patients than in normals. All patients were drug free at the time of testing. Magaro (1972) carried out a study on 72 schizophrenic patients divided into acute versus chronic and 'good' versus 'poor' (Phillips, 1953). The patients were on different amounts of medication but a correlational analysis showed no significant relation between basal conductance and level of medication. Results, on examination of the tonic level data show a significant poor–good effect 'due to the "poors" exhibiting a higher basal level than the "goods" which was mainly due to an exceedingly high conductance exhibited by the acute "poors"'. Evidence since 1965 from well-conducted studies thus tends to point to a higher than normal level of skin conductance in some schizophrenics. Nevertheless, the literature undoubtedly contains evidence which suggests that the skin conductance of some schizophrenic patients is lower than normal. Some of the earliest studies by Syz (1926), Syz & Kinder (1928), report lower than normal SCLs in catatonic patients. This type of finding is in general accord with the findings of low sympathetic tonus in schizophrenics reported in the Russian literature which is reviewed by Lynn (1963).

There would seem to be at least three possible explanations for the discrepant findings in this area. One is suggested by Lykken & Maley (1968) who on finding that both 'the maximum and minimum SC values produced by the schizophrenics were some 70 to 80 per cent higher than those of non-psychotic patients' suggested that 'the schizophrenics were simply less relaxed during the rest periods and more excited during the stress periods than were the control subjects'. The first possiblity, therefore, is that the schizophrenic reacts more markedly to the conditions of the experimental situation than the normal. All that we know about subject–experimenter interaction in experimentation with normal subjects (see Chapter 3) may be magnified with schizophrenics. The second possibility is that the relation of SCL to the objective impact of the situational and stimulus parameters of the testing situation is non-linear. In other words that the SCL decreases after a certain point as stress increases. This is a point of view which follows directly from a Pavlovian interpretation of the schizophrenic as being characterized by a 'weak nervous system' and consequently being prone to develop protective inhibition and consequently to show 'paradoxical effects'. This has been found in the case of work using reaction time measures to a range of stimuli of varying intensity by Venables & Tizard (1956; 1958) where on the first occasion of testing with visual stimuli slower RTs were made to higher than to moderate intensity stimuli. Gruzelier, Lykken & Venables (1972) provide data which shows the paradoxical lowering of skin conductance level with increased activation very clearly. In two experiments, skin conductance level, skin potential level, heart rate and two flash threshold were measured in chronic schizophrenic patients, divided into paranoids and non-paranoids and in a male nurse control group; both patient groups were on phenothiazine medication. Measurements were taken under three activation conditions, rest, pedalling an exercise bicycle under no load, and pedalling under load. Heart rate increased linearly over the three activation conditions in patients and normals and this was also the case with skin potential; however, while the SCL for normals and paranoid schizophrenics increased over activation conditions, that for the non-paranoid patients fell so that while the SCL under resting conditions did not distinguish any patients from controls, the SCL of non-paranoid schizophrenics under high activation conditions was much lower than that of normals or paranoids. It is noteworthy that the fall in SCL in non-paranoid schizophrenics occurs in conditions of high muscular activity, and it is in the case of catatonic patients where there is major muscular involvement that the early studies show low values of SCL.

The third possiblity for the interpretation of inconsistent SCL results with schizophrenic patients, which is not incompatible with the two suggestions which have been made previously, is that of sampling. It has already been shown, for instance, in the Bernstein (1970) data that his high MRS patients not on drugs showed a higher than normal SCL in comparison to low MRS patients not on drugs (when the same types of patients were under pheno-thiazine medication, however, the low MRS patients had SCLs below normal, while the high MRS patients did not differ from normals).

Recent data (Gruzelier & Venables, 1972; Gruzelier, 1973a) has indicated, however, that differences in SCL may occur within a schizophrenic sample and not be related to sub-classifications commonly employed in clinical practice. It was found that in a large heterogeneous group of schizophrenics, both institutionalized and non-institutionalized, that approximately half showed no SC orienting response to moderate intensity non-signal tones. The other half of the experimental population showed orienting responses but these, in contrast to those of normal subjects, did not habituate within the 15 present-ations during which all normals habituated to a criterion of three consecutive zero responses. The two groups of 'non-responding' and 'responding' schizo-phrenic patients did not differ in age, length of institutionalization, degree of medication or in terms of any of the usually employed psychiatric sub-categories. The SCLs of the two groups did, however, differ markedly. The non-institutionalized and institutionalized responders had SCLs higher than normal, although this was not significant in the case of the latter group, both types of non-responders, however, had significantly lower SCLs than normal. Although not differing on routine psychiatric categories it was found that on Wittenborn (1968) scale ratings the responder group was significantly higher on anxiety, psychotic beligerence, attention-demanding and assaultive be-haviour; they were also rated as being more manic. The groups did not differ on the withdrawal scale; but this contains items referring to both passive and active withdrawal and the results may thus be ambiguous; neither did they differ on the scales of flatness of affect and apathy which may characterize schizophrenics in general. It may be that the two groups are best distinguished on behavioural activity and interaction with the environment which may parallel the distinction between Bernstein's high MRS (responder) and low MRS (non-responder) groups. On the other hand, within the total institutionalized group, all of whom were on phenothiazines, there were positive correlations between aspects of schizophrenic behaviour (Wittenborn ratings) and skin conductance levels suggesting that the more severe the illness the higher the SCL. These correlations with SCL were hebephrenia 0.54, silliness 0.63; resistance 0.60; motoric 0.48; all being significant with $P < 0.05$.

12.3.1.2. Phasic activity

There are several aspects of the phasic response. The parameters of the response itself are latency, time to peak amplitude, recovery time (or rate) and amplitude, while other measures are concerned with the extent to which the response habituates over successive evocations. In general it may be said that there is a conflict in the results reported in the literature. As examples, two sets of studies carried out on apparently comparable groups of patients tend to draw opposite conclusions. These are the experiments of Bernstein (1964; 1969; 1970) and Zahn (1964), and of Zahn et al. (1968).

Bernstein (1964) describes a study carried out on 60 'regressed' and 60 'remitted' schizophrenics and 48 normal controls. Half of each of the schizophrenic groups was on phenothiazines and half were not. The subjects were presented with a 1-sec flash of light repeated 10 times at intervals of between 15 and 60 sec, half the subjects received 5-ft-candle intensity and half 25-ft-candle flashes. Regressed schizophrenics showed impaired reactivity, half of this group failing to respond at all to the first trial. Both remitted and regressed groups of schizophrenics habituated more rapidly than controls although the remitted schizophrenics were otherwise not differentiated from controls. There was no difference in OR reactivity which was attributable to medication. Bernstein's findings were extended (1969, 1970) by an examination of the OR to auditory stimuli of three intensities 60, 75 and 90 dB. As with the earlier experiment only half the sicker patients (now called 'confused') showed an OR on the first presentation of the 60 dB tone although 89 per cent responded to the first presentation of a 75 dB tone, and at 90 dB there was no difference between the early trial responsivity of schizophrenics or controls. The less sick patients (now called 'clear') were indistinguishable from the controls in early responsivity. However, both clear and confused patients in general habituated more rapidly than did controls over the range of intensities studied. The dichotomy 'clear vs confused' extended over the diagnostic range although there were more paranoids in the former category and more hebephrenics in the latter. However, Bernstein makes the point that the electrodermal hyporeactivity is related to 'confusion' and not to a particular diagnostic subcategory. It should also be noted that it is only in phasic reactivity that impairment is found, as outlined earlier in Sction 12.3.1.1, unmedicated schizophrenics showed greater *tonic* responsivity than normal (Bernstein, 1967). It is thus apparently only to specific discrete signals that 'confused' chronic schizophrenics are under-active, tonic reactivity suggests that they are able to 'maintain sensitivity towards the general demand characteristics of their environment' (Bernstein, 1970).

In contrast to these findings of Bernstein; Zahn and his colleagues (1964, 1968) report in studies carried out under very similar conditions and with patients similar to those of Bernstein that the most striking finding with regard to specific (orienting) electrodermal responses was their '*slow habituation in the schizophrenic group*' (reviewers italics). Zahn's experiments involved 52 chronic schizophrenic patients none of whom were medicated and examined their electrodermal (and heart rate) responses to 1 sec presentations of a 15-W red bulb or a 300-Hz, 72-dB tone. The report states that the stimuli were presented at 30-sec intervals, and it is possible in this that the difference between the Zahn and the Bernstein results lie. While Bernstein's presentation of stimuli was at irregular times, that of Zahn, being regular, may have brought about a temporal conditioning which maintained responsivity. Zahn did note that there was a dichotomy among his patients with some who gave few and some many responses. However, on matching a group of schizophrenics to a group of controls on mean and range of total response frequency the habituation rate was still slower for the schizophrenics than the controls. It is also interesting to note that somewhat similarly to Bernstein, Zahn *et al.* (1968) report that the percentage of subjects giving trial ORs to the light are 55 per cent for the patients and 50 per cent for the controls, and for the tone 67 per cent for the patients and 95 per cent for the controls. Also in accord with Bernstein, Zahn *et al.* report that responsivity was highest among paranoids and least among hebephrenics, respectively over- and under-represented in Bernstein's 'clear' and 'confused' categories. In contrast to Bernstein, however, Zahn *et al.* suggest that 'there are several indications in the present data that the schizophrenics 'advantage' in responsivity is greater when the stimuli are *weak*', in that the normals habituate more quickly to a weak stimuli.

The data presented by Gruzelier (1973a) and Gruzelier & Venables (1972, 1973) provide a resolution, of a kind, for the conflicting data presented by Zahn & Bernstein. These data have been introduced in the previous section; in short, in a heterogeneous group of schizophrenics approximately half show orienting to tones of 75 dB, or 85 dB intensity (1000 Hz, 1-sec duration) and these patients showed no habituation over the 15 stimulus presentations during which normals habituated. The other 50 per cent of schizophrenic patients showed no orientation at all, neither to the first nor to subsequent stimuli. Equally represented among both 'responders' and 'non-responders' were non-institutionalized (mean hospitalization 0·8 years) and institutionalized patients (mean hospitalization 17·1 years) both groups being on phenothiazine medication at dosage levels which did not distinguish the groups. Subdiagnostic differences did not distinguish the responders from the nonresponders. In a later experiment Gruzelier & Venables (1973), after an habituation experiment had been carried out with the above results, tones of two frequencies were presented to the subject. One indicated that a bar press was required and was designated as a signal tone, the other required no action and was designated as neutral. Subjects were designated as responders or non-responders on the basis of their performance on an initial habituation series of tones. It was found that although still not responding (or only minimally) to the neutral tone, the non-responders did in fact respond to the signal tone while the responders of course continued to respond. This experiment suggests that the lack of responsivity to the neutral tone in the non-responding group is in no way due to peripheral factors. One explanation for diminished responsivity which has been suggested in the past (e.g., Venables, 1964) has been the invocation of the 'law of initial value', however, the finding, previously reported (in Section 12.3.1.1) of a lower SCL in the non-responding group would refute this explanation in its usual form.

These experiments suggest that a resolution of the Zahn and Bernstein finding is possibly a matter of sampling, and possibly a matter of the significance with which their patients endowed the stimuli which were presented. The influence of instructions is very strong. To achieve the finding of 50 per cent of responders and 50 per cent non-responders the patients were instructed just to listen to the tones and do nothing. It was found that if otherwise non-responding patients for instance counted the number of stimuli presented they tended to give responses to these stimuli. In spite of the apparent discrepancy between the Zahn and Bernstein studies it is worth noting that they both report a degree of initial non-responsiveness which is similar to that reported by Gruzelier & Venables. The extent to which there is, or is not, subsequent habituation of responses to non-signal stimuli may be a function of the extent to which re-orientation is possible, this may very well depend on the availability of extraneous stimulation in the testing situation and may also, as is suggested earlier, be related to the extent to which anticipatory response are facilitated by regular rather than irregular sequences of stimuli. Neither Zahn nor Bernstein reported on any of the temporal characteristics of the responses in their studies. Gruzelier & Venables (1972, 1973) measured latency of responses and showed that schizophrenics had shorter latencies than normal with non-institutionalized patients having shorter latencies than chronic patients within the schizophrenic group.

One of the characteristics of apparent potential usefulness in distinguishing schizophrenics from normals is the recovery time of the response, which bearing in mind that the decay is exponential, is usually measured as the time taken for the responses to recover from half of its peak amplitude. This is a measure which has been used by Mednick & Schulsinger (1968) to distinguish in a prospective study among those children in schizophrenic mothers those who in later years would suffer a schizophrenic breakdown from those who would not. Ax & Bamford (1970) report that chronic schizophrenic patients, like the 'breaking-down' children in the Mednick & Schulsinger study, had a faster rate of recovery than normal. Gruzelier & Venables (1972) reported a faster recovery in non-institutionalized schizophrenics than controls, the institutionalized patients had a slightly faster recovery rate than normals but this was not significant. A similar result is also reported by Gruzelier & Venables (1973). The availability of responses on which to measure recovery rate means that they are characteristic of the group of patients who show slow habituation. Working with normals, Edelberg (1970) reports the significant association of slow habituation with fast electrodermal recovery. If, as Bagshaw, Kimble & Pribram (1965) suggest, the SCR is an index of registration of stimulus material in a 'Sokolovian' (Sokolov, 1963) neural model, then a short period of registration which might be indicated by an SCL with a fast recovery would bring about a slower build-up of the neural model with greater possibilities for re-orientation and apparently slower habituation. On the other hand, Edelberg (1972) and Furedy (1972) provide data which indicates that a long recovery occurs in situations where a 'defensive', 'closed attentional gate' posture is taken by the subject. The reverse of this is an 'open attentional gate' position which might be indicated by a fast recovery limb and would suggest that the mechanisms by which slow habituation occurs in conjunction with fast recovery is that too wide a range of attention brings about continual mismatch with the neural model and consequently continuing orientation. A fast recovery limb indicating an 'open gate' position would accord with those theorists, e.g. Broen (1966, 1968), McGhie (1969), Venables (1971) who suggest an over-wide range of attention as a characteristic of schizophrenia.

12.3.1.3. Spontaneous activity

Depue & Fowles (1973) suggest, in addition to rate of habituation of responses being a measure which indicates that chronic schizophrenics are over-aroused, that frequency of spontaneous activity yields consistent results. In general, the data which they cite does show a higher level of spontaneous activity in schizophrenics than in normals and will not be reiterated here. Again, however, the results of the study by Gruzelier & Venables (1972) show a difference with the schizophrenic sample divided into responders and non-responders on the basis of their elicited phasic activity. The 'responding' patients had higher spontaneous fluctuation frequencies than controls who again had higher spontaneous fluctuation frequencies than 'non-responders'. It is necessary, however, to bear in mind that all the patients in the Gruzelier & Venables (1972) study were on phenothiazines. While the average dosages of medication for the responder and non-responder groups did not differ, it may be that the extent to which the medication was effective did distinguish the groups and that spontaneous fluctuation frequency, as well as tonic SCL was lowered in the non-responder group by the action of phenothiazines as outlined in Section 2.1.

12.3.1.4. Lateral asymmetry in activity

Syz (1926) noted an asymmetry of electrodermal activity of catatonic schizophrenics which was twice as high as normal controls, the direction of the asymmetry was not reported. Dykman, Reese, Galbrecht, Ackerman & Sunderman (1968) also reported a tendency towards larger than normal bilateral differences in skin resistance levels in a heterogeneous group of schizophrenic patients; the asymmetry was found to be in both directions.

Gruzelier (1973b) as part of the series of studies already reported investigated the phenomena of asymmetry of electrodermal activity. Subjects were divided as before into responders and non-responders, and into non-institutionalized patients. Fewer responses were found from the left hand in the institutionalized responder group and in three patients there was a mixed pattern with absence of response from the left hand and response from the right which were slow to habituate. In the case of skin conductance level SCL was higher on the right for the responder group and on the left for the non-responders. There were no differences in lateral incidence of spontaneous fluctuations. Under the conditions of the experiment bilateral differences in orienting response frequency and SCLs were not shown in the normal control group. Gruzelier & Venables (1973) in the experiment previously reported on responses to signal versus neutral tones, found that there were higher rates of responding on the right hand to signal tones in the non-responder group (so defined on the basis of their non-response to neutral tones) and to neutral tones in the responder group. Laterality differences, on the whole, were less pronounced when the tones had signal value, suggesting possibly that the signal value of the tone required particular involvement of an otherwise less involved hemisphere. Alternatively, it may be suggested (e.g., Murphy & Venables, 1971) that direction of laterality of function is related to the general 'arousal' level of the subject and that the reason why SCL was higher on the left hand in the non-responder group was that they had an overall lower level of SCL than the responder group. In fact, in the experiment with signal tones (Gruzelier & Venables, 1973) all SCLs were higher than in the earlier experiment and under these circumstances both responders and non-responders had higher right hand than left hand SCLs.

12.3.2. Skin potential

Although in many cases skin potential is treated as an indicant of electro-dermal activity that is closely parallel to skin conductance, consideration of the mechanisms involved (Venables & Christie, 1973) suggests that there are marked differences particularly in peripheral factors and in the extent to which hormonal activity may be involved.

The study of Gruzelier, Lykken & Venables (1972) showing that the skin potential and skin conductance levels of non-paranoid schizophrenics behave in a very different way under states of behavioural activity underlines this point. Whereas the SCL of non-paranoid patients tended to fall with increased activation the SPL continued to rise. It is evident, therefore, that statements which group SCL and SPL as though they were the same may be erroneous.

In the case of phasic activity there may, however, not be such a clear distinction, while the SPR, being multiphasic, is difficult to quantify, it rarely appears in in absence of a concomitant SCR.

12.3.2.1. Tonic levels

There are no data to suggest that schizophrenics differ from normals on measures of SPL. The data in Venables (1963) show that the SPL of two groups of non-paranoid, and one group of paranoid chronic schizophrenics and two groups of normal subjects are not significantly different from each other. Lykken & Maley (1968) present data showing SPLs in a group of schizophrenics which do not differ from those of a group of controls (non-schizoprenic patients). Gruzelier, Lykken & Venables (1972) also provide data which suggest that no difference in SPL exists between schizophrenics and normals, as do Ax *et al.* (1970). Within the schizophrenic group, however, the picture is different. Venables & Wing (1962) replicated the results of three earlier unpublished studies, in showing that SPL was positively related to withdrawal (Venables, 1957) in non-paranoid patients. SPL and withdrawal, however, were inversely related in coherently deluded paranoid patients. The finding with non-paranoid patients was independently replicated by Spain (1966) using the same measures. Crider, Grinspoon & Maher (1965) published data which appears to be at variance with these findings. They reported a correlation of $+0.62$ between SPL and pre-morbid adjustment measured by the Phillips (1953) scale. In so far as one might expect the least adjusted to be also the most withdrawn patients, this result is the reverse of that of Venables and his colleagues. The possibility of the effect of drug dosage is considered by Crider *et al.*, but no significant relation between drug dosage and other measures is reported.

12.3.2.2. Phasic activity

Little data appears to be available on the SPRs of schizophrenics. Venables (1960) presents an experiment on a group of chronic schizophrenic patients divided into four groups on the basis of nurses' ratings of paranoid tendency and withdrawal (Venables & O'Connor, 1959). The experiment involved the presentation of discrete, fairly intense auditory or visual stimuli, in the presence or absence of additional background stimulation. More and bigger responses with shorter latency were given by patients who were not withdrawn, under non-stimulating conditions; the responses of the groups in the presence of background stimulation were, however, indistinguishable from those of a withdrawn group in non-stimulating conditions. The study which should probably be replicated using SCR measures clearly points to the sensitivity of patient subjects to the ongoing ambient level of stimulation against which discrete stimuli are presented; and also to the need to recognize that not all schizophrenic subjects behave in the same way to the background stimulation.

12.3.3. Cardiovascular activity

By far the greatest bulk of data in this area is concerned with heart rate (HR) and other cardiovascular measures will not be considered.

12.3.3.1. Tonic levels of activity

Lang & Buss's (1965) review points to a consistent finding that levels of HR are raised in schizophrenics as compared with controls. Data since 1965 certainly support this view. Spohn *et al.* (1971) in their study, which has already been discussed (Section 2.4), reported that even when phenothiazine medication (which elevates HR) had been withdrawn, the HR of patients remained significantly higher than normal. Zahn, Rosenthal & Lawlor (1968) in the study which has previously been outlined (Section 3.1.2) also report elevated HR in the chronic unmedicated schizophrenics. Fenz & Velner (1970) also report higher than normal HRs in process and reactive schizophrenic patients, however, their patients were receiving phenothiazine medication and elevated HR may be due in part to this factor. Gruzelier & Venables (1975) report on HR levels of their patients who are also on phenothiazines. The HRs of both the SC responder and non-responder schizophrenic groups were higher than normal. These data provide a tentative resolution of the possibility that the division into SC responders and non-responders is based on the extent to which apparently equal doses of phenothiazines are differently metabolized in one group as compared to the other. If the high SCL and large spontaneous SC fluctuation frequency in the responder group was due to lack of phenothiazine influence in this group then it might be expected that the HR of this group would be lower than that of the non-responder group in whom SC activity was depressed by effectively acting phenothiazines. In so far as the HR of the responder group is, however, higher than that of the non-responder group the drug differential hypothesis appears to receive little support.

12.3.3.2. Heart rate responsivity

There is surprisingly little data in this area, in view of the rather large amount of effort that has been expended in exploring the characteristics of the HR response in normals (e.g., Graham & Clifton, 1966; Lacey, 1967). Studies with normals in general show a close connection between the perceptual or attentional status of the subject and his HR response; the generally accepted point of view that attentional deficits are found in schizophrenic patients (e.g., Venables, 1964; McGhie, 1969) would seem to suggest that more detailed studies of the HR response in schizophrenics should be undertaken. Smith (1967) in an unpublished thesis reports post-stimulus HR increases in schizophenics that were higher in withdrawn than in non-withdrawn patients. The stimuli in this case were tones ranging from 70–110 dB. Zahn *et al.* (1968) report no HR response to the very low intensity light flashes used in their experiment, however, they did report responses to their 72-dB, 300-Hz tones.

'The most usual type of response was an acceleration which peaked somewhere between the fourth and eighth beat after the stimulus, this rise was usually prededed by a deceleration over the first 1–3 beats after the stimulus'. Their data were analysed as the difference between the lowest point during the initial deceleration and the highest point of the acceleration. The data indicated a larger mean acceleration for the patients as compared to normals, which was significant only on later trials. Dykman *et al.* (1968) recorded HR and electrodermal responses to 12 repetitions of an 800-Hz, 5-sec, 60-dB tone. Following Lacey (e.g., 1967) they classify patterns of responses as 'open'—'a GSR > 800 Ω coupled with deceleration' in HR; 'closed'—'negligible decrease in SR paired with acceleration in HR' and 'alerting'—'a GSR > 800 Ω in conjunction with acceleration in HR'. The schizophenics tended to show initial 'alerting' changing to a 'closed' pattern, i.e. they tended to show a continuing acceleratory HR pattern. The normal subjects in this experiment (in this case students) also showed a preponderance of 'alerting' patterns but showed more 'open' than 'closed' patterns as compared to the schizophrenics. Russian work reported by Lynn (1963) also suggests following the reports above that in general schizophrenics give acceleratory responses to auditory stimuli which are more pronounced than is the case with normal subjects.

In the case of visual stimuli as shown earlier, Zahn *et al.* (1968) report no HR responses. Spohn *et al.* (1971), however, who examined only five beats post-stimulus report a HR deceleration in both normals and schizophrenics to visual stimuli; in this case, however, the visual material consisted of slides which undoubtedly had more attentional value than the light used by Zahn.

Gruzelier (1973a) again using the SC responders–non-responders dichotomy reports that after an initial post-stimulus deceleration over the first one or two beats shown by all subjects, there was a secondary acceleration in the SC responder groups whether 85- or 75-dB tones were used as stimuli. In non-responder groups after the initial, first component, deceleration there was a gradual return to pre-stimulus level, i.e. no response was shown. In non-schizophrenics, whose SCR habituated normally, there was a second component deceleration, which might be thought of as a normal OR. These data, therefore, seem to be in line with the rest of the literature in that when a response to tone is shown by schizophrenic patients it tends to be acceleratory. The results of work by Lobstein (1974) are in contrast to those already described. He used 1000-Hz, 1-sec, 85-dB stimuli, but in contrast to those of Gruzelier in which the rise time was uncontrolled, the rise and fall time was now 25 msec. Hatton, Berg & Graham (1970) have provided data on normal subjects which suggests that high intensity fast onset tones produce acceleration and slow onset tones deceleration. Lobstein's schizophrenics could be divided into non-responders and responders on the basis of their SCRs but the latter category also included some who both responded and habituated to criterion; all were on pheno-thiazines.

In contrast to Gruzelier's (1973a) data, SC non-responders did give HR responses, in this case marked deceleration followed by minor insignificant acceleration at beat 10. The SC responders, however, while showing significant initial deceleration also showed significant secondary acceleration at beats 10 and 11. This pattern of responding was still present in the SC responder group at the 15th trial. The most striking deviation from previous results is shown when HR responsivity to 100-dB, 1000-Hz controlled rise-time tones is examined. In this case both SC responders and non-responders show marked deceleratory patterns. In the case of the SC non-responders deceleration is immediate, in the case of the SC responders, however, there is a minor deceleration to beat 6 after which there is a major deceleration which is still present at beat 20. The response of normal subjects to an identical tone is an initial two beat acceleration followed by an acceleration to beat 6 and a subsequent small deceleration to beat 12.

These unusual findings are interpreted by Lobstein as possibly indicating a paradoxical inhibition of sympathetic activity in the schizophrenic, and especially the SC non-responding patients. If his result is replicated it suggests that HR activity indicates an unusually 'open' pattern in schizophrenics to some forms of high intensity noise, and this possibly provides a parallel to the suggestion in Section 3.1.2 that the short recovery SCRs found in schizophrenics also indicate an 'openness' to the environment.

12.3.4. Cortical activity

It is not practicable to consider work using electroencephalographic techniques in quite the same way as has been the case with electrodermal and heart-rate measures. Analysis of tonic activity is conveniently included in the consideration of the continuous EEG record, whether by traditional, 'clinical' eye-ball methods or by more sophisticated techniques. Examination of phasic activity, while including experiments in which 'alpha-blocking' is the variable under consideration, conveniently includes studies of the averaged evoked response (AER) and the 'contingent negative variation' (CNV) although this may not be taken to imply equivalence of these 'phasic' aspects. It is impossible in a chapter of this size to cover studies using AER techniques in a more than cursory fashion. A measure of the extent of the field can be made by reference to the recent review of the area by Shagass (1972).

12.3.4.1. 'The continuous EEG record'

The statement of Kiloh & Osselton (1961) that 'no particular EEG pattern can be regarded as typical of schizophrenia' is perhaps initially calculated to preclude further examination of this area. However, Davis (1942) and Hill (1957) had reported more fast or 'choppy' EEG records from schizophrenics than from a normal population. Hill had suggested that this type of record indicated the 'presence of intense continuous and abnormal activation of the cortex by sub-cortical mechanisms'.

In Section 12.2.3, the Drohocki (1948) method of integrating the continuous

EEG record which was used by Goldstein and his colleagues was described. Two measures are derived from this method, one a measure of 'mean energy content' the other a measure of the variation of this value. While the mean energy content (MEC) measure which is a function of the mean voltage of the EEG over time and summed over frequencies might seem to be a measure which would most directly be related to 'cortical arousal' (if it is cortical arousal which might distinguish schizophrenics from normals), in practice the coefficient of variation (CV) of the MEC which gives the better discrimination between schizophrenics and normals.

In one of the early studies, Goldstein, Murphree, Sugerman, Pfeiffer & Jenney (1963) showed that in a group of normal subjects the coefficient of variation of 15·4 per cent was significantly larger than that of a group of process schizophrenics where it was 8·0 per cent. In a later more extensive study, Goldstein, Sugerman, Stolberg, Murphree & Pfeiffer (1965) examined the MEC and CV of the EEG of 104 normals and 101 chronic schizophrenic patients. There were no significant differences in MEC between male normals and male patients, however, normal females showd a significantly smaller MEC than all groups. The CV was significantly smaller in schizophrenics (9·1) than normals (18·5) and was smaller in catatonics than in other schizophrenics. There were no significant trends in relation to age or length of illness. None of the patients in the study had received any medication for at least one month prior to the experiment.

Using a slightly different integrating system, Marjerrison, Krause & Keogh (1968) carried out a study very similar to those of Goldstein et al. (1963, 1965). Groups of chronic and acute schizophrenics and normals were not distinguished by a 'mean integrated amplitude' measure (the equivalent of MEC) but were significantly different on the CV measure, the normals having a higher CV than the acute schizophrenics and these in turn had a higher CV than the chronic schizophrenics. Some of the patients were on drugs and among the chronic patients drug states produced no significant effect. However, in the acute group those without medication had a higher CV than those receiving medication, but this could be an artefact of sampling. CV was shown to be consistently lower among those patients who were hallucinating than among those who were not.

The relationship of the measures used in these studies to the construct of 'arousal' is implied by for instance the study of Murphree, Jenney & Pfeiffer (1962) showing a decrease of 20 per cent in MEC and 35 per cent in CV in normal subjects under dextro-amphetamine medication. It is, of course, also in accord with the standard clinical evaluation of the EEG in which alpha desynchronization can be indicative of arousal, and it also relates to the position of Hill (1957), cited earlier, in which he suggests that the fast EEG of the schizophrenic is related to intense and *continuous* (i.e., non-variant) activation from sub-cortical centres.

Lifshitz & Gradijan (1972) point out that a decrease in alpha activity and, hence lowered MEC, is also seen with decreasing arousal from a waking state as in the initial stages of drowsiness. They, therefore, carried out a study in which analysis of delta band activity was undertaken in addition to an analysis similar to that of Goldstein and Marjerrison. They quote data from Lubin, Johnson & Austin (1969) showing that delta band activity is monotonically related to levels of arousal from sleep to wakefulness. Their study was carried out on a group of largely chronic unmedicated schizophrenics and age-matched normal controls. Their data confirm those of the earlier workers in showing a smaller CV in patients than in controls for EEG collected from occipitally placed electrodes, but not for data from other sites. They also show that there is a significant positive relation between their measure equivalent to CV and delta band intensity and that this relation is more marked in schizophrenics than controls. In considering their data as a whole, Lifschitz & Gradijan come to the opposite conclusion to the preceding workers in the field and suggest that schizophrenics are less than normally aroused and show diminished movement between the different spectral bands of the EEG and hence to either higher *or* lower levels of cortical arousal.

Using frequency analysis methods, Volovka, Matousek & Roubicek (1966) compared the EEG of a group of unmedicated schizophrenics and normal controls. They showed greater theta and alpha activity among the schizophrenics than the controls and no significant difference in the coefficient of variation of the activity in these or other bands between the two groups. This reversal of the other results described could, however, be explained by the fact that the schizophrenics were tested lying down in a quiet laboratory and the normals sitting in a 'less tranquil' laboratory. It should also be noted that of the 42 patients in this study 22 were paranoid and consequently might be excepted to produce rather different results from other non-paranoid patients. The two groups were not distinguished in the analysis of the data.

Salamon & Post (1965) while reporting no difference in alpha abundance between schizophrenics and normals when using conventional methods of measurement do show greater baseline alpha activity in schizophrenics using a more refined method. No effect of medication was shown with these patients. The data provide some support for Volovka *et al.* (1966) but overall the conclusion that must be drawn is that more or less conventional analyses of the EEG resulting in statements about 'resting' levels of activity, whether or not frequency analysis is undertaken, lead to equivocal results.

The data in this area just reviewed have not been so much concerned with voltage levels as with the extent of activity within particular frequency bands. However, although the data on integrated voltage levels is equivocal there is some tendency to suggest a lower voltage among patients than among normals. Some support for this latter position comes from work by Bruck (1964) showing that in schizophrenics having apparently normal EEGs there was a tendency for lower than normal voltages to be recorded. Serafetinides (1972, 1973) showed that improvement in clinical status of schizophrenics was accompanied by an increase in EEG voltage from left-sided leads, but not from right-sided leads; it should be noted in this context that the studies of the integrated EEG reviewed above all employed left lead placements. It can, on the basis of these studies then be suggested that perhaps the EEG index of normality using these techniques is for a variable, responsive, record. Furthermore, because greater variability can imply a greater possibility of higher amplitude activity; a higher voltage record, particularly from that hemisphere responsible for speech is also indicative of normality. Clearly, much more work could valuably be undertaken in this area.

12.3.4.2. Phasic activity: 'alpha blocking'

Analyses in terms of variability measures do provide promise in showing a lower CV among patients than controls. To extend these data, some of the limited numbers of papers on alpha-blocking will be reviewed.

McMahon & Walter first described, in 1938, two cases of schizophrenia with non-responsive alpha-activity during visual stimulation. Liberson (1945) reported less reduction in alpha in response to a light flash in schizophrenics than among neurotic patients. In contrast, Hein, Green & Wilson (1962) reported no differences in the latency and duration of alpha blocking between a group of chronic schizophrenics and a group of controls. Blum (1957) reported diminished alpha responsiveness in schizophrenics as compared to normals and that this was not related to medication status, he also reported no difference between patients and controls in the presence of resting alpha rhythm. The work of Salamon & Post (1965) has already been mentioned earlier in relation to baseline alpha activity; they also showed that schizophrenic patients in comparison to normals 'demonstrated significantly less alpha blocking, both in terms of number of alpha waves produced during stimulation and in terms of per cent alpha blocking'. In considering the effect of drugs they showed that 'the differences in the degree of alpha blocking are, for the most part, due to the lower rate of alpha blocking in those patients who had received drugs prior to the EEG'.

While, as stated above, Hein, Green & Wilson (1962) showed no difference in alpha blocking latency between schizophrenics and normals; Cromwell & Held (1969) reported that the latency of alpha blocking was slower in schizophrenics than normals while there was no difference in the RT of the two groups. However, these authors screened and rejected 23 patients who had abnormal wave patterns and per cent time alpha under 50 per cent. The seven patients who remained in the study must thus be considered highly selected. In an extension of this work, Nideffer, Deckner, Cromwell & Cash (1971) showed no relation between alpha status and RT in groups of schizophrenics and normals who did not differ on the latter variable. However, they did show that whether the eyes were open or not was a greater determinant of alpha state for schizophrenics than for normals, and that schizophrenics have only one quarter as much alpha as normals in the eye open condition. Clearly, this is an important variable and needs to be taken into account in work using

EEG measures particularly but possibly also in studies using other psycho-physiological techniques.

12.3.4.3. Phasic activity: Averaged evoked responses

As with so much work in psychology and psychiatry, work in this area tends to be concentrated in particular laboratories and the topics investigated have something of an idiosyncratic flavour. Added to this the use of different systems of nomenclature for labelling different components of the averaged evoked response (AER) do not make cross comparisons of data an easy undertaking. It is generally recognized that short latency components are reflections of primary sensory activity while the longer latency components are less specific to particular sensory modalities and may be related to other more 'psychological' variables (e.g., Wilkinson, 1967). To some extent, therefore, an examination of studies divided on the basis of the latency of the components investigated is one means of possible classification.

Pioneer work, using short latency components as the bases of analyses, has been carried out by Shagass and his colleagues, e.g. Shagass & Schwartz (1961, 1962; 1963a, b, c; 1965). Shagass, Overton & Straumanis (1972) and summarized in Shagass (1968, 1972). Two types of measurement are involved, one of these, the recovery cycle, is determined by administering pairs of stimuli separated by varying intervals, the relative size of the second compared to the first response of a pair indicates the extent to which the system has recovered its capacity to respond after a given interval. The second type of measurement, the intensity–response relation examines the mean amplitude of the AER in relation to stimulus intensity.

Work on the recovery cycle has used the primary component of the somatosensory AER as a basis, this component has an initial negative feature with a latancy of about 20 msec followed by a positive peak at 25 msec. The recovery cycle has a biphasic form in normal persons, 100 per cent recovery being present at about 20 msec followed by diminished recovery until a second phase of full recovery which peaks at about 120 msec.

Shagass & Schwartz (1963a, b) showed that recovery of the early primary somatosensory AER at 20 msec was markedly depressed in schizophrenics, psychotic depressives, and patients classed as personality disorders. A similar type of study using the visual AER was carried out by Speck, Dim & Mercer (1966). In this the difference in amplitude of the positive wave at 50–60 msec latency, and the negative wave at 70–90 msec latency was used as basis for analysis. The recovery ratio of 80 per cent of non-patients showed supernormal peaks at 35 msec and 100 msec with an intermediate sub-normal dip. In an analagous manner to that of Shagass & Schwartz the amount of recovery at 35 msec was used as a method to compare groups. Schizophrenic patients showed significantly smaller-than-normal recovery, but they were not distinguished by this means from other patient groups, a finding which again supports those of Shagass & Schwartz. Further work using this type of technique has been carried out on the visual AER by Floris, Morcutti, Amabile, Bernardi, Rizzo & Vasconetto (1967), and Vasconetto, Floris & Morcutti (1971). Using the amplitude of the third (negative) component at 70–90 msec latency these workers showed that there was a phase of super-normality of recovery between 50 and 250 msec in normal subjects and that no facilitation was seen in schizophrenic or neurotically depressed patients. The data from these three laboratories are summed up by Vasconetto *et al.* (1971) who say, 'these data suggest that the psychiatric population has some defect in the facilitatory mechanisms'.

The other measurement pioneered by Shagass and his colleagues is that of the intensity-response curve. Stimuli used were shocks stimulated by electrodes placed over the ulnar nerve at the wrist. Threshold was determined and intensity increased in 10-V steps from the threshold, 'pain was not elicited in any intensity'. The early primary components of the somatosensory AER were again used for measurement. The data (Shagass & Schwartz, 1963, b, c) show that schizophrenics and all other patients excluding 'dysthymics' exhibit a higher intensity–response relation than normal over all intensities used; dysthymics did not differ from normal. In summing up their findings Shagass & Schwartz (1963c) suggest that they may indicate impairment of controlling mechanisms which normally restrict the degree of nervous response.

In a rather different theoretical context a number of studies have been carried out which examine intensity–response relations, where the 'response' is one of the later AER components. The theoretical background for these studies is that of Silverman (1964, 1967, 1972) in which, following the work of Petrie (1967), subjects are assessed as falling along the dimension of 'augmentation' or 'reduction' to the extent that they exert 'stimulus intensity control', and appear either to augment or reduce the effect of incoming sensory stimuli. In an early study Buchsbaum & Silverman (1968) showed that a group of unmedicated non-paranoid male schizophrenics showed a reduction in the amplitude of component 4 (latency 100–140 msec) of the visual AER as stimulus intensity increased. This reduction was greater than in a group of normals designated on the basis of the AER patterns as 'reducers'. On the other hand, Inderbitzin, Buchsbaum & Silverman (1970) examined similar data from acute reactive paranoid and chronic process non-paranoid patients, all of whom were on phenothiazine medication and all showed an 'augmenting' pattern, that is, that AER component 4 increased in amplitude as visual stimulus intensity increased. There was a tendency for the patients in the paranoid group to show greater augmentation than those in the non-paranoid group. In addition to mean values of amplitudes of AER components their variability was also measured. Patients who showed greater increases in AER amplitudes with increasing stimulus intensity had more stable evoked responses, these patients also performed with relatively high accuracy on the rod and frame test. Contrasting this study with the earlier one (Buchsbaum & Silverman, 1968) the authors suggest that 'phenothiazines inhibit reduction behaviour and induce augmentation behaviour both perceptually and neurophysiologically'. The high variability of the AER in those patients showing patterns of response which were most in the 'reduction' direction and hence possibly those patients diagnosed as process non-paranoid in whom pheno-thiazines were least effective may set the context of a series of studies by Callaway and his colleagues. Jones, Blacker, Callaway & Layne (1965); Callaway, Jones & Layne (1965) provided data which suggested that if two tones at 600 Hz and 1000 Hz were presented, schizophrenic subjects would give different responses to these tones even though they did not indicate any different outcome, while normal subjects would not maintain a differential responsivity to tones which were trivially different. The difference in AER to the tones shown by the patients was indicated by a lower correlation between the two AERs from the patients than from the normals. This promising finding was, however, later shown (Callaway, Jones & Donchin, 1970; Donchin, Callaway & Jones, 1970) to be a result of the greater AER variability shown by the schizophrenic patients, a useful finding in itself, but one which did not fit so neatly with the 'segmental set' ideas of Shakow (1962) which had been invoked as an explanation of the earlier 'maintenance of trivial difference' findings.

The finding of greater AER variability is also demonstrated in a very comprehensive study by Saletu, Saletu & Itil (1973) where other work by this group is also reviewed. They showed that in comparison to schizophrenics (chronic, non-medicated), normal subjects showed longer latencies, higher amplitudes and lower intra-individual variability of auditory AERs. Within the schizophrenic group the more severe the psychopathology of the patient, the shorter the latency, the smaller the amplitude and the higher the variability of his AER. The components measured in this study were P_1 (c. 50 msec), N_1 (c. 100 msec) and P_2 (150–190 msec), later components were also measured but were variably represented in patients and controls. Looking more closely at the data the authors suggest that the greater the AER variability the more there is disturbance in thought processes and higher mental functions, and that low AER amplitudes are correlated with 'preoccupation, ideas of influence, unsystematized delusions, auditory hallucination, hypoactivity and with-drawal'.

One of the most interesting aspects of the work of this group is that concerned with the division of patients into therapy-responsive versus therapy-resistant on the basis of their clinical response to various tranquillizing medications. The most consistent finding is that of a marked increase in latency of late AER components in the responsive patients while the non-responsive patients show only a small increase in latency or even a decrease during medication. Amplitude changes were not so consistent.

Finally, a study by Roth & Cannon (1972) must be mentioned, particularly in so far as of all the studies using EEG techniques it probably has the greatest affinity with the studies in the earlier part of the review on electrodermal and heart rate activity. This study is particularly concerned with the third positive going component of the AER to auditory stimuli, P_3 (c. 210 msec in this study). This component occurs under circumstances 'when the subject's attention is focused on a difficult-to-detect stimulus, when a stimulus delivers relevant information or when a stimulus is novel or unexpected' (Roth and Cannon, 1972). These authors suggest that when P_3 occurs in a situation where it is a response to unpredictably occurring stimuli it can be regarded as a component of the orienting response. Their data with normal subjects show that it behaves as such in so far as it shows a high initial amplitude which habituates. In the schizophrenic the component was difficult to identify, variable, and of low amplitude; no indication of habituation could be seen. In contrast P_2 (c. 150 msec) could be detected, but was of lower amplitude than normal. Whereas the amplitude of P_2 was significantly related to drug dosage, that of P_3 was not, a finding which is in line with those presented earlier (Sections 12.2.1, 12.2.2) which suggested that the orienting response (electrodermal or cardiovascular) was not affect by medication.

Work on the CNV (contingent negative variation or expectancy wave) in schizophrenics has been limited. A fairly definitive study by Small & Small (1971) suggests that there is no consistent wave in schizophrenics, who, as is usual, are characterized more by the variability of their responses than anything else. The finding is in general agreement with that of McCallum & Walter (1968).

An overall summing of the work using EEG measurements is obviously impossible. There does, however, seem to be a superficial inconsistency in the findings that needs discussion. In the field of tonic activity high intra-individual variability is indicative of health whereas in the case of AER measurements the reverse is true. Clearly, in the first instance variability indicates a varied repertoire of responsivity to the environment, while in the second, variability indicates inconsistency of response to particular stimuli. The other finding which appears with some consistency is that greater amplitude of response, or greater possibility of amplitude of response is an indication of health. The complexity of the data reviewed, however, suggest that summary statements such as these should not be taken as other than very loose general indications.

The work reviewed in Section 12.3 has been confined to studies on adult schizophrenic patients. Little attempt has been made in these studies to define the stage of the illness at which they were carried out in other than the crudest dichotomous fashion. With patients exhibiting a variety of clinical manifestations the extent to which there is any consistency in the data is surprising. With is in mind, it seems important now to turn to the data from 'high risk' studies (cf. Section 12.1.3), although, because of the long-term nature of these studies the data is necessarily incomplete.

12.4. PSYCHOPHYSIOLOGICAL WORK WITH 'HIGH-RISK' SUBJECTS

The potential value of the use of psychophysiological techniques in work with 'high risk' subjects has been outlined in Section 12.1.3.

By the very nature of prospective studies, results are not readily publishable and few have appeared in the literature. Perhaps the best known study for which data is available is that started by Mednick and Schulsinger in Copenhagen in 1962. The high-risk subjects of this study were children of schizophrenic mothers. Their mean age at time of testing was approximately 15 years; they were therefore sufficiently old for psychiatric disturbance to appear in a major way within the next 10 years, an important consideration in an initial study in this area. Two hundred children each with a severely-ill schizophrenic mother, and 100 children with normal parents were examined in 1962. In addition to psychiatric, neurological and psychological assessment, psychophysiological data was collected. These were skin conductance (actually resistance), heart rate and EMG measures in response to a tape-recorded orientation conditioning, generalization and extinction sequence. The EMG data have never been analysed (nor are likely to be, in so far as they were recorded in an un-integrated form). The SC data, however, have been subjected to extensive analysis and the HR data to substantial but less complete investigation. In general the pattern of results shows (Mednick & Schulsinger, 1968, 1973; Mednick, 1970) that of the 207 high-risk children 20 have broken down in some psychiatric fashion (data at 1970), these are called the 'sick' group. The remainder continue normal, and are called the 'well' group. The low risk group of 100 children remain normal. The 'sick' group can be distinguished on basis of the 1962 psychophysiological data by showing, in general, a higher non-habituating SC responsivity and particularly a shorter SC recovery than the well group, a pattern of responses that is typical of one class of adult schizophrenics (*cf.* Section 12.3.4.2). This pattern is particularly characteristic of the 75 per cent of the 'sick' group who experienced perinatal birth complications. Only 15 per cent of the high risk 'well' group, and 33 per cent of the low-risk group experienced similar complications (Mednick, 1970).

Herman (1972) examined the heart rate data from this study; she was able to show that the sick group, in comparison to the control low-risk group, showed better conditioning and generalization and faster time to peak acceleration, the well group also showed both conditioning and generalization but did not reach peak acceleration as quickly as the sick subjects.

The relative success of this study has prompted two further ones in this field. The first, is based on a series of 9006 completely recorded births in Copenhagen during 1959–1961. Samples of children with high and low genetic risk have been drawn from this birth recorded population (Mednick, Mura, Schulsinger & Mednick, 1971). Again, in addition to full psychological and psychiatric assessments, psychophysiological data has been collected. This consists of SC, measured from the right and left hands, SP and EKG, and is being analysed by Mednick & Venables and their colleagues. Normative data from this work will be available in the foreseeable future, but final analysis of the data collected on 11-year-old children will obviously not be available for some time.

The second study which follows the original 1962 experiment has been initiated on the island of Mauritius. In this case the selection of the 'high risk' children is being made solely on the basis of the the patterning of their psychophysiological responses. Skin conductance SP and HR data have been collected on 1800 3- to 4-year-old children. From this sample 200 children have been selected. These are divided into four groups of 50, 36 of each group at the time of testing exhibited responses which are akin to those shown by the high risk children in Denmark and also by adult schizophrenics; the remaining 14 children exhibit 'normal' responsivity. Two groups of 50 are being invited to participate in two special nursery schools and the other two groups will continue through the traditional patterns of child care and schooling as controls for the specially selected groups. It is hoped that by closer attention to the behaviour of the potentially high-risk children in the nursery schools that some interventive measures may be introduced which will attenuate tendencies to abnormal behaviour. It is evident that no definitive experimental data will appear for about 20 years, however, a considerable amount of normative data is available and re-testing of the 200 children is being continued bi-annually so that considerable longitudinal material will become available. Parallel developmental psychological data has been collected by Sutton-Smith; the psychophysiological data has been collected by Bell and Venables in co-operation with Mednick, Schulsinger and Raman. EEG data has been collected from a sample of the total group of 1800 by Ulett and Itil.

The investment of effort in high risk studies is to some extent a matter of faith, in so far as the time taken for the results to come to fruition is so extended. Difficulties also arise because of the bulk of data that has to be collected to cover a relatively small eventual psychiatric population, nevertheless, it may be that this sort of study has more potential for the production of really informative material on the topic of schizophrenia than work on the adult patient. In the context of this volume it is, as has been suggested in Section 12.1.3, the point at which psychophysiology can make its best contribution.

12.5. CONCLUSIONS

The data presented in the earlier sections have indicated a not-too-inconsistent pattern in the range of psychophysiological data on schizophrenia which has been examined. What is perhaps disappointing is the comparative lack of attempt to use data from the psychophysiology of normal subjects in the design of studies on schizophrenics. New data from normal work is continuously appearing, however, and there are signs in work now being undertaken that findings from this literature are being used to inform work on patients. It is clear that psychophysiological studies on schizophrenia will continue necessarily to be imperfect for many of the reasons that have been outlined. However, perhaps the weight of evidence from the widest possible range of sources will eventually provide an approach to a consistent picture.

12.6. ACKNOWLEDGMENT

This chapter was prepared while the author was in receipt of Grants G971/736 and G972/984 from the Medical Research Council.

12.7. REFERENCES

Acker, C. W. An exploration of the autonomic effects of phenothiazines. *Psychopharmacologia (Berl.)*, 1965, **7**, 150–158.

Ax, A. F. & Bamford, J. L. The GSR recovery limb in chronic schizophrenia, *Psychophysiology*, 1970, **7**, 145–147.

Ax, A. F., Bamford, J. L., Beckett, P. G. S., Fretz, N. F. & Gottlieb, J. G. Autonomic conditioning in chronic schizophrenia. *Journal of Abnormal Psychology*, 1970, **76**, 140–154.

Bagshaw, M. H., Kimble, D. P. & Pribram, K. H. The GSR of monkeys during orienting and habituation and after ablation of the amygdala, hippocampus, and inferotemporal cortex. *Neuropsychologia*, 1965, **3**, 111–119.

Bernstein, A. S. The galvanic skin response orienting reflex among chronic schizophrenics. *Psychonomic Science*, 1964, **1**, 391–392.

Bernstein, A. S. Electrodermal base level, tonic arousal, and adaptation in chronic schizophrenics. *Journal of Abnormal Psychology*, 1967, **72**, 221–232.

Bernstein, A. S. The electrodermal orienting responses in chronic schizophrenia: manifest confusion as a significant dimension. In Siva Sankar, D. V. (Ed.), *Schizophrenia current concepts in research*. Hicksville, P. J. D. Publications, 1969.

Bernstein, A. S. Phasic electrodermal orienting response in chronic schizophrenics. *Journal of Abnormal Psychology*, 1970, **75**, 146–156.

Blum, R. H. Alpha-rhythm 'responsiveness' in normal, schizophrenic, and brain damaged persons. *Science*, 1957, **126**, 749–750.

Broen, W. E. Response disorganization and breadth of observation in schizophrenia. *Psychological Review*, 1966, **73**, 579–585.

Broen, W. E. *Schizophrenia research and theory*. New York: Academic Press, 1968.

Brown, G. W. Length of hospital-stay and schizophrenia: A review of statistical studies. *Acta Psychiatrica et Neurologica Scandinavica*, 1960, **35**, 414–430.

Bruck, M. A. A method of determining average voltage of the EEG. *EEG Clinical Neurophysiology*, 1962, **12**, 580–582.

Bruck, M. A. Synchrony and voltage in the EEG of schizophrenics. *Archives of General Psychiatry*, 1964, **10**, 454–468.

Buchsbaum, M. & Silverman, J. Stimulus intensity control and the cortical evoked response. *Psychosomatic Medicine*, 1968, **30**, 12–22.

Callaway, E., Jones, R. T. & Donchin, E. Auditory evoked potential variability in schizophrenia. *EEG Clinical Neurophysiology*, 1970, **29**, 421–428.

Callaway, E., Jones, R. T. & Layne, R. S. Evoked responses and segmental set of schizophrenia. *Archives of General Psychiatry*, 1965, **12**, 83–89.

Chapman, L. T. The problem of selecting drug-free schizophrenics for research. *Journal of Consulting Psychology*, 1963, **27**, 540–542.

Ciganek, L. The effect of largactil on the electroencephalographic response (evoked potential) to light stimulus in man. *EEG Clinical Neurophysiology*, 1959, **11**, 65–71.

Connor, W. N. & Lang, P. J. Cortical slow-wave and cardiac rate responses in stimulus orientation and reaction time conditions. *Journal of Experimental Psychology*, 1969, **82**, 310–320.

Crider, A. B., Grinspoon, L. & Maher, B. A. Autonomic and psychomotor correlates of premorbid adjustment in schizophrenia. *Psychosomatic Medicine*, 1965, **27**, 201–206.

Cromwell, R. & Held, J. M. Alpha blocking latency and reaction time in schizophrenics and normals. *Perceptual and Motor Skills*, 1969, **29**, 195–201.

Curry, S. H. Chlorpromazine: Concentrations in plasma, excretion in urine and duration of effect. *Proceedings of the Royal Society of Medicine*, 1971, **64**, 285–289.

Davis, P. A. Comparative study of the EEG of schizophrenic and manic depressive patients. *American Journal of Psychiatry*, 1942, **99**, 210–217.

Depue, R. A. & Fowles, D. C. Electrodermal activity as an index of arousal in schizophrenics. *Psychological Bulletin*, 1973, **79**, 233–328.

Donchin, E., Callaway, E. & Jones, R. T. Auditory evoked potential variability in schizophrenia. II. The application of discriminant analysis. *EEG Clinical Neurophysiology*, 1970, **29**, 429–440.

Drohocki, Z. L'integrateur de l'éléctroproduction cérébrale par l'encephalographie quantitative. *Revue Neurologique (Paris)*, 1948, **80**, 619–624.

Dykman, R. A., Reese, W. G., Galbrecht, C. R., Ackerman, P. T. & Sunderman, R. S. Autonomic responses in psychiatric patients. *Annals of the New York Academy of Science*, 1968, **147**, 237–303.

Edelberg, R. The information content of the recovery limb of the electrodermal response. *Psychophysiology*, 1970, **6**, 527–539.

Edelberg, R. Electrodermal recovery rate, goal-orientation, and aversion. *Psychophysiology*, 1972, **9**, 512–520(a).

Epstein, S. Toward a unified theory of anxiety. In Maher, B. A. (Ed.), *Progress in experimental personality research (4)*, New York: Academic Press, 1967.

Epstein, S. Anxiety, reality and schizophrenia. *Schizophrenia*, 1970, **2**, 11–35.

Epstein, S. & Coleman, M. Drive theories of schizophrenia. *Psychosomatic Medicine*, 1970, **32**, 113–149.

Fenz, W. D. & Velner, J. Physiological concomitants of behavioural indexes in schizophrenia. *Journal of Abnormal Psychology*, 1970, **76**, 27–35.

Fink, M. Quantitative electroencephalography in human pharmacology: Drug patterns. In Glaser, G. (Ed.), *EEG and behaviour*, New York: Basic Books, 1963.

Fink, M. The electroencephalogram in clinical psychiatry. Chapter 14. In Mendels, J. (Ed.), *Biological psychiatry*. New York: Wiley, 1973.

Floris, V., Morcutti, C., Amabile, G., Bernardi, G., Rizzo, P. A. & Vasconetto, C. Recovery cycle of visual evoked potentials in normal and schizophrenic subjects. *EEG Clinical Neurophysiology*, 1967, Suppl. **26**, 74–81.

Forrest, F. M., Forrest, I. S. & Mason, A. S. Review of rapid urine tests for phenothiazine and related drugs. *American Journal of Psychiatry*, 1961, **118**, 300–307.

Foulds, G. A. & Owen, A. Are paranoids schizophrenic? *British Journal of Psychiatry*, 1963, **109**, 674–679.

Furedy, J. J. Electrodermal recovery time as a supra-sensitive autonomic index of anticipated intensity of threatened shock. *Psychophysiology*, 1972, **9**, 281–282.

Goldstein, L., Murphree, H. B., Sugerman, A. A., Pfeiffer, C. C. & Jenney, E. H. Quantitative electroencephalographic analysis of naturally occurring (schizophrenic) and drug induced psychotic states in human males. *Clinical Pharmacology and Therapeutics*, 1963, **4**, 10–21.

Goldstein, L., Sugerman, A. A., Stolberg, H., Murphree, H. B. & Pfeiffer, C. C. Electrocerebral activity in schizophrenics and non-psychotic subjects: Quantitative EEG amplitude analysis. *EEG Clinical Neurophysiology*, 1965, **19**, 350–361.

Goldstein, M. J. & Acker, C. W. Psychophysiological reactions to films by chronic schizophrenics. II. Individual differences in resting levels and reactivity. *Journal of Abnormal Psychology*, 1967, **72**, 23–29.

Goldstein, M. J., Acker, C. W., Crockett, J. T. & Riddle, J. J. Psychophysiological reactions to films by chronic schizophrenics. I. Effects of drug status. *Journal of Abnormal Psychology*, 1966, **71**, 335–344.

Goldstein, M. J., Rodnick, E. H., Jackson, N. P., Evans, J. R., Bates, J. E. & Judd, L. L. The stability and sensitivity of measures of thought, perception and emotional arousal. *Psychopharmacologia (Berl.)*, 1972, **24**, 107–120.

Graham, F. K. & Clifton, R. K. Heart rate changes as a component of the orienting response. *Psychological Bulletin*, 1966, **65**, 305–320.

Gruzelier, J. H. The investigation of possible limbic dysfunction in schizophrenia by psychophysiological methods. Unpublished Ph.D. thesis, University of London, 1973(a).

Gruzelier, J. H. Bilateral asymmetry of skin conductance orienting activity and levels in schizophrenics. *Biological Psychology*, 1973, **1**, 21–42(b).

Gruzelier, J. H., Lykken, D. T. & Venables, P. H. Schizophrenia and arousal revisited. Two flash thresholds and electrodermal activity in activated and non-activated conditions. *Archives of General Psychiatry*, 1972, **26**, 427–432.

Gruzelier, J. H. & Venables, P. H. Skin conductance orienting activity in heterogenous sample of schizophrenics. *Journal of Nervous and Mental Disease*, 1972, **155**, 277–287.

Gruzelier, J. H. & Venables, P. H. Skin conductance responses to tones with and without attentional significance in schizophrenic and non-schizophrenic psychiatric patients. *Neuropsychologia*, 1973, **11**, 211–230.

Gruzelier, J. H. & Venables, P. H. Evidence of high and low levels of physiological arousal in schizophrenics. *Psychophysiology*, 1975, **12**, 66–73.

Hatton, H. H., Berg, W. K. & Graham, F. K. Effects of acoustic rise time on heart rate response. *Psychonomic Science*, 1970, **19**, 101–103.

Hein, P. L., Green, R. L. & Wilson, W. P. Latency and duration of photically elicited arousal responses in the electroencephalograms of patients with chronic regressive schizophrenia. *Journal of Nervous and Mental Disease*, 1962, **135**, 361–364.

Heninger, G. & Speck, L. B. Visual evoked responses and status of schizophrenics. *Archives of General Psychiatry*, 1966, **15**, 419–426.

Herman, T. M. Heart rate functioning in children with schizophrenic mothers. Unpublished doctoral dissertation. New School for Social Research, New York, 1972.

Herron, W. G. The process-reactive classification of schizophrenia. *Psychological Bulletin*, 1962, **59**, 329–343.

Higgins, J. & Peterson, J. C. Concept of process-reactive schizophrenia: A critique. *Psychological Bulletin*, 1966, **66**, 201–206.

Hill, D. Electroencephalogram in schizophrenia. In Richter, D. (Ed.), *Schizophrenia: Somatic aspects.* New York: Pergamon, 1957.

Inderbitzin, L. B., Buchsbaum, M. & Silverman, J. EEG averaged evoked response and perceptual variability in schizophrenics. *Archives of General Psychiatry*, 1970, **23**, 438–444.

Itil, T. M., Keskiner, A. & Fink, M. Therapeutic studies in therapy resistant schizophrenic patients. *Comprehensive Psychiatry*, 1966, **7**, 488–493.

Johannsen, W. J., Friedman, S. H., Leitschuch, T. H. & Ammons, H. A study of certain schizophrenic dimensions and their relationship to double alternation learning. *Journal of Consulting Psychology*, 1963, **27**, 375–382.

Johnson, L. C. & Lubin, A. Spontaneous electrodermal activity. *Psychophysiology*, 1966, **3**, 8–17.

Jones, R. T., Blacker, K. H., Callaway, E. & Layne, R. S. The auditory evoked responses as a diagnostic and prognostic measure in schizophrenia. *American Journal of Psychiatry*, 1965, **122**, 33–41.

Kiloh, L. G. & Osseleton, J. W. *Clinical electroencephalography.* London: Butterworth, 1961.

Kraepelin, E. *Psychiatrie.* Leipzig: Barth, 1913.

Lacey, J. I. Somatic response patterning and stress: Some revision of activation theory. In Appley, M. H. & Trumbull, R. (Eds.), *Psychological Stress.* New York: Appleton–Century–Crofts, 1967.

Lang, P. J. & Buss, A. Psychological deficit in schizophrenia. II. Interference and activation. *Journal of Abnormal Psychology*, 1965, **70**, 77–106.

Liberson, W. T. Functional electroencephalography in mental disorders. *Diseases of the Nervous System*, 1945, **5**, 357–364.

Lifshitz, K. & Gradijan, J. Relationships between measures of the coefficent of variation of the mean absolute EEG, voltage and spectral intensities in schizophrenic and control subjects. *Biological Psychiatry*, 1972, **5**, 149–163.

Lobstein, T. J. Heart rate and skin conductance activity in schizophrenia. Unpublished Ph.D. thesis, University of London, 1974.

Lubin, A., Johnson, L. C. & Austin, M. T. Discrimination among states of consciousness using EEG spectra. *Psychophysiology*, 1969, **6**, 122–132.

Lykken, D. T. & Maley, M. Autonomic versus cortical arousal in schizophrenic and non-psychotics. *Journal of Psychiatric Research*, 1968, **6**, 21–32.

Lykken, D. T. & Venables, P. H. Direct measurement of skin conductance: A proposal for standardization. *Psychophysiology*, 1971, **8**, 656–672.

Lynn, R. Russian theory and research in schizophrenia. *Psychological Bulletin*, 1963, **60**, 486–498.

McCallum, W. C. & Walter, W. G. The effects of attention and distraction on the contingent negative variation in normal and neurotic subjects. *EEG and Clinical Neurophysiology*, 1968, **25**, 319–329.

McGhie, A. *Pathology of Attention*. Harmondsworth: Penguin, 1969.

MacMahon, J. F. & Walter, W. G. The electroencephalogram in schizophrenia. *Journal of Mental Science*, 1938, **84**, 781–787.

Magaro, P. A. Base Level and reactivity in schizophrenia as a function of premorbid adjustment, chronicity and diagnosis. *Journal of Genetic Psychology*, 1972, **120**, 61–73.

Magaro, P. A. Skin conductance basal level and reactivity in schizophrenia as a function of chronicity, premorbid adjustment, diagnosis and medication. *Journal of Abnormal Psychology*, 1973, **81**, 270–281.

Marjerrison, G., Krause, A. E. & Keogh, R. P. Variability of the EEG in schizophrenia: Quantitative analysis with a modulus voltage integrator. *EEG Clinical Neurophysiology*, 1968, **24**, 35–41.

Mednick, S. A. Breakdown in individuals at high risk for schizophrenia: possible predispositional perinatal factors. *Mental Hygiene*, 1970, **54**, 50–63.

Mednick, S. A. & McNeil, T. F. Current methodology in research on the etiology of schizophrenia. Serious difficulties which suggest the use of high-risk group method. *Psychological Bulletin*, 1968, **70**, 681–693.

Mednick, S. A., Mura, E., Schulsinger, F. & Mednick, B. Perinatal conditions and infant development in children with schizophrenic parents. *Social Biology*, 1971, **18**, Supplement, 103–113.

Mednick, S. A. & Schulsinger, F. Some pre-morbid characteristics related to breakdown in children with schizophrenic mothers. In Rosenthal, D. & Kety, S. S. (Eds.), *The transmission of schizophrenia*. New York: Pergamon Press, 1968.

Mednick, S. A. & Schulsinger, F. A learning theory of schizophrenia: thirteen years later. Chap. 18 in M. Hammer, K. Salzinger, S. Sutton (Eds.), *Psychopathology*, New York: Wiley, 1973.

Montagu, J. D. The measurement of electrodermal activity: an instrument for recording log skin admittance. *Biological Psychology*, 1973, **1**, 161–166.

Murphree, H. B., Jenney, E. H. & Pfeiffer, C. C. Quantitative electroencephalographic analysis of the effects of lysergic and diethylamide (LSD-25) and D-amphetamine in man. *Federation Proceedings*, 1962, **21**, 337.

Murphy, E. H. & Venables, P. H. The effects of caffeine citrate and white noise on ear asymmetry in the detection of two clicks. *Neuropsychologia*, 1971, **9**, 27–32.

Nideffer, R. M., Deckner, C. W., Cromwell, R. & Cash, T. F. The relationship of alpha activity to attentional sets in schizophrenia. *Journal of Nervous and Mental Disease*, 1971, **152**, 346–352.

Pavlov, I. P. *Conditioned reflexes and psychiatry*. Translated by W. H. Gantt. New York: International University Press, 1941.

Petrie, A. Individuality in pain and suffering. Chicago: University of Chicago Press, 1967.

Phillips, L. Case history data and prognosis in schizophrenia. *Journal of Nervous and Mental Disease*, 1953, **117**, 515–525.

Pugh, L. A. Respone time and electrodermal measures in chronic schizophrenia: The effects of chlorpromazine. *Journal of Nervous and Mental Disease*, 1968, **146**, 62–70.

Rackow, L. L., Napoli, P. J., Klebanoff, S. G. & Schillinger, A. A. A group method for rapid screening of chronic psychiatric patients. *American Journal of Psychiatry*, 1953, **109**, 561–566.

Roth, W. T. & Cannon, E. H. Some features of the auditory evoked response in schizophrenics. *Archives of General Psychiatry*, 1972, **27**, 466–471.

Salamon, I. & Post, J. Alpha blocking and schizophrenia. *Archives of General Psychiatry*, 1965, **13**, 367–374.

Saletu, B., Saletu, M. & Itil, T. M. The relationship between psychopathology and evoked response before, during, and after, psychotropic drug treatment. *Biological Psychiatry*, 1973, **6**, 45–74.

Saletu, B., Saletu, M., Itil, T. M. & Marasa, J. Somatosensory evoked potential changes during haloperidol treatment of chronic schizophrenics. *Biological Psychiatry*, 1971, **3**, 299–307.

Serafetinides, E. A. Laterality and voltage in the EEG of psychiatric patients. *Diseases of the Nervous System*, 1972, **33**, 622–623.

Serafetinides, E. A. Voltage laterality in the EEG of psychiatric patients. *Diseases of the Nervous System*, 1973, **34**, 190–191.

Shagass, C. Averaged somatosensory evoked responses in various psychiatric disorders. In Wortis, J. (Ed.), *Recent advances in biological psychiatry*. New York: Plenum, 1968.

Shagass, C. *Evoked brain potentials in psychiatry*. New York: Plenum, 1972.

Shagass, C., Overton, D. A. & Straumanis, J. J. Sex differences in somatosensory evoked responses related to psychomatic illness. *Biological Psychiatry*, 1972, **5**, 295–309.

Shagass, C. & Schwartz, M. Reactivity cycle of somatosensory cortex in humans with and without psychiatric disorder. *Science*, 1961, **134**, 1757–1759.

Shagass, C. & Schwartz, M. Excitability of the cerebral cortex in psychiatric disorders. In Roessler, R. & Greenfield, N. S. (Eds.), *Physiological correlates of psychological disorder*. Madison: University of Wisconsin Press, 1962.

Shagass, C. & Schwartz, M. Psychiatric correlates of evoked cerebral cortical potentials. *American Journal of Psychiatry*, 1963, **119**, 1055–1061(a).

Shagass, C. & Schwartz, M. Psychiatric disorder and deviant cerebral responsiveness to sensory stimulation. In Wortis, J. (Ed.), *Recent advances in biological psychiatry*, 5. New York: Plenum, 1963(b).

Shagass, C. & Schwartz, M. Cerebral responsiveness in psychiatric patients. *Archives of General Psychiatry*, 1963, **8**, 177–189(c).

Shagass, C. & Schwartz, M. Visual cerebral evoked response characteristics in a psychiatric population. *American Journal of Psychiatry*, 1965, **121**, 879–987.

Shakow, D. Segmental set. *Archives of General Psychiatry*, 1962, **6**, 1–17.

Shakow, D. Psychological deficit in schizophrenia. *Behavioural Science*, 1963, **8**, 275–305.

Shakow, D. Some observations on the psychology (and some fewer, on the biology) of schizophrenia. *Journal of Nervous and Mental Disease*, 1971, **153**, 300–316.

Shaw, J. C. Quantification of biological signals using integration techniques. Chapter 12, In Venables, P. H. & Martin, I. (Eds.), *A manual of psychophysiological methods*. Amsterdam: North-Holland, 1967.

Silverman, J. The problem of attention in research and theory in schizophrenia. *Psychological Review*, 1964, **71**, 352–379.

Silverman, J. Variation in cognitive control and psychophysiological defense in the schizophrenias. *Psychosomatic Medicine*, 1967, **29**, 225–251.

Silverman, J. Stimulus intensity modulation and psychological disease. *Psychopharmacologia* (Berl.), 1972, **24**, 42–80.

Small, J.G. & Small, I. F. Contingent negative variation (CNV) correlations with psychiatric diagnoses. *Archives of General Psychiatry*, 1971, **25**, 550–554.

Smith, B. D. Habituation and spontaneous recovery of skin conductance and heart rate in schizophrenics as a function of repeated tone presentations. Unpublished doctoral dissertation, University of Massachusetts, 1967.

Smith, D. B. D. & Strawbridge, P. J. Stimulus duration and the human heart rate response. *Psychonomic Science*, 1968, **10**, 71–72.

Smith, D. B. D. & Strawbridge, P. J. The heart rate response to a brief auditory and visual stimulus. *Psychophysiology*, 1969, **6**, 317–329.

Sokolov, E. N. *Perception and the conditioned reflex*. New York: Macmillan, 1963.

Spain, B. Eyelid conditioning and arousal in schizophrenic and normal subjects. *Journal of abnormal Psychology*, 1966, **71**, 260–266.

Speck, L. B., Dim, B. & Mercer, M. Visual evoked responses of psychiatric patients. *Archives of General Psychiatry*, 1966, **15**, 59–63.

Spiegel, D. E. & Keith-Spiegel, P. The effects of carphenazine, trifluoperazine and chlorpromazine on ward behavior, physiological functioning and psychological test scores in chronic schizophrenic patients. *Journal of Nervous and Mental Disease*, 1967, **144**, 111–116.

Spohn, H. E., Thetford, P. E. & Cancro, R. The effects of phenothiazine medication on skin conductance and heart rate in schizophrenic patients. *Journal of Nervous and Mental Disease*, 1971, **152**, 129–139.

Sugarman, A. A., Goldstein, L., Murphree, H. B., Pfeiffer, C. C. & Jenney, E. H. EEG and behavioural changes in schizophrenia. *Archives of General Psychiatry*, 1964, **10**, 340–344.

Syz, H. C. Psychogalvanic studies in schizophrenia. *Archives of Neurology and Psychiatry*, 1926, **16**, 747–758.

Syz, H. C. & Kinder, E. F. Electrical skin resistance in normal and in psychotic subjects. *Archives of Neurology and Psychiatry*, 1928, **19**, 1026–1035.

Tecce, J. J. & Cole, J. D. Psychophysiologic responses of schizophrenics to drugs. *Psychopharmacologia* (Berl.), 1972, **24**, 159–200.

Tizard, J. & Venables, P. H. The influence of extraneous stimulation on the reaction time of schizophrenics. *British Journal of Psychology*, 1957, **48**, 299–305.

Uno, T. & Grings, W. W. Autonomic components of orienting behaviour. *Psychophysiology*, 1965, **1**, 311–321.

Vasconetto, C., Floris, V. & Morcutti, C. Visual evoked responses in normal and psychiatric subjects. *EEG Clinical Neurophysiology*, 1971, **31**, 77–83.

Venables, P. H. A short scale of rating 'activity-withdrawal' in schizophrenics. *Journal of Mental Science*, 1957, **103**, 197–199.

Venables, P. H. The effect of auditory and visual stimulation on the skin potential response of schizophrenics. *Brain*, 1960, **83**, 77–92.

Venables, P. H. The relationship between level of skin potential and fusion of paired light flashes in schizophrenic and normal subjects. *Journal of Psychiatric Research*, 1963, **1**, 279–287.

Venables, P. H. Input dysfunction in schizophrenia. Chapter 1. In Maher, B. (Ed.), *Advances in experimental personality research 1*. Academic Press: New York, 1964.

Venables, P. H. Partial failure of cortical–subcortical integration as a factor underlying schizophrenic behaviour. In J. Romano (Ed.), *Origins of Schizophrenia*. Excerpta Medica: Amsterdam, 1967.

Venables, P. H. Schizophrenia as a disorder of input processing. *Vest. Akad. med. Nauk SSSR*, 1971, **5**, 10–12. (In Russian).

Venables, P. H. & Christie, M. J. Mechanisms, instrumentation, recording techniques and quantification of responses. Chapter 1. In Prokasy, W. F. & Raskin, D. C. (Eds.), *Electrodermal activity in psychological research*. New York: Academic Press, 1973.

Venables, P. H. & O'Connor, N. A short scale for rating paranoid schizophrenia. *Journal of Mental Science*, 1959, **105**, 815–818.

Venables, P. H. & Tizard, J. Paradoxical effects in the reaction time of schizophrenics. *Journal of Abnormal and Social Psychology*, 1956, **33(2)**, 220–224.

Venables, P. H. & Tizard, J. The effect of auditory stimulus intensity on the reaction time of schizophrenics. *Journal of Mental Science*, 1958, **104**, 437, 1160–1164.

Venables, P. H. & Wing, J. K. Level of arousal and the sub-classification of schizophrenia. *Archives of General Psychiatry*, 1962, **7**, 114–119.

Volovka, J., Matousek, M. & Roubicek, J. EEG frequency analysis in schizophrenia. *Acta psychiatrica Scandinavica*, 1966, **42**, 237–245.

Wang, G. H. The galvanic skin reflex. A review of old and recent works from a physiologic point of view. Part I. *American Journal of Physical Medicine*, 1957, **36**, 295–320.

Wang, G. H. The galvanic skin reflex. A review of old and recent works from a physiologic point of view. Part II. *American Journal of Physical Medicine*, 1958, **37**, 35–37.

Wilkinson, R. T. Evoked response and reaction time. *Acta Psychologica*, 1967, **27**, 235–245.

Wittenborn, J. R. *Manual of Wittenborn Psychiatric Rating Scales*. Slough: National Foundation for Educational Research, 1968.

Zahn, T. P. Autonomic reactivity and behavior in schizophrenia. *Psychiatric Research Report*, 1964, **19**, 156–173.

Zahn, T. P., Rosenthal, D. & Lawlor, W. G. Electrodermal and heart rate orienting reactions in chronic schizophrenia. *Journal of Psychiatric Research*, 1968, **6**, 117–134.

Chapter 13

Psychopathy

ROBERT D. HARE

University of British Columbia
Vancouver, Canada

13.1. INTRODUCTION

13.1.1. Definition of psychopathy

The term psychopathy has had a variety of meanings over the years (see Craft, 1965; Maughs, 1941), and is still a source of confusion to much of the general public who often consider it to be more or less synonymous with mental disturbance and/or criminality. Among clinicians and behavioural scientists, however, there is a growing tendency to restrict its use to a particular disorder. The World Health Organization (1968) and the American Psychiatric Association (1968) refer to this disorder as category 301.7, antisocial personality: 'This term is reserved for individuals who are basically unsocialized and whose behaviour pattern brings them repeatedly into conflict with society. They are incapable of significant loyalty to individuals, groups or social values. They are grossly selfish, callous, irresponsible, impulsive and unable to feel guilt or to learn from experience and punishment. Frustration tolerance is low. They tend to blame others or offer plausible rationalizations for their behaviour. A mere history of repeated legal or social offences is not sufficient to justify this diagnosis ...' (American Psychiatric Association, 1968, p. 43).

More extensive clinical descriptions of the psychopathic (or sociopathic) individual have been given in Cleckley's influential book, *The Mask of Sanity* (1964). This book, along with the work of Arieti (1967), provides a useful conceptual framework for psychopathy (see Hare, 1970, for a more extended discussion).

Cleckley (1964) lists the main features of psychopathy as including (i) superficial charm and good intelligence; (ii) absence of delusions and other signs of irrational thinking; (iii) absence of nervousness or other neurotic manifestations; (iv) unreliability; (v) untruthfulness and insincerity; (vi) lack of remorse or shame; (vii) antisocial behaviour without apparent compunction; (viii) poor judgment and failure to learn from experience; (ix) pathologic egocentricity and incapacity for love; (x) general poverty in major affective reactions; (xi) specific loss of insight; (xii) unresponsiveness in general interpersonal relations; (xiii) fantastic and uninviting behaviour with alcohol; (xiv) sex life impersonal, trivial, and poorly integrated; (xv) failure to follow any life plan.

13.1.2. Secondary and dysocial 'psychopathy'

The individual described so far is often referred to as a *primary* or *classical* psychopath. He can be distinguished from others whose antisocial behaviour is essentially symptomatic of some underlying emotional disturbance (neurotic, secondary, or symptomatic 'psychopathy') or is the result of membership in a subculture whose rules of conduct and morality are in conflict with society at large (dysocial 'psychopath'). However, as has been argued elsewhere (Hare, 1970, 1971) that the terms neurotic and dysocial psychopathy may be misleading since they imply that the individuals involved are basically psychopaths. A more appropriate term for neurotic or secondary 'psychopaths' may be *acting-out neurotic* or *neurotic delinquent*, since the motivations behind their behaviour, their personality structure, life history, response to treatment, etc., are probably quite different from those of the psychopath. Moreover, unlike psychopaths, they seem quite able to experience guilt and remorse and to form sincere affectional relationships with others. Similarly, the term *subcultural delinquent* may be preferable to dysocial psychopath, since the individuals involved also seem capable of guilt and remorse, as well as strong loyalties and warm relationships within the context of their own group.

13.1.3. Selection of subjects

One of the problems that any investigator in this area has is trying to ensure that his method of selecting subjects (Ss) is reasonably consistent with the conception of psychopathy that underlies his research. Since many behavioural scientists more or less begin with the Cleckley conception of psychopathy, it seems appropriate that his list of criteria (discussed above) should provide a useful basis for selecting Ss. In our own research programme we usually begin a study by discussing Cleckley's conception of psychopathy with the professional staff of the institution we happen to be working in, and asking them to submit the names of inmates whom they feel do or do not fit the descriptions given. On the basis of whatever information we can obtain, including institutional files, behavioural ratings by others, interviews, etc., we make two or three global assessments (on a 7-point scale) of the extent to which we are confident that each inmate does or does not fit our criteria for psychopathy. Psychopaths (P) are defined as those Ss who receive a rating of 1 or 2, and nonpsychopaths (NP) as those with a rating of 6 or 7. Sometimes a 'mixed' group (M) is used, consisting of inmates with a rating of from 3–5; many of the Ss in the group would probably have been placed in Group P had more information on them been available (see Hare, 1971). In earlier studies the global rating was preceded by a 15-item checklist of criteria derived from Cleckley (and originally used by Lykken, 1957). However, we found that the checklist was not really necessary, since ratings with and without it usually lead to the result, partly because there seems to be a large halo effect involved in filling it out—each item is not independent of the others. Our experience has been that the checklist is useful in helping to keep the concept of psychopathy clearly in mind when making global clinical assessments. In any case, the result of our selection procedure is the identification of Ss (Group P) that probably represent the extreme of the psychopathy dimension (see Hare, 1970, pp. 11–12) as it exists among criminals. We recognize that while the groups so selected may be relatively homogeneous with respect to the core attributes defining psychopathy, a considerable amount of diversity in behaviour patterns and personality structure no doubt exists. It is likely that future research will find a common set of psychophysiological processes associated with psychopathy in general, as well as other processes that are specific to the various subtypes of psychopathy that may exist—for example, Karpman's (1961) aggressive–predatory and passive–parasitic types, and Arieti's (1967) simple and complex types (see Hare, 1970).

Although the use of these global ratings has produced theoretically meaningful and reasonably replicable results in a series of experiments by the author and his colleagues, it could be argued that the subjective element involved makes direct comparisons with the research of other investigators difficult. There have been several attempts to make the selection of Ss more objective by operationally defining them in terms of scores on various psychometric inventories, including the MMPI (Dahlstrom & Welch, 1960), several factor analytically derived scales developed by Quay and his associates (e.g., Quay & Parsons, 1971), the Activity Preference Questionnaire or APQ (Lykken & Katzenmeyer, 1968) and the Gough Delinquency (De) scale (Cough & Peterson, 1952). Research is needed to assess the extent to which these various selection procedures might be measuring the same thing. Until this research is carried out, it will be difficult to compare the results of different studies.

Before discussing some of the recent research literature, it should be pointed out that most of the research has been done with adult, male, inmates of penal institutions. The extent to which the results of this research can be generalized to nonincarcerated psychopaths, including female ones, is unknown. Research with the more socially successful psychopath is badly needed, although it is recognized that there are real difficulties involved in obtaining suitable Ss. An additional need, and ultimately the most important, is for research in the developmental aspects of psychopathy.

13.2. AUTONOMIC CORRELATES OF PSYCHOPATHY

Because of space limitations coverage of the research literature will be somewhat selective, with emphasis being placed on research with Ss who most closely fit the Cleckley conception of psychopathy. More extended discussions, particularly of the earlier literature, are available in Hare (1968, 1970, 1971).

13.2.1. Tonic autonomic activity

Clinical acccounts of psychopathy generally make reference to a relative lack of anxiety, emotional tension, or arousal, particularly in situations that would ordinarily be considered stressful by normal individuals. Most of the empirical evidence relevant to this view comes from studies in which electrodermal and cardiovascular activity are monitored while Ss are engaged in a variety of tasks. In general, the results have been fairly consistent, particularly among studies in which we can be reasonably certain that psychopathic Ss were involved.

13.2.1.1. Electrodermal activity

A number of studies has found that the tonic skin conductance (SC) of psychopathic inmates is significantly lower than that of other inmates or noncriminal control Ss (Blankstein, 1969; Dengerink, 1972; Hare, 1965a, 1968, 1972a; Hare & Quinn, 1971; Mathis, 1970; Schalling, Lidberg, Levander & Dahlin, 1973). Others have obtained a similar, though nonsignificant trend (Hare & Craigen, 1973; Schalling, Lidberg, Levander & Dahlin, 1968). A few studies found no differences between groups (Borkover, 1970; Schmauk, 1970; Sutker, 1970); however, there is some doubt that the Ss included psychopaths as defined here. There is some evidence that when the experimental procedures are somewhat monotonous, the differences between psychopathic and nonpsychopathic Ss increase, largely because the tonic SC of the former tends to decrease from the initial 'resting' period at the beginning of the experiment (Hare, 1968; Hare & Quinn, 1971; Schalling, et al., 1973). For example, Figure 13.1(a) shows tonic SC during an experiment (Hare, 1968) involving

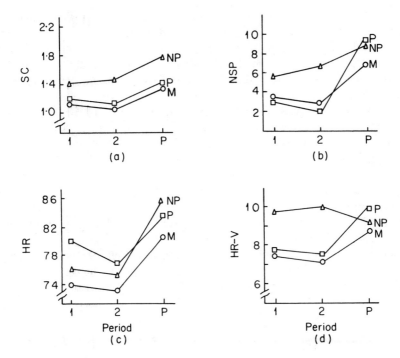

FIGURE 13.1. Mean tonic skin conductance (a), nonspecific fluctuations in skin conductance (b) heart rate (c), and heart rate variability (d) during an initial rest period (1), after 15 repetitive tones (2), and during solution of arithmetic problems. P = psychopaths; M = mixed group; NP = non-psychopaths. (Hare, R. D. Psychopathy, autonomic functioning and the orienting response, *Journal of Abnormal Psychology, Monograph Supplement,* **73,** 1968 (3, pt. 2). Copyright 1968 by the American Psychological Association and reproduced by permission.)

the repetitive presentation of tones. The three measurements were taken after a 15-min rest period at the beginning of the experiment (Period 1), after a series of 15 80-dB, 900-Hz tones had been presented over a 15-min period (Period 2) and during the solution of a series of arithmetic problems (Period P). It is evident that during repetitive stimulation the tonic SC of the psychopaths (P) and 'mixed' group of Ss (M) tended to decrease. However, it also appears these Ss were quite capable of sharp increases in SC during the cognitive activity required to solve arithmetic problems. Incidentally, as noted earlier, our Group M Ss probably included a high proportion of psychopaths, which would account for the physiological similarities between Groups P and M in this study and others described below.

If the experimental procedure is somewhat stressful or involves important interpersonal interactions, the differences between groups may also increase, primarily because the SC of nonpsychopathic Ss increases considerably more than does that of psychopathic ones (Hare, 1972a) for example, found that the stress associated with injections of saline and adrenaline produced a large increase in the tonic SC of nonpsychopaths and relatively little change in psychopaths and a "mixed" group of *S*s. A study by Dengerink (1972) obtained similar results (his selection procedures were identical to ours, and his *S*s came from the same inmate population), except that rather than injections of adrenalin the tasks involved administration of shocks to another *S* for errors made.

Results similar to those obtained with tonic SC have also been found with spontaneous or nonspecific fluctuations in skin conductance (NSP). Thus, in a variety of experimental conditions, psychopaths tend to exhibit less NSP activity than do other *S*s (Hare, 1968; Hare & Quinn, 1971; Schalling *et al.*, 1973; Schalling *et al.*, 1968). Figure 13.1(b) indicates that the differences between groups may increase during the monotonous (repetitive tones) phase of an experiment (similar results were obtained by Schalling *et al.*, 1973) and that cognitive activity may decrease or erase these differences. Incidentally, the increase in tonic SC and NSP activity shown by the nonpsychopathic *S*s (Group NP) during monotonous stimulation [see Figures 13(a) and (b)] is consistent with the finding by London & Schubert (1972) that boredom can produce an increase in arousal in normal *S*s. Apparently such is not the case with psychopaths.

13.2.1.2. Cardiovascular activity

Most studies have failed to find any significant relationship between psychopathy and tonic heart rate (Blankstein, 1969; Fenz, 1971; Hare, 1968, 1972a; Hare & Craigen, 1973)—see Figure 13.1(c) for example. An exception is the study by Dengerink, referred to above. Although there were no group differences in tonic heart rate (HR) at the beginning of the experiment, the HR of the nonpsychopathic *S*s decreased slightly throughout the session, while that of the psychopaths remained more or less the same. As a result, the tonic HR of the psychopathic *S*s was slightly (less than 2 bpm), though significantly, higher at the end of the session than that of the other *S*s. In a somewhat similar (though less complex) task (discussed below) in which pairs of *S*s administered shocks to one another, tonic HR was unrelated to the diagnosis of the *S*s (Hare & Craigen, 1973). It may be, therefore, that Dengerink's results reflect some unusual interaction between psychopathy and the particular nature of the task he used.

Several studies [e.g., see Figure 13.1(d)] have found that the mean amplitude of 'spontaneous' fluctuations in HR tends to be somewhat smaller in psychopathic *S*s than in other *S*s (Fenz, 1971; Hare, 1968; Hare & Quinn, 1971). Like the other index of spontaneous autonomic variability already discussed, *viz.* NSP activity, the group differences in HR variability tend to disappear when the *S*s are engaged in the cognitive activity associated with solving arithmetic problems [see Figure 13.1 (d)].

One other measure of cardiovascular variability, fluctuations in digital pulse amplitude, is apparently unrelated to psychopathy (Schalling *et al.*, 1973).

13.2.1.3. Some Interpretations

One way of interpreting the above data is to assume that most of the experimental situations typically used in research do not have the same emotional
impact upon psychopathic Ss as they do upon others Ss. This interpretation
relies, to a large extent, upon the fact that autonomic (especially electrodermal)
activity is associated with (among other things) emotional arousal. However,
there is also evidence that autonomic activity may have important effects upon
cortical arousal. Lacey & Lacey (1958), for example, have postulated that
fluctuations in autonomic activity may have excitatory effects upon the cortex.
Similarly, others have suggested that fluctuations in skin conductance reflect
the operation of an internal arousing mechanism (Lader, 1965) or of a cortical–
subcortical regulatory system (Venables, 1967), which helps to maintain an
optimal level of cortical arousal. What this suggests is that the relatively little
spontaneous autonomic variability observed in psychopaths reflects a chronic
tendency towards both autonomic and cortical hypoarousal. Elsewhere (Hare,
1968, 1970, 1971) it has been noted that there is a considerable amout of physiological and behavioural evidence (some of it discussed in later sections) that
also leads to the hypothesis that psychopaths are cortically underaroused,
particularly in situations that are monotonous or tedious. One interesting
behavioural implication of this cortical underarousal is that psychopaths
probably need an inordinate amount of stimulation in order to maintain a
level of cortical arousal that is optimum for the particular task at hand (cf.
Quay, 1965; Zuckerman, 1969).

13.2.2. Phasic physiological activity

In this section a selection of studies concerned with unconditioned physiological responses to simple, discrete stimuli is briefly considered.

13.2.2.1. Electrodermal responses

In several earlier accounts (e.g., Hare, 1971) it was noted that the evidence
concerning electrodermal responsivity in psychopaths was equivocal, with
some studies finding that they were hyporesponsive and others that they were
normally responsive. Part of the problem is that in several of the studies reporting negative results there is some doubt about the diagnosis of the Ss used.
Further in some studies in which responses to electric shock were measured,
the shock was preceded by a warning signal, i.e. a classical conditioning
paradigm was used. Kimmel (1966) has reviewed evidence indicating that
when a conditioned stimulus (CS) is followed by an unconditioned stimulus
(UCS) such as shock, the CS may eventually come to exert an inhibitory
influence on the unconditioned response (UCR) elicited by the shock. That
is, the response to a shock preceded by a signal may be smaller than it would
have been had the shock been presented alone. This means that in those studies
of psychopathy which used a signal–shock combination, electrodermal

responsivity to shock may have been confounded with the inhibitory influence of the signal. Whether this inhibitory influence is greater or less than normal in psychopaths is unknown; however, the extent of this inhibitory process may be dependent upon some interaction between psychopathy and the particular nature of the experimental task involved, thus making comparisons between studies difficult. In spite of these problems, it is beginning to appear as though a reasonable hypothesis is that psychopaths are electrodermally hyporesponsive to stimuli that are intense or that would ordinarily be considered to be stressful. Thus, although psychopaths were found to be normally responsive to 80-dB tones (Hare, 1968), Blankstein (1969) found that they gave comparatively small skin conductance and skin potential responses to 100-dB tones. In classical conditioning experiments Lykken (1957), Hare & Quinn (1971) and Hare & Craigen (1973) found that psychopathic Ss gave significantly smaller SC responses to electric shock than did other Ss. They also gave smaller SC responses to the insertion of hypodermic needles during intramuscular infusion of saline and adrenaline solutions (Hare, 1972a). Using pictorial stimuli Mathis (1970) found that psychopathic inmates tended to give smaller SC responses than did noncriminal Ss; the differences between groups were larger when slides of severe facial injuries were used than when less stressful slides were used. Pictorial stimuli were also used in the classical conditioning study by Hare & Quinn (1971). Slides of nude females elicited relatively small SC responses from the psychopathic inmates; however, the differences between groups did not attain significance.

Although the hypothesis of electrodermal hyporesponsivity in psychopaths has been confined to intense or stressful stimulation, it is possible that the hypothesis may be too restrictive. Lykken, Rose, Luther & Maley (1966) have argued that comparisons of autonomic responsivity may be more meaningful when individual differences in the range of activity possible are taken into account. They suggested that an appropriate way of correcting SC responses is to express each S's response as a proportion of the range between his maximum and minimum SC level. This suggestion was followed in the study reported above (Hare, 1968) in which, it will be recalled, the amplitude of uncorrected SC responses to tones was unrelated to the diagnosis of the Ss. Correction for range (see Hare, 1968, Table 4) using the maximum and minimum levels of SC during the experiment, resulted in psychopaths giving somewhat smaller SC responses to the novel tones in the series than those given by the other Ss; however, only the difference in response to the novel 16th tone approached significance ($P < 0.10$). A real problem with this procedure is that an adequate estimate of an individual's range is difficult to determine. Recently Lykken & Venables (1971) have suggested that a more appropriate correction procedure might be to express each SC response as a proportion of the maximum response given during the experiment. This procedure was therefore used in a reanalysis of the SC responses to the 1st and 16th tones. The results indicated that the psychopathic Ss gave significantly smaller range-corrected SC responses to both the 1st tone ($P < 0.05$) and the 16th tone ($P < 0.005$).

Whether correction for range would similarly affect the SC response data of the other studies reported in this section is unknown. If subsequent reanalyses of data do produce similar results, the hypothesis that psychopaths are electrodermally hyporesponsive to intense stimuli would be further strengthened, and could be extended to other forms of stimulation as well.

The psychopath's tendency to give small SC responses to noxious stimulation could readily be interpreted to mean that such stimulation has relatively little emotional consequence for him. On the other hand, Bagshaw, Kimble & Pribram (1965) have reviewed evidence that SC responses may signify the central registration of stimuli required for the nervous system to develop neuronal models of these stimuli. The development of these neuronal models is associated with habituation of the orienting response (Sokolov, 1963). According to this position, then, the small SC responses of psychopaths could indicate that these neuronal models are slow to develop, with the result that habituation of the OR should be retarded. Some supportive evidence for this suggestion is presented in the next section.

Before concluding this section, some unpublished data are presented which have a bearing on Edelberg's (1970, 1972) hypothesis that the rate at which an electrodermal response recovers increases during mobilization for goal-directed behaviour. Recovery rates for the electrodermal responses to each of the 16 tones in the Hare (1968) study were computed by determining the number of seconds required to reach 50 per cent recovery ($t/2$ or 'recovery half-time') and then converting the obtained values into their reciprocals. There were no significant differences between groups in the mean recovery rates of the responses to the first 15 tones in the series. However, the psychopathic Ss showed a slower recovery rate ($P < 0.05$) to the novel 16th tone (lower in frequency and intensity than the preceding 15) than did the nonpsychopathic Ss. Edelberg (1972) has reported that recovery rate and level of electrodermal arousal are positively correlated. Consistent with this relationship is the finding that the slow recovery rate of the psychopaths to the 16th tone occurred at a time when their level of electrodermal arousal was relatively low. The slow recovery rate of the psychopaths may also indicate that they were relatively unprepared for involvement in goal-oriented behaviour.

13.2.2.2. Cardiovascular responses

The relatively few studies of cardiovascular responses in psychopaths have been more concerned with the role played by such responses in the modulation of sensory input than with their implications for emotional behaviour. The conceptual framework for this research is based largely upon (i) recent theory and research indicating that the orienting response (OR) to novel stimulation is associated with HR deceleration and cephalic vasodilation, while the defensive response (DR) to intense or disturbing stimulation includes HR acceleration and cephalic vasoconstriction (e.g., see Graham & Clifton, 1966; Hare, 1972b; Sokolov, 1963); and (ii) Lacey's (1967) hypothesis that sensory-intake is associated with HR deceleration, and sensory-rejection with HR acceleration.

In the Hare (1968) study it will be recalled that electrodermal and cardio-vascular responses were recorded while Ss heard a repetitive series of 15 80-dB tones, followed by one presentation of a 70-dB tone. As already noted, the diagnosis of the Ss was unrelated to the size of the SC responses elicited; it was also unrelated to the rate at which habituation of these responses occurred. On the other hand, as Figure 13.2 indicates, there were group differences in the size of the cardiac OR (deceleraion) elicited by the tones that could be considered most novel, *viz.* Tones 1 and 16, and that the response habituatcd more rapidly in the nonpsychopathic Ss. The small cardiac ORs given by the psychopathic Ss suggests that they may be less sensitive and/or responsive to small changes in environmental stimulation than are normal individuals.

Since psychopaths may be unusually tolerant of strong stimulation (Hare & Thorvaldson, 1970), we might expect that the shift from a cardiac OR (deceler-ation) to a cardiac DR (acceleration) would require more intense stimulation for them than it would for normal persons. In support of this prediction,

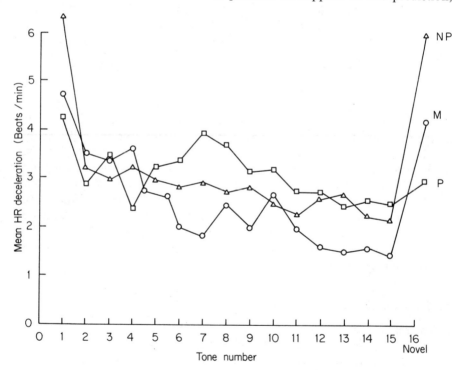

FIGURE 13.2. Mean cardiac deceleration in response to repetitive (Tones 1–15) and novel (Tone 16) stimulation. P = psychopaths; M = mixed group; NP = non-psychopaths. (Hare, R. D. Psychopathy, autonomic functioning and the orienting response, *Journal of Abnormal Psychology, Monograph Supplement,* **73,** 1968, (3, pt. 2). Copyright 1968 by the American Psychological Association and reproduced by permission.)

Blankstein (1969) found that the initial 100-dB tone in a series produced a biphasic accelerative–decelerative response in nonpsychopaths, but only a decelerative response in psychopaths. When intense electric shocks are used, it appears that psychopaths, like normal Ss, respond with cardiac acceleration (Hare & Craigen, 1973; Hare & Quinn, 1971). Incidentally, Blankstein's data could also be interpreted to mean that nonpsychopaths have a lower threshold for the elicitation of a startle response than do psychopaths. Hatton, Berg & Graham (1970), for example, have shown that auditory stimuli not quite intense enough to elicit a cardiac DR will elicit a decelerative response when stimulus onset is relatively slow, but that the same stimulus may elicit a biphasic accelerative–decelerative response when its onset is very sudden. To what extent startle and defensive responses are related is not known. However, research is obviously needed in which the effects of acoustic rise-time on cardiac responses of psychopaths are systematically investigated.

Several studies have been concerned with cardiovascular responsivity to drug injections rather than to discrete stimuli. Schachter & Latane (1964) reported that adrenaline produced a larger heart rate increase in psychopaths than in nonpsychopaths. This finding was based upon only four Ss in each group, and would hardly seem to justify the author's conclusion that psychopaths are autonomically hyperresponsive. It seems that even Schachter (1971) is no longer entirely convinced of the soundness of this conclusion or of the data upon which it was based. A more recent study (Hare, 1972a) with considerably more Ss (16) in each group found no differences between psychopaths and other inmates in either the size or the duration of HR response to injected adrenaline.

In addition to HR, several studies have taken measures of vasomotor activity. The general finding is that psychopaths do not differ from other Ss in their digital vasomotor response (constriction) to tones of moderate intensity (Hare, 1968; the responses of the former were somewhat more resistant to habituation, however), slides of nude females (Hare & Quinn, 1971) or injections of adrenaline (Hare, 1972a). Cephalic vasomotor responses were recorded in one study (Hare & Quinn, 1971), with rather strange results— psychopaths responded to electric shock with cephalic vasodilation rather than the more appropriate vasoconstriction. Whether this was simply a chance finding, or whether it is indicative of some cardiovascular anomaly in psychopaths is unknown.

Some comment is needed here on the rather unusual pattern of autonomic response habituation observed in the Hare (1968) study. It will be recalled that there were no group differences in rate of SC habituation to repetitive tones, but that the cardiovascular ORs (HR deceleration and digital vasoconstriction) of the psychopaths were relatively slow to habituate. Earlier the author sugges-ted that results such as these would be consistent with the position that neuronal models of stimulation develop slowly in psychopaths. In this regard it is interesting that somewhat similar autonomic response patterns to repetitive stimulation have been observed in drowsy Ss (McDonald, Johnson & Hord,

1964) and brain-damaged adults (Holloway & Parsons, 1971). In each case one could argue that the cortical mechanisms required for the development of neuronal models are unable to operate efficiently, with the result that habituation is retarded.

13.2.3. Conditioning and avoidance learning

13.2.3.1. Anticipatory responses

Several studies have found that specific instructions that an aversive stimulus is about to be received produce less anticipatory electrodermal activity in psychopaths than in other Ss (Hare, 1965a; Lippert & Senter, 1966; Schalling & Levander, 1967). For example, Figure 13.3 shows the mean log SC of psychopathic (P) and nonpsychopathic (NP) criminals and noncriminal Ss (C) while they were watching the consecutive numbers 1–12 appear in the window of a memory drum; after the first trial they had been told that from now on each time the number 8 appeared, they would receive a strong electric shock. It is evident that during both the second and the sixth (last) trials, Group P showed less of an anticipatory increase in SC than did the other groups; moreover, the total increase in SC from stimulus 1 to stimulus 8, an increase which includes both the anticipatory activity and the response to the shock itself, was significantly less for Group P than for Group NP. The fact that the nonpsychopathic Ss gave large anticipatory responses, even before shock had been received for

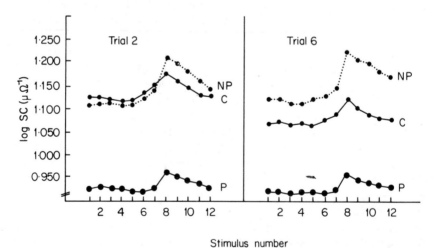

FIGURE 13.3. Mean log (skin conductance) as a function of anticipated shock (administered at stimulus number 8). P = psychopathic criminals; NP = nonpsychopathic criminals; C = normal noncriminals. (Hare, R. D. Temporal gradient of fear arousal in Psychopaths. *Journal of Abnormal Psychology*, **70**, 1965, 442. Copyright 1965 by the American Psychological Association and reproduced by permission.)

the first time, may reflect the ability of most people to cognitively reinstate earlier associations between warning cues and aversive events. With psychopaths, however, these earlier associations presumably were either not made with sufficient strength to generate emotional responses and/or failed to generalize to the experimental situation. In any case, these and related findings are consistent with the hypothesis that psychopaths exhibit a relatively steep temporal gradient of fear arousal (Hare, 1965a, 1965c, 1971). In other words, unless warning cues are in very close temporal proximity to an expected aversive event, little anticipatory fear is elicited in psychopaths.

The more traditional classical conditioning paradigms also indicate that psychopaths do not acquire anticipatory electrodermal responses readily (Hare, 1965b; Hare & Quinn, 1971; Lykken, 1957). Consider, for example, the study by Hare & Quinn (1971), in which Ss were presented with a series of three different tones or conditioned stimuli (CS), each 10-sec long. One tone (the Cs^s) was always followed by an aversive unconditioned stimulus (UCS), electric shock; one tone (the CS^p) was always followed by a more pleasant UCS, a 2-sec glimpse of a coloured slide of a nude female; the remaining tone (the CS$^-$) was not followed by anything. Each CS, followed by the appropriate UCS, was presented 16 times in random order. An increase in SC that began between 1 and 4 sec after CS onset was considered to be an orienting response (OR), while a SC response beginning between 4 and 11 sec after CS onset was defined as an anticipatory response (AR). The mean electrodermal ARs elicited by each CS are plotted in Figure 13.4. The differences between groups were dramatic, particularly when shock was the UCS. The non-psychopaths (Group NP) gave very large electrodermal ARs to the CS^s, whereas the other Ss gave very small responses. The differences between groups were somewhat smaller when nude pictures were involved. Similar results were obtained when the ORs to each CS were analysed—the ORs given by Group NP to both CS^s and the CS^p increased sharply over trials, while those of the other groups did not.

Since the above study was published several additional (unpublished) analyses of the data were undertaken. In view of the argument by Lykken & Venables (1971) that electrodermal responses may be more meaningful if corrected for individual differences in range, each AR preceding shock (i.e., elicited by the CS^s) was expressed as a proportion of the response elicited by the shock. The result of this correction for range was to reduce somewhat the difference between groups; however, Group P still gave significantly smaller responses than did Group NP. A further analysis was carried out to determine whether the small ARs given by Group P were partially the result of having included in the original analysis Ss who failed to give a measurable response— since somewhat more failures to respond occurred in Group P than in Group NP, one could argue that the size of the responses of those Group P Ss who did respond was underestimated. However, a trial-by-trial analysis of the data of only those Ss who did give a measurable response indicated that the responses

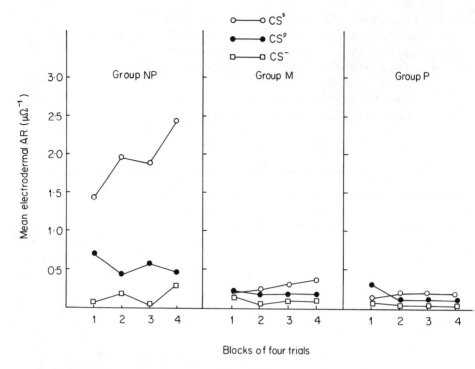

FIGURE 13.4. Mean electrodermal anticipatory responses elicited by 10-sec tones presented alone (CS^-) or followed by either shock (CS^s) or a slide of a nude female (CS^p). P = psychopaths; M = mixed group; NP = nonpsychopaths. (Hare, R. D. & Quinn, M. Psychopathy and autonomic conditioning. *Journal of Abnormal Psychology*, **77**, 1971, 223–239. Copyright 1971 by the American Psychological Association and reproduced by permission.)

of Group NP were still much larger than those of Group P. Similar results were obtained with respect to the AR elicited by the CS^p.

Taken together with the results of other studies, then, these data indicate that psychopaths do not develop conditioned electrodermal responses readily, especially where the responses are anticipatory to an aversive stimulus.

13.2.3.2. Avoidance learning

The psychopath's difficulty in acquiring conditioned electrodermal responses bears a conceptual relationship to his apparent inability to avoid punishment and to perform well in tasks mediated by fear or anxiety (Lykken, 1957; Rosen & Schalling, 1971; Schachter & Latane, 1964; Schoenherr, 1964; Schmauk, 1970). Mowrer (1947) has suggested that learning to avoid punishment involves two stages, the classical conditioning of fear to cues associated with the punishment, and the reinforcement, by fear reduction, of responses that remove the person from the fear-producing cues. If we assume that anticipatory electrodermal activity prior to noxious stimulation is a reasonable indicant of fear arousal, then the psychopath's apparent inability to avoid punishment or to anticipate the negative consequences of his own behaviour may be a reflection of the failure of cues (physical, symbolic, etc.) to generate sufficient anticipatory fear for the instigation and reinforcement of avoidance behaviour. As I've indicated earlier, the psychopath's inability to experience the anticipatory fear required for avoidance behaviour is probably most evident when the expected aversive event is temporally remote. This doesn't necessarily mean that he is intellectually incapable of anticipating the future consequences of his own behaviour, only that he is not sufficiently motivated to do so. As Arieti has put it, the psychopath ' . . . knows theoretically that he may be caught in the antisocial act and be punished. But . . . this punishment is a possibility concerning the future and, therefore, he does not experience the idea of it with enough emotional strength to change the course of his present actions' (1967, p. 248).

13.2.3.3. Dissociation of conditioned electrodermal and cardiovascular responses

The model of psychopathy in which electrodermal conditioning and avoidance learning are linked largely depends upon the assumption that the extent to which electrodermal responses occur in the interval prior to an aversive event is a reflection of the degree of apprehension or anticipatory fear experienced. However valid this assumption may be, it seems reasonable to ask what some of his other physiological systems are doing while the psychopath is anticipating an aversive event. The answer seems to be, at least in so far as cardiovascular activity is concerned, more or less what occurs with normal Ss. For example, in the Hare & Quinn (1971) study, described above, the psychopathic Ss were just as proficient as the other Ss in the acquisition of anticipatory cardiac and digital vasomotor responses. That is, while the psychopaths were very poor electrodermal conditioners, they were good cardiovascular ones. Similar results were obtained in a recent study by Hare & Craigen (1974) in which pairs of Ss (A and B) were required to take turns in administering shocks to themselves and to one another. A 10-sec tone (CS) preceded each shock, so that it was possible to evaluate physiological activity prior to reception of shock received by self (direct shock) and by the other Ss (vicarious shock). We found that the psychopathic inmates (P) gave smaller anticipatory SC responses than that did the nonpsychopathic ones (NP), particularly when they themselves were about to receive the shock. Similar results were obtained for the ORs elicited by CS onset. However, when cardiac responses were considered, the psychopaths turned out to be the better conditioners. Figure 13.5 shows the mean sec-by-sec changes in HR following onset of the CS preceding shock to self (S) and the CS preceding shock to the other S (O); the data are averaged over the eight trials involved. The anticipatory HR response was primarily accelerative in nature, giving way to a decelerative phase just prior to shock. The size and form of the response were much the same whether shock was

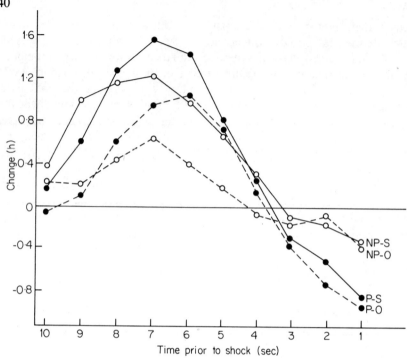

FIGURE 13.5. Mean sec-by-sec changes in heart rate shown by psychopaths (P) and nonpsychopaths (NP) to the tones preceding shock to self (S) and shock to the other *S*, averaged over eight trials. (From Hare & Gaigen, 1974)

about to be received directly (S) or vicariously experienced (O). However, both the accelerative and decelerative components were significantly larger in Group P than in Group NP. The most dramatic difference between groups, a difference partially obscured through the averaging of data across trials, occurred on the very first trial. As Figure 13.6 indicates, the anticipatory HR responses of Group P on Trial 1 consisted primarily of marked acceleration during the first 5 or 6 sec after CS onset, while those of Group NP were small and slightly decelerative. On the second trial, Group P developed a secondary decelerative component, while Group NP's responses were similar to those given by Group P on the first trial. On subsequent trials the response patterns of each group became more and more similar to one another.

These findings, when considered along with those from a previous study (Hare & Quinn, 1971) again suggest that psychopaths may be poor electrodermal conditioners but good cardiovascular ones. It appears that much the same can be said for vicariously conditioned responses, since the anticipatory electrodermal and HR responses of Group P were more or less the same when others were about to receive shock as when it was about to be directly experienced. In some respects this could be considered surprising, since psychopaths are generally considered to lack empathy and concern for the welfare of others.

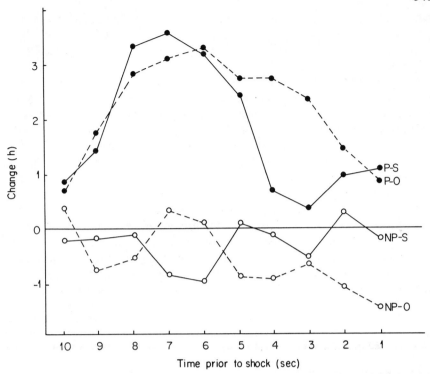

FIGURE 13.6. Mean sec-by-sec changes in heart rate shown by psychopaths (P) nonpsychopaths (NP) to the tones preceding shock to self (S) and shock to the other S (O) on Trial 1. (From Hare & Craigen 1974)

However, a discrepancy arises only if anticipatory HR activity is assumed to be primarily related to some form of emotional arousal. While such may be the case, there is increasing evidence that cardiovascular activity either influences or at least is associated with the modulation of sensory input and with transactions with the environment (e.g., Graham & Clifton, 1966; Hare, 1972b, 1973; Lacey, 1967; Raskin, Kotses & Bever, 1969). Thus, it is possible that the anticipatory HR responses of the Ss in the present study were more related to defensive behaviour than to emotional arousal in the usual sense. Since the tones preceding shock functioned as warning signals, the initial period of HR acceleration may have been part of a defensive response (DR) to cues that had acquired aversive properties. Presumably this DR served to reduce the aversiveness of the situation and helped the Ss to cope with it (Lacey, 1967; Lykken, 1968; Sokolov, 1963). The decelerative component that followed this initial period of acceleration may have been partly due to 'vagal rebound' (Obrist, Wood & Perez-Reyes, 1965). Dronsejko (1972) has suggested that this decelerative phase may also reflect the operation of a mechanism for coping with the forthcoming stressor.

If anticipatory HR responses are, in fact, related to the efficiency with which *S*s modulate aversive cues and cope with an impending stressor, the present results support the hypothesis (Hare, 1968, 1970; Lykken, 1968) that psychopaths may be relatively adept at the process. Both the accelerative and decelerative components were generally larger in Gorup P than in Group NP. The fact that Group P gave large accelerative responses on the first trial, while Group NP did not, is of special interest here. It appears that, whereas Group NP required a considerable amount of actual experience with the stimuli and contingencies involved in the experiment before conditioned HR responses appeared, the pre-experimental instructions were largely sufficient for Group P.

One way, then, of explaining the dissociation of conditioned electrodermal and cardiovascular responses in psychopaths is to assume that small electrodermal responses preceding aversive stimuli reflect the relative absence of fear arousal, while anticipatory cardiac activity is a protective response that serves to reduce the emotional impact of the situation. The implications that this would have for the behaviour of psychopaths probably depends upon the particular characteristics of the situation they happen to find themselves in. For example, they should perform poorly on tasks in which fear and/or arousal have facilitating effects, and efficiently on tasks in which fear and/or arousal have disrupting effects.

13.3. CORTICAL CORRELATES OF PSYCHOPATHY

13.3.1. EEG studies

Very few studies have been primarily concerned with the brain-wave activity of psychopaths. In most cases, the electroencephalogram (EEG) is obtained as part of a general survey of psychiatric patients, many of them of somewhat uncertain diagnosis. Nevertheless, the results have been reasonably consistent (see review by Hare, 1970). Briefly, it appears that anywhere between 30 and 60 per cent of diagnosed 'psychopaths' exhibit some form of EEG abnormality, most usually widespread slow-wave activity (e.g., Arthurs & Cahoon, 1964; Ellingson, 1954; Hill & Watterson, 1942; Knott, Platt, Ashby & Gottlieb, 1953). In some cases, the highly aggressive forms of psychopathy may be associated with temporal abnormalities consisting of either slow-wave (Hill, 1952) or positive-spike (Kurland, Yeager & Arthur. 1963) activity.

These data can be interpreted in several ways. For example, the generalized slow-wave activity frequently found in psychopaths is consistent with the hypothesis that they tend to be cortically underaroused (Hare, 1968, 1970; Quay, 1965) and that they tend to become quickly bored and drowsy in situations that are dull and unexciting, including routine EEG procedures (Forssman & Frey, 1953). Since the psychopath's slow-wave activity is somewhat similar to that of normal children, it has been suggested that psychopathy may be related to delayed maturation of cortical processes (see Kiloh & Osselton, 1966). In spite of some difficulties with this maturational retardation hypothesis (see Hare, 1970), some indirect support is available. For instance, histologic studies of the nervous system indicate that the maturation of cortical mechanisms is roughly correlated with a shift from the slow-wave activity of childhood to the faster rhythms of adulthood (Lindsley, 1964; Scheibel & Scheibel, 1954). Gibbens, Pond & Stafford-Clark (1955) found that psychopaths with EEG abnormalities have a better prognosis than those with normal EEGs. Similarly, Robins (1966) found that the behaviour of about one-third of a group of psychopaths became less grossly antisocial between the ages of 30 and 40. Since EEG data were not available, it is not known whether this improvement in behaviour was associated with increasing normality of brain-wave activity. Obviously what is required here is a developmental study in which behavioural and psychophysiological measures are taken over an extended period.

In an earlier paper (Hare, 1971) it was suggested that the highly impulsive behaviour of individuals with EEG abnormalities localized in the temporal lobes could be interpreted in terms of McCleary's (1966) concept of response perseveration. This concept is based upon studies in which lesions in limbic inhibitory mechanisms may result in perseveration of the most dominant response in any given situation, even though this response would ordinarily be inhibited. With respect to psychopathy, we might assume that the activity of these inhibitory mechanisms is periodically dampened, perhaps during states of high drive produced by sexual arousal, anger, etc. As a result, the dominant response in that particular situation (e.g., sexual or aggressive behaviour) would occur, regardless of the consequences.

13.3.2. Cortical evoked potentials

Very few data are available on the relationship between cortical evoked potentials and psychopathy. Shagass & Schwartz (1962) determined neural recovery rates in psychiatric patients by comparing them on the size of the somatosensory evoked response to the second of two stimuli presented closely together in time. They reported that both normal and neurotic Ss had faster recovery rates than did schizophrenic and psychopathic ones, suggesting that the latter two disorders are characterized by reduced cortical excitability. Similar results were recently reported by Shagass & Canter (1972), although in both studies the criteria for selection of Ss are not outlined.

13.3.3. Contingent negative variation

McCallum & Walter (1968) reported that the only Ss for whom the contingent negative variation (CNV) during the foreperiod of a reaction-time study was absent or greatly reduced in magnitude was a group of psychopaths. However, the Ss involved were apparently not psychopaths in the sense that the term is used here. More recently, Syndulko, Parker, Maltzman, Jens & Ziskind (1972) obtained CNV recordings from psychopathic and normal Ss while they were engaged in several different reaction-time tasks. They found that during standard task conditions—a warning signal followed by a low intensity 70-dB tone) imperative stimulus—reaction-time and the amplitude of the CNV were the same in both groups. When the intensity of the imperative stimulus was increased to 95-dB, the CNV of the normal Ss increased in size while their reaction-time decreased. The psychopaths also showed a decrease in reaction-time to the more intense stimulus; however, there was not a corresponding increase in CNV amplitude.

13.3.4. Brain mechanisms in conditioning

Stein (1964) has suggested that the facilitation or inhibition of ongoing behaviour is associated with the elicitation of classically conditioned anticipatory responses that activate reward or punishment mechanisms in the hypothalamus. More recently (Gray, 1971, 1972) has proposed that the reward mechanism consists of the septal area, the medial forebrain bundle, and the lateral hypothalamus, while the punishment mechanisms is to be found in the medial frontal cortex, the medial septal nuclei, and the hippocampus. Like Stein, Gray suggests that these mechanisms are activated by expectations of rewards and punishments, i.e. by classically conditioned anticipatory responses. Psychopaths, according to Gray, are neurotic extraverts, and as such their behaviour is seen as the result of a relative sensitivity to rewards and a relative insensitivity to punishment and threatening stimuli. One difficulty with this argument is that, if anything, the psychopath is more like a stable extravert than a neurotic one (Hare, 1968). Moreover, clinical and research evidence suggest that psychopaths are relatively unaffected by both threats of punishment and promises of reward, particularly when these events are temporally remote (Hare, 1965c, 1971). Further, Gray's model would be more applicable to psychopathy if the *temporal integration* of anticipated rewards and punishments were taken into account (Renner, 1964). That is, it may be true that a psychopathic person will take an immediate reward when the aversive consequences for doing so are somewhere in the future; on the other hand, however, it is unlikely that he will accept some immediate discomfort for the sake of some promised future reward. Elsewhere (Hare, 1971) it has been suggested that the ability of promises of reward and threats of punishment to activate reward and punishment mechanisms in the brain decreases with temporal remoteness, with the rate of decrease being greater for psychopathic than for nonpsychopathic persons. Whether a given response would be initiated or inhibited would then depend upon the relative remoteness of expected rewards and punishments, and upon the relative degree to which the corresponding reward and punishment mechanisms were activated.

13.4. ACKNOWLEDGMENT

Preparation of this manuscript and some of the research reported were supported by Grant MA-4511 from the Medical Research Council of Canada, and by the Canadian Mental Health Association.

13.5. REFERENCES

American Psychiatric Association. *Diagnostic and Statistical Manual: Mental Disorders.* Washington, D.C.: Author, 1968.

Arieti, S. *The intrapsychic Self.* New York: Basic Books, 1967.

Arthurs, R. G. & Cahoon, E. B. A clinical and electroencephalographic survey of psychopathic personality. *American Journal of Psychiatry,* 1964, **120,** 875–882.

Bagshaw, M. H., Kimble, D. P. & Pribram, K. H. The GSR of monkeys during orienting and habituation and after ablation of the amygdala, hippocampus and inferotemporal cortex. *Neuropsychologia,* 1965, **3,** 111–119.

Blandstein, K. R. Patterns of autonomic functioning in primary and secondary psychopaths. Unpublished Master's thesis. University of Waterloo, 1969.

Borkovec, T. Autonomic reactivity to sensory stimulation in psychopathic, neurotic and normal juvenile delinquents. *Journal of Consulting and Clinical Psychology,* 1970, **35,** 217–222.

Cleckley, H. *The Mask of Sanity* (4th Ed.). St. Louis, Mo.: Mosby, 1964.

Craft, M. J. *Ten studies into psychopathic personality.* Bristol: John Wright, 1965.

Dahlstrom, W. G. & Welch, G. S. *An MMPI handbook.* Minneapolis: University of Minnesota Press, 1960.

Dengerink, H. A. & Bertilson, H. S. Psychopathy, aggression and arousal. Presented at Workshop in Sociopathy, Society for Psychophysiological Research meeting, Boston, 1972.

Dronsejko, K. Effects of CS duration and instructional set on cardiac anticipatory responses to stress in field dependent and independent subjects. *Psychophysiology,* 1972, **9,** 1–13.

Edelberg, R. The information content of the recovery limb of the electrodermal response. *Psychophysiology,* 1970, **6,** 527–539.

Edelberg, R. Electrodermal recovery rate, goal-orientation and aversion. *Psychophysiology,* 1972, **9,** 512–520.

Ellingson, R. J. Incidence of EEG abnormality among patients with mental disorders of apparently nonorganic origin: A criminal review. *American Journal of Psychiatry,* 1954, **111,** 263–275.

Fenz, W. Heart rate responses to a stressor: A comparison between primary and secondary psychopaths and normal controls. *Journal of Experimental Research in Personality,* 1971, **5,** 7–13.

Forssman, H. & Frey, T. S. Electroencephalograms of boys with behaviour disorders. *Acta Psychiat. Neurol. Scand.,* 1953, **28,** 61–73.

Gibbens, T. C., Pond, D. A. & Stafford-Clark, D. A follow-up study of criminal psychopaths. *British Journal of Delinquency,* 1955, **5,** 126–136.

Gough, H. G. & Peterson, D. R. The indentification and measurement of predispositional factors in crime and delinquency. *Journal of Consulting Psychology,* 1952, **16,** 207–212.

Graham, F. & Clifton, R. Heart rate change as a component of the orienting response. *Psychological Bulletin,* 1966, **65,** 305–320.

Gray, J. A. *The psychology of fear and stress.* New York: McGraw-Hill, 1971.

Gray, J. A. The psychophysiological nature of introversion–extraversion: A modification of Eysenck's theory. In V. D. Nebylitsyn & J. A. Gray (Eds.), *Biological bases of individual behaviour.* New York: Academic Press, 1972, pp. 182–205.

Hare, R. D. Temporal gradient of fear arousal in psychopaths. *Journal of Abnormal Psychology,* 1965, **70,** 442–445(a).

Hare, R. D. Acquisition and generalization of a conditioned fear response in psychopathic and nonpsychopathic criminals. *Journal of Psychology,* 1965, **59,** 367–370(b).

Hare, R. D. A conflict and learning theory analysis of psychopathic behaviour. *Journal of Research in Crime and Delinquency,* 1965, **2,** 12–19(c).

Hare, R. D. Psychopathy, autonomic functioning and the orienting response. *Journal of Abnormal Psychology*, Monograph Supplement, 1968, **73**, (3, Pt. 2).

Hare, R. D. *Psychopathy: Theory and Research*. New York: Wiley, 1970.

Hare, R. D. Psychopathic behaviour: Some recent theory and research. In H. Adams & W. Boardman (Eds). *Advances in experimental clinical psychology*. New York: Pergamon, 1971, pp. 1–46.

Hare, R. D. Psychopathy and sensitivity to adrenalin. *Journal of Abnormal Psychology*, 1972, **79**, 138–147(a).

Hare, R. D. Cardiovascular components of orienting and defensive responses. *Psychophysiology*, 1972, **9**, 606–614(b).

Hare, R. D. Psychophysiological studies of psychopathy. Presented at Ninth Annual Conference on Current Concerns in Clinical Psychology, University of Iowa, November, 1972.

Hare, R. D. & Craigen, D. Psychopathy and physiological activity in a mixed-motive game situation. *Psychophysiology*, 1974, **11**, 197–206.

Hare, R. D. & Quinn, M. Psychopathy and autonomic conditioning. *Journal of Abnormal Psychology*, 1971, **77**, 223–239.

Hare, R. D. & Thorvaldson, S. A. Psychopathy and sensitivity to electrical stimulation. *Journal of Abnormal Psychology*, 1970, **76**, 370–374.

Hatten, H., Berg, W. & Graham, F. Effects of acoustic rise time on heart rate response. *Psychonomic Science*, 1970, **19**, 101–103.

Hill, D. EEG in episodic psychotic and psychopathic behaviour: A classification of data. *EEG and Clinical Neurophysiology*, 1952, **4**, 419–442.

Hill, D. & Watterson, D. Electroencephalographic studies of the psychopathic personality. *Journal of Neurology and Psychiatry*, 1942, **5**, 47–64.

Holloway, F. A. & Parsons, O. A. Habituation of the orienting reflex in brain damaged patients. *Psychophysiology*, 1971, **8**, 623–634.

Karpman, B. The structure of neurosis: With special differentials between neurosis, psychosis, homosexuality, alcoholism, psychopathy and criminality. *Archives of Criminal Psychodynamics*, 1961, **4**, 599–646.

Kiloh, L. & Osselton, J. *Clinical electroencephalography*, Washington: Butterworth, 1966.

Kimmel, H. D. Inhibition of the unconditioned response in classical conditioning. *Psychological Review*, 1966, **73**, 232–240.

Knott, J. R., Platt, E. B., Ashby, M. C. & Gottlieb, J. S. A familial evaluation of the electroencephalogram of patients with primary behaviour disorder and psychopathic personality. *EEG and Clinical Neurophysiology*, 1953, **5**, 363–370.

Kurland, H. D., Yeager, C. T. & Arthur, R. J. Psychophysiologic aspects of severe behavior disorders. *Archives of General Psychiatry*, 1963, **8**, 599–604.

Lacey, J. I. Somatic response patterning and stress: Some revisions of activation theory. In M. H. Appley & R. Trumbell (Eds.), *Psychological Stress: Issues in research*. New York: Appleton–Century–Crofts, 1967, pp. 14–44.

Lacey, J. I. & Lacey, B. C. The relationship of resting autonomic activity to motor inpulsivity. In *The brain and human behavior*. Baltimore: Williams & Wilkins, 1958, pp. 144–209.

Lader, M. H. The effects of cyclobarbitone on spontaneous autonomic activity. *Journal of Psychosomatic Research*, 1965, **9**, 201–207.

Lindsley, D. B. The ontogeny of pleasure: Neural and behavioural development. In R. G. Health (Ed.), *The role of pleasure in behaviour*. New York: Harper & Row, 1964, pp. 3–22.

Lippert, W. W. & Senter, R. J. Electrodermal responses in the sociopath. *Psychonomic Science*, 1966, **4**, 25–26.

London, H., Schubert, D. S. & Washburn, D. Increase of autonomic arousal by boredom. *Journal of Abnormal Psychology*, 1972, **80**, 29–36.

Lykken, D. T. A study of anxiety in the sociopathic personality. *Journal of Abnormal and Clinical Psychology*, 1957, **55**, 6–10.

Lykken, D. T. Neuropsychology and psychophysiology in personality research. In E. Borgotta & W. Lambert (Eds.), *Handbook of personality theory and research*. Chicago: Rand McNally, 1968.

Lykken, D. T. & Katzenmeyer, G. Manual for the Activity Preference Questionnaire (APQ). Research Report No. PR-68-3, Department of Psychiatry, University of Minnesota, 1968.

Lykken, D. T., Rose, R., Luther, B. & Maley, M. Correcting psychophysiological measures for individual differences in range. *Psychological Bulletin*, 1966, **66**, 481–484.

Lykken, D. T. & Venables, P. H. Direct measurement of skin conductance: A proposal for standardization. *Psychophysiology*, 1971, **8**, 656–672.

Mathis, H. I. *Emotional responsivity in the antisocial personality*. (Doctoral dissertation, The George Washington University) Ann Arbor, Mich.: University Microfilms, 1970.

Maughs, S. B. Concept of psychopathy and psychopathic personality. Its evolution and historical development. *Journal of Criminal Psychopathology*, 1941, **2**, 329–356.

McCallum, W. C. & Walter, W. G. The effects of attention and distraction on the contingent negative variation in normal and neurotic subjects. *EEG and Clinical Neurophysiology*, 1968, **25**, 319–329.

McCleary, R. Response-modulating functions of the limbic system: Initiation and suppression. In E. Stellar & J. Sprague (Eds.), *Progress in physiological psychology*. Vol. 1, New York: Academic Press, 1966, pp. 209–272.

McDonald, D., Johnson, L. & Hord, D. Habituation of the orienting response in alert and drowsy subjects. *Psychophysiology*, 1964, **1**, 163–173.

Mowrer, O. H. On the dual nature of learning: A reinterpretation of 'conditioning' and 'problem-solving'. *Harvard Educational Review*, 1947, **17**, 102–148.

Obrist, P. A., Wood, D. M. & Perez-Reyes, M. Heart-rate conditioning in humans: Effects of UCS intensity, vagal blockade, and adrenergic block of vasomotor activity. *Journal of Experimental Psychology*, 1965, **70**, 32–42.

Quay, H. Psychopathic personality as pathological stimulation seeking. *American Journal of Psychiatry*, 1965, **122**, 180–183.

Quay, H. C. & Parsons, L. B. *The differential behavioural classification of the juvenile offender*. Washington, D.C.: Bureau of Prisons, 1971.

Raskin, D., Kotses, H. & Bever, J. Cephalic vasomotor and heart rate measures of orienting and defensive reflexes. *Psychophysiology*, 1969, **6**, 149–159.

Renner, K. E. Conflict resolution and the process of temporal integration. *Psychological Reports*, 1964, **15**, 423–438.

Robins, L. N. *Deviant children grown up*. Baltimore: Williams & Wilkins, 1966.

Rosen, A. & Schalling, D. Probability learning in psychopathic and non-psychopathic criminals. *Journal of Experimental Research in Personality*, 1971, **5**, 191–198.

Schachter, S. *Emotion, obesity and crime*. New York: Academic Press, 1971.

Schachter, S. & Latane, B. Crime, cognition and the autonomic nervous system. In M. R. Jones (Ed), *Nebraska Symposium on Motivation*. Lincoln: University of Nebraska Press, 1964, pp. 221–275.

Schalling, D. & Levander, S. Spontaneous fluctuations in EDA during anticipation of pain in two delinquent groups differing in anxiety proneness. Report No. 238 from the Psychological Laboratory, University of Stockholm, 1967.

Schalling, D., Lidberg, L., Levander, S. & Dahlin, Y. Relations between fluctuations in skin resistance and digital pulse volume and scores on the Gough De Scale. Unpublished manuscript, University of Stockholm, 1968.

Schalling, D., Lidberg, L., Levander, S. & Dahlin, Y. Spontaneous activity as related to psychopathy. *Biological Psychology*, 1973, **1**, 83–98.

Scheibel, M. E. & Scheibel, A. B. Some neural substrates of postnatal development. In M. Hoffman & L. Hoffman (Eds), *Review of child development research*. Vol. 1. New York: Russell Sage Foundation, 1954, pp. 481–519.

Schmauk, F. J. A study of the relationship between kinds of punishment, autonomic arousal, subjective anxiety and avoidance learning in the primary sociopath. *Journal of Abnormal Psychology*, 1970, **76**, 325–355.

Schoenherr, J. C. *Avoidance of noxious stimulation in psychopathic personality*. (Doctoral dissertation, University of California, Los Angeles) Ann Arbor, Mich.: University Microfilms, 1964, No. 64-8334.

Shagass, C. & Canter, A. Cerebral evoked responses and personality. In V. D. Nebylitsyn & J. A. Gray (Eds), *Biological bases of individual behaviour*. New York: Academic Press, 1972, 111–127.

Shagass, C., & Schwartz, M. Observations on somatosensory cortical reactivity in personality disorders. *Journal of Nervous and Mental Disease*, 1962, **135**, 44–51.

Sokolov, E. H. *Perception and the Conditioned reflex*. New York: MacMillan, 1963.

Stein, L. Reciprocal action of reward and punishment mechanisms. In R. Heath(Ed). *The role of pleasure in behavior*. New York: Harper & Row, 1964, pp. 113-139.

Sutker, P. Vicarious conditioning and sociopathy. *Journal of Abnormal Psychology*, 1970, **76**, 380–386.

Synduldo, K., Parker, D., Maltzman, I., Jens, R. & Ziskind, E. The effects of noxious stimulation on the CNV in sociopaths and controls. Presented at Workshop on Sociopathy, Society for Psychophysiological Research meeting, Boston, 1972.

Venables, P. H. Partial failure of cortical-subcortical integration as a factor underlying schizophrenic behaviour. In *The origins of schizophrenia*, Amsterdam: Exerpta Medica International Congress Series No. 151, 1967, pp. 42–53.

World Health Organization. *International Classification of diseases*. Eighth Revision, Geneva, 1968.

Zuckerman, M. Theoretical formulations: I. In J. P. Zubek (Ed), *Sensory deprivation: Fifteen years of research*. New York: Appleton–Century–Crofts, 1969, pp. 407–432.

SECTION 3

Psychology and Psychophysiology

Chapter 14

The Sensitivity of the Evoked Potential to Psychological Variables

SAMUEL SUTTON and PATRICIA TUETING

Biometrics Research,
New York State Department of Mental Hygiene

Some years ago—and to some extent this is still true—it was very common for papers on human average evoked potentials* to refer to the high degree of inter- and intra-subject variability. This is particularly emphasized for the later components of the average evoked potential. Our own experience in this area—and this has been shared by some other laboratories—is that much of this variability is due to the lack of experimental control over psychological variables of a fairly complex nature. We have found that to the extent that one is successful in exerting precise experimental control over these psychological variables, variability is substantially reduced. The later components of the evoked potential are also at least as reliable as the earlier components. In addition, these later components are found to have systematic relationships to complex psychological variables (Donchin, Kubovy, Kutas, Johnson & Herning, preprint; Hillyard, Squires, Bauer & Lindsay, 1971; Paul & Sutton, 1972; Ritter, Simson & Vaughan, 1972; Tueting, Sutton & Zubin, 1971).

There are basically two reasons why the last statement should occasion any surprise. The first reason arises from the fact that in humans the electrical activity of the brain is recorded at the scalp which is at some distance, physically and electrically, from the underlying cortex. Related to this is the fact that the detection of evoked potentials depends on the averaging of activity over many trials. Consequently, since we are using a relatively gross tool for measurement, it is not self-evident that the output of such measurements should be so sensitive to complex psychological variables.

The second reason arises from the history of the development of our knowledge of the physiology of the nervous system. Even in this day of increasing use of implanted electrodes for studying the brain in awake animals, the overwhelming bulk of our information about the electrophysiology of the nervous system is a result of work with anaesthetized animals. Anaesthetized animals are not capable of much in the way of complex psychological function. Even

---

*The evoked potential is the sequence of voltage changes recorded from scalp in awake human subjects upon presentation of a stimulus. In order to reduce the influence of background noise, averages are taken across many trials at each point in time following stimulus onset.

awake animals are incapable of giving us the clues which can be provided by verbal self-report in humans. Nor are animal subjects sensitive, without elaborate training, to subtle nuances and complexities of instructions. By contrast, one can tell the human subject that a rather intense stimulus is task irrelevant—for example, that it is an artifact of our experimental apparatus— while an otherwise identical stimulus presented at liminal intensity is all-important to his task. The influence of such variables on physiological measurements will be developed below.

Even in human psychological experiments, the subject's experience, as evidenced by his verbal report, is often taken too little into account. It is on the whole too easy to assume, for example, that because the stimulus is a pair of light flashes separated by a dark interval, the subject's ability to discriminate the presence of a dark interval implies that the nature of his experience is a perception of 'flick' or discontinuity. However, when a verbal report was obtained after each discrimination (Kietzman & Sutton, 1968), we found that even at a dark interval long enough to yield a 90 per cent level of accuracy, less than one-third of the correct discriminations were associated with a report of 'flick'. A somewhat larger proportion of trials elicited a report of 'longer duration', and the balance of trials elicited a report of 'colour difference' and a variety of other percepts.

It has been argued elsewhere (Sutton, 1969) that in physiological experiments with awake humans one must always consider the relations among three classes of variables: the stimuli, or physical events; the physiological events; and the psychological events, as evidenced by the behaviour of the subject. One can to only a very limited degree pose with respect to the awake human subject experimental questions of a kind that raise no problem in the anaesthetized animal: for example, what is the waveform of electrophysiological activity associated with light flashes? At the very least, the results of such an experiment will be reported as having a high degree of 'variability'.

The balance of this chapter is devoted to presenting examples of the extreme sensitivity of the average evoked potential in awake humans to psychological manipulation. In all cases, it will be shown that the way in which the task defines the role of the stimulus is a key determinant of the evoked potential waveform. Further, since these effects are reliable, one can gain some appreciation of the hazards involved in ignoring these psychological variables when designing experiments.

In Figure 14.1 are shown the average evoked potential waveforms in an experiment in which a subject is detecting the presence or absence of a click at a threshold level of intensity (Tueting & Sutton, 1973). The experiments are based on a signal detection theory paradigm: the stimulus may be either present or absent and the subject may report for either case a judgment of present or absent. This generates four categories of trials: hit trials, where the click is present and the subject correctly reports its presence; correct rejection trials, where the click is absent and the subject correctly reports its absence; miss trials, where the click is present but the subject incorrectly reports that it is

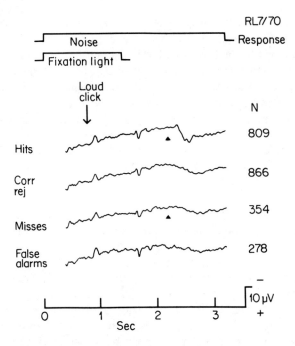

FIGURE 14.1. Average evoked potential waveforms for one subject recorded from vertex to earlobe (amplifier half-amplitude points, 0·0165 and 20 Hz). Data for the early portion of the trial, the evoked response to noise and fixation light onset, are not shown. The subject's response is made at the offset of the noise. The occurrence of the threshold click is shown as a triangle below the waveforms for hits and misses. The number of trials in the average is shown at the right of the waveform. (Adapted from Tueting & Sutton in S. Kornblum (Ed.), *Attention and performance. IV*. New York: Academic Press, 1973, pp. 185–207, with permission.)

absent; and false alarm trials, where the click is absent and the subject incorrectly reports it to be present. A separate average evoked potential is obtained for each category beginning in time from the simultaneous onset of a noise and fixation light which indicate the beginning of the trial. As can be seen in the average for the hits trials (top curve), a rather large average waveform occurs shortly after the presentation of the threshold level click (which is symbolized by the black triangle) about 2·2 sec after trial onset.

The importance of the role of the stimulus is clear when one compares, in the hit trials, the average evoked response waveform to this threshold-intensity click with the average evoked response waveform which occurs about 0·8 sec after trial onset. This earlier and much smaller average waveform is obtained to a click which is 30-dB more intense than the threshold level click. The amplitude of the response to the more intense click is only one-third the size of the response obtained to the threshold level click. Other experiments, by contrast, have shown a monotonic relationship between stimulus intensity and amplitude of the average evoked potential waveform—increasing amplitude with increasing intensity (Davis & Zerlin, 1966; Nelson, 1970).

The explanation is quite simple. In this experiment, subjects were told that the first click was a kind of artifact of our apparatus. It was described to the subject as a 'reference' click for the experimenter and had no relationship to the subject's task. On the other hand, the subject's detection of the presence or absence of the threshold click was presented as the *raison d'être* of the experiment.

The second aspect of these findings is perhaps less predictable, but may be no less important. It should be noted that the threshold-level click is physically present in both the hit trials and the miss trials, and physically absent in both the false alarms and the correct rejections. Yet the evoked potential to the threshold click is found only in the hit trials.* In an earlier study (Hakerem & Sutton, 1966), we had observed similar findings for average pupillary responses to light flashes of threshold intensity. These findings are illustrated in Figure 14.2. In both studies, we found that a response is not obtained unless two conditions are fulfilled: the stimulus must be present and it must be correctly detected. We have speculated elsewhere as to the interpretation of these findings (Sutton & Paul, in press).

In the experiment illustrated in Figure 14.1, the intense stimulus is irrelevant to the task while the threshold level stimulus is relevant. In the next illustration, the two stimuli to be compared are physically identical and are both relevant to the task, but in different ways. In Figure 14.3 are shown results for four subjects from an experiment by Jenness at our laboratory (Jenness, 1972). These waveforms are obtained from an experiment in which the subjects were making a very difficult absolute judgment of the pitch characteristics of supra-threshold intensity clicks. If the subject makes a correct judgment, the identical click is repeated later in the trial as feedback. The pairs of superimposed waveforms represent average responses to identical stimuli: the dotted lines are the average response to the click when it is to be discriminated (task click), the solid lines are the average response to the click when it informs the subject that his discrimination was correct (feedback click). As can be seen, the two waveforms are dramatically different as a function of the role of the stimulus.

In the balance of the examples, the subject's task is to guess rather than to make a discrimination. The stimuli whose evoked potentials we study serve the role of telling the subject whether his guess was right or wrong. In a number of such experiments, we have shown that the average evoked potential— paticularly a component which has a latency of about 300 msec which is

---

*However, recent data indicate (Squires, Hillyard & Lindsay, preprint) that an average evoked potential may be found in the high confidence false alarms.

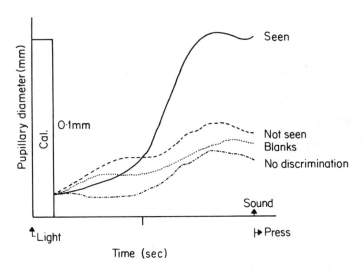

FIGURE 14.2. Average waveforms of relative pupillary diameter arbitrarily superimposed at onset of stimulation. The curves labelled 'seen' and 'not seen' were obtained with identical stimulus energy (0·010 sec at 6×10^{-5} mL). The curve labelled 'blanks' was obtained with a stimulus energy which was one-tenth of that value (0·001 sec at 6×10^{-5} mL). The curve labelled 'no discrimination', in which the subject was instructed to press on all trials (or not to press on all trials), included both stimuli and blanks. (Adapted from Hakerem & Sutton, *Nature*, 1966, **212**, 485–486, by permission of Macmillan (Journals) Ltd.)

generally known as P_3—is quite different as a function of the subject's foreknowledge as to the stimulus which will be presented. It is much larger when the subject does not have foreknowledge, so that its occurrence resolves his uncertainty with respect to its identity (Sutton, Braren, John, & Zubin, 1965a). In Figure 14.4 average evoked potential waveforms to click stimuli are presented for five subjects from an experiment in which they are guessing whether clicks or light flashes will be presented.

This finding is completely reliable. During the last several years we have run over one hundred subjects in various versions of this paradigm. The amplitude of P_3 is always larger when the stimulus resolves an uncertainty.

In a variation of this design, in which the subject is asked to guess whether a single or a double click will be presented, the average evoked potential to the single click (regardless of the guess) shows a response at the point in time at which the second click could have appeared (Sutton, Tueting, Zubin & John, 1967). This response is an emitted or endogenous potential, which signals the non-appearance of the second click. In Figure 14.5 data are presented for single clicks only. The waveform at the top is to single clicks in the certain condition, in which the subject has been told in advance that the stimulus will be a single click. The second and third waveforms are to single clicks in the uncertain condition, in which the subject made a guess. He did not know in

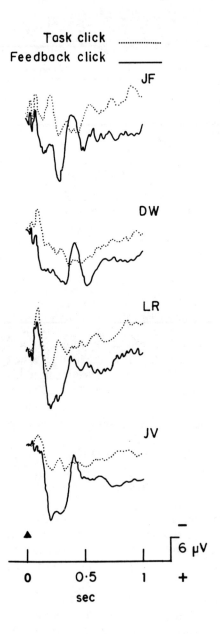

FIGURE 14.3. Average evoked potential waveforms for four subjects to physically identical clicks—task clicks, which were to be discriminated, and feedback clicks which were presented only when the subjects made a correct discrimination. (Adapted from Jenness, *Physiology and Behavior*, 1972, **9,** 141–148, by permission of Brain Research Publication Inc.)

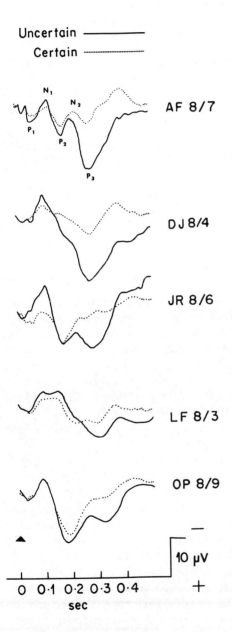

FIGURE 14.4. Average evoked potential waveforms for five subjects to physically identical clicks (triangle)— 'certain' condition clicks when the subject was told in advance when a click would be presented, and 'uncertain' condition clicks when the subject guessed and the clicks informed him of the correctness or incorrectness of his guess. (Adapted from Sutton, Braren, Zubin & John, *Science*, 1965, **150,** 1187–1188. Copyright 1965 by the American Association for the Advancement of Science.)

358

Single sound

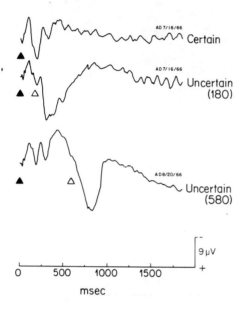

FIGURE 14.5. Average evoked potential waveforms for one subject to psychically identical single clicks (filled triangles) in three conditions: 'certain', when the subject was told in advance that a single click would be presented, 'uncertain, 180' and 'uncertain, 580', when the subject guessed whether or not a second click would occur at the points in time indicated by the unfilled triangle. (Adapted from Sutton, Teuting, Zubin & John, *Science*, 1967, **155**, 1436–1439. Copyright 1967 by the American Association for the Advancement of Science.)

advance whether the stimulus would be a single or a double click. The filled triangle shows the point in time at which the first click occurred. The second, unfilled, triangle shows the point in time at which the second click might have been presented, but in the trials used for this average, was not presented. The interval for the double click in the experiment from which the second waveform was obtained was 180 msec. The conditions for the third waveform were the same as for the second, except that the interval in that experiment was 580 msec. The large positive (downward) deflection is shifted in latency and follows the point in time when the second click might have been presented.

Quite similar findings are obtained with single and double flashes (Ruchkin & Sutton, in press). This is illustrated in Figure 14.6.

The response to absent stimuli appears to be the way the brain says 'I distinctly heard that clock not strike.' But the brain only bothers to give this message when 'not striking' is task relevant. This is illustrated in an experiment in which there were four possible stimuli: a single click at a soft or loud intensity, and a double click (the interval was 580 msec) at the same soft or loud intensities (Sutton *et al.*, 1967). While any one of these four stimuli varying along these two dimensions could occur at random in any trial, the subject was told to guess with respect to only one dimension in any given block of trials. That is, in some blocks the subject was told to guess whether the stimulus would be loud or soft, and that his guess would be considered correct or incorrect in terms of that dimension—whether it was single or double was irrelevant. In other blocks the subject was told to guess whether the stimulus would be single or double—whether it was loud or soft was irrelevant. As can be seen in Figure

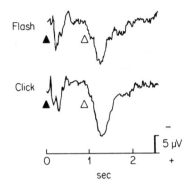

Flash

Click

5 µV

0   1   2   +

sec

FIGURE 14.6. Average evoked potential waveforms to single clicks or light flashes in the uncertain condition. Triangles as in Figure 5. (Adapted from Ruchkin & Sutton, *Bulletin of the Psychonomic Society*, in press. Reported by permission.)

14.7, when singleness *vs* doubleness is the criterion, there is a large waveform locked in time to the second 'click', whether it is present or absent. This waveform in response to the present or absent second click is not seen when loudness *vs* softness is the relevant crietrion.

However, the fact that the emitted potential is found when stimulus absence is relevant, but not found when stimulus absence is not relevant, does not necessarily generalize to other experimental paradigms. For example, in the threshold data shown in Figure 14.1, no emitted potential is apparent in the absence of the threshold click, i.e., in the false alarms or in the correct rejections. Similarly in the experiment by Jenness (1972) for which feedback for correct detections is shown in Figure 14.3, no emitted potential is found for absent feedback clicks. In that experiment, a feedback click was not delivered when the subject's detection was inaccurate. Taken together, the data on emitted potentials show a number of contradictions which cannot yet be resolved (see also Klinke, Fruhstorfer & Finkenzeller, 1968; Picton, Hillyard & Galambos, in press; Squires *et al.*, preprint; Weinberg, Walter & Crow, 1970). The generality of the task relevance finding must for the present be limited to these experiments in which the presence or absence of a click delivers information with respect to the correctness of a guess.

With respect to the second criterion in the experiment shown in Figure 14.7, the relevance of the loudness–softness dimension appears to be indicated in these waveforms by the amplitude of P_3 to the *first* click. This makes sense since even if a second click is present, all of the information with respect to intensity is available at the first click. It can be seen that for all four stimuli, P_3 to the first click is larger when loudness–softness is the relevant dimension, than when singleness–doubleness is the relevant dimension. Whether the first click is loud or soft appears to be carried by the relative amplitude of the evoked potential, larger for the more intense click. On the other hand, the loudness or softness of the second click—whose informational value is redundant with respect to intensity—produces no systematic effects on the amplitude of the evoked potential to that click.

Finally, it can be shown that the amplitude of the evoked potential is sensitive to the subject's motivational state. This can be manipulated by using different amounts of payoff for correct guesses in different blocks of trials (Sutton,

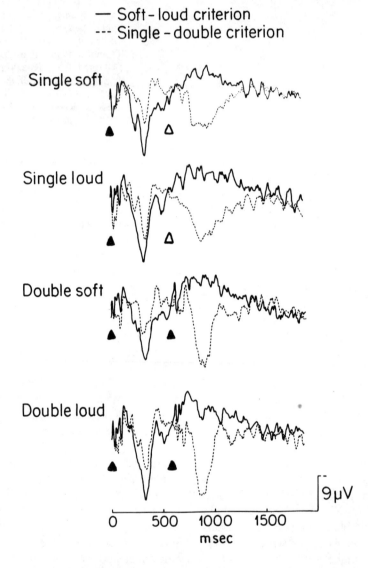

FIGURE 14.7. Average evoked potential waveforms obtained to four types of clicks (as labelled at left) for one subject. (——), Waveforms obtained when the subject is guessing soft versus loud; (- - - -), Waveforms obtained when the subject is guessing single versus double; (▲), points at which clicks were delivered; (△), points at which clicks might have been, but were not, delivered. (Adapted from Sutton, Teuting, Zubin & John, *Science*, 1967, **155**, 1436–1439. Copyright 1967 by the American Association for the Advancement of Science.)

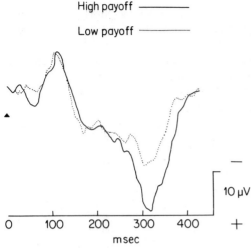

High payoff ————

Low payoff ··············

FIGURE 14.8. Average evoked potential waveforms for one subject. Solid line is for correctly guessed clicks when being correct means that the subject has won ten cents. Dashed line is for correctly guessed clicks when being correct means that the subject has won 2 cents. Triangle indicates Time of click occurrence

Braren & Zubin, 1965b). In Figure 14.8 are sample data for one subject. The waveforms are shown for correct guesses only. The solid line is obtained when subject receives 10¢ for each correct guess; the dashed line when the subject receives 2¢ for each correct guess.

SUMMARY

We have argued that in evoked potential research with awake human subjects it is at least inadvisable, and may even lead to incorrect conclusions, to conduct the experiment without reference to the subject's psychological relation to the stimulus. This has been supported by data which show that the evoked potentials are reliably sensitive to manipulations of psychological variables.

Illustrations have been given which lead to several conclusions. In the threshold experiments we found that:

(i) A correctly detected stimulus at absolute threshold yields a larger evoked potential than a much more intense, but irrelevant stimulus.

(ii) For both evoked potential and pupillary data, clear responses are found at absolute threshold only when a stimulus is present *and* it is detected to be present.

(iii) Identical stimuli yield very different evoked potentials when they are the stimuli to be detected as compared to when they deliver feedback about the correctness of the detection.

In the guessing experiments we found that:

(i) A stimulus whose identity is not known in advance yields larger evoked potentials than a stimulus whose identity is known in advance.

(ii) Even an absent stimulus (whether sound or light) yields an evoked

362

potential related to the point in time at which its absence is noted. However the evoked potential to an absent stimulus only occurs when its absence is task relevant.

(iii) When intensity of the stimulus is task relevant, the evoked potential is larger than when its intensity is not task relevant.

(iv) A stimulus that confirms a high payoff guess yields a larger evoked potential than a stimulus which confirms a low payoff guess.

It is assumed that psychological variables which are illustrated in the above experiments can enter as factors in experiments in which they are not controlled. Thus, for example, when simply instructed to watch repetitive and monotonous light flashes, subjects will vary in their degree of alertness, their degree of motivation, and their interpretation of the meaning of the task. Subjects may even invent tasks, e.g. counting the stimuli, to reduce boredom. When subjects are given material to read and told to ignore the stimuli, their attention may back and forth from the reading material to the stimuli. All such factors will influence the amplitude and shape of the waveform being studied. Unless such factors can be guaranteed to 'average out' because they are random—a rather large assumption—they can lead to variable or even spurious results.

ACKNOWLEDGMENTS

Based on a talk presented at the meetings of the American EEG Society, September, 1970, Washington, D.C. This work was supported by grants MH 14580, MH 0776, and MH 07997 from the National Institute of Mental Health, United States Public Health Service. We are indebted to Muriel Hammer and Joseph Zubin for a critical reading of the manuscript; to Margery Braren, Gad Hakerem, Marion Hartung, David Jenness, Dina Doré Paul, and Daniel S. Ruchkin for assistance with the experiments; to Marion Hartung for editorial and drafting assistance; to Robert Laupheimer and Raymond Simon for the design and building of the instrumentation. We wish to thank Dr M. Wallach, Director of Brooklyn State Hospital for providing facilities for carrying out this research.

REFERENCES

Davis, H. & Zerlin, S. Acoustic relations of the human vertex potential. *Journal of the Acoustical Society of America*, 1966, **39**, 109–116.

Donchin, E., Kubovy, M., Kutas, M., Johnson, R., Jr. & Herning, R. Graded changes in evoked response (P_{300}) amplitude as a function of cognitive activity. Preprint.

Hakerem, G. & Sutton, S. Pupillary response at visual threshold. *Nature*, 1966, **212**, 485–486.

Hillyard, S. A., Squires, K. C., Bauer, J. W. & Lindsay, P. H. Evoked potential correlates of auditory signal detection. *Science*, 1971, **172**, 1357–1360.

Jenness, D. Stimulus role and gross differences in the cortical evoked response. *Physiology and Behaviour*, 1972, **9**, 141–146.

Kietzman, M. L. & Sutton, S. The interpretation of two-pulse measures of temporal resolution in vision. *Vision Research*, 1968, **8**, 287–302.

Klinke, R., Fruhstorfer, H. & Finkenzeller, P. Evoked responses as a function of external and stored information. *Electroencephalography and Clinical Neurophysiology*, 1968, **25**, 119–122.

Nelson, D. A. *Interactive effects of recovery period and stimulus intensity on the human auditory evoked vertex response*. (Doctoral dissertation, University of Minnesota) Ann Arbor, Mich.: University Microfilms, 1970. No. 71–8191.

Paul, D. D. & Sutton, S. Evoked potential correlates of response criterion in auditory signal detection. *Science*, 1972, **177**, 362–364.

Picton, T. W., Hillyard, S. A. & Galambos, R. Cortical evoked responses to omitted stimuli. In M. W. Livanov (Ed), *Major problems in brain electrophysiology*. Moscow: USSR Academy of Science, in press.

Ritter, W., Simon, R. & Vaughan, H. G., Jr. Association cortex potentials and reaction time in auditory discrimination. *Electroencephalography and Clinical Neurophysiology*, 1972, **33**, 547–555.

Ruchkin, D. S. & Sutton, S. Visual evoked and emitted potentials and stimulus significance. *Bulletin of the Psychonomic Society*, in press.

Squires, K. C., Hillyard, S. A. & Lindsay, P. H. Vertex potentials evoked during auditory signal detection: relation to decision criteria. Preprint.

Sutton, S. The specification of psychological variables in an average evoked potential experiment. In E. Donchin & D. B. Lindsley (Eds), *Average evoked potentials—Methods, results, and evaluations*. Washington, D.C.: NASA, 1969, pp. 237–262.

Sutton, S., Braren, M., John, E. R. & Zubin, J. Evoked potential correlates of stimulus uncertainty. *Science*, 1965, **150**, 1187–1188(a).

Sutton, S., Braren, M. & Zubin, J. Sensory, conceptual and emotional components of the evoked response to sound stimuli in man. Paper presented at the meetings of the Psychonomic Society, Chicago, 1965(b).

Sutton, S. & Paul, D. D. Evoked potential correlates of the dectability of low intensity signals. *Proceedings of the conference, Average evoked potentials and their conditioning in psychiatry and psychology*, (Tours), in press.

Sutton, S., Tueting, P., Zubin, J. & John, E. R. Information delivery and the sensory evoked potential. *Science*, 1967, **155**, 1436–1439.

Tueting, P. & Sutton, S. The relationship of pre-stimulus negative shifts and post-stimulus components of the averaged evoked potential. In S. Kornblum (Ed.), *Attention and performance*. IV. New York: Academic, 1973, pp. 185–207.

Tueting, P., Sutton, S. & Zubin, J. Quantitative evoked potential correlates of the probability of events. *Psychophysiology*, 1971, **7**, 385–394.

Weinberg, H., Walter, W. G. & Crow, H. J. Intracerebral events in humans related to real and imaginary stimuli. *Electroencephalography and Clinical Neurophysiology*, 1970, **29**, 1–9.

Chapter 15

Psychophysiology and Conditioning

IRENE MARTIN

Institute of Psychiatry, London

15.1. HUMAN CONDITIONING STUDIES

' 'Tis all in pieces, all cohesion gone,' lamented John Donne when the stranglehold of the Aristotelian Schoolmen was broken and the 'solid, walled-in universe of the middle ages lay in shambles, exposed to the speculative depravations of hosts of Paracelsians, Gilbertians, Copernicans and Galileans' (Koestler, 1964). It might be judged (or hoped!) that a similar state of 'creative anarchy' describes contemporary attacks on the structure of traditional conditioning and learning theory. In the present period of questioning and search for a more 'human' psychology, conditioning is often selected for attack because of its alleged mechanistic and anti-humanistic bias. Clinical psychologists applying behaviour modification techniques face inevitable difficulties, and question the validity and inflexibility of traditional paradigms. But a tight S–R reflexology hardly reflects the current position in conditioning research, which within itself flourishes with new debates. Learning theorists themselves feel that formulations about conditioning have been too strongly shaped by conventional and convenient experimental procedures, and too little influenced by the whole framework of information-processing concepts and response strategies. Much of the reintegration which is being attempted is stimulated by insights concerning 'higher mental processes' on the one hand and by clinical experience on the other.

Research into human conditioned responses has diverse origins. One set of studies has been carried out within conventional conditioning theory and typified by work on the conditioned eyelid response. The second has been carried out within the general rubric of psychophysiological research and includes the conditioning of many types of autonomic responses. The third, more at home in brain research and EEG laboratories than elsewhere, is the study of the CNV (contingent negative variation). Research in these areas is typically published in different journals and has followed distinctively different paths. This diversity has the welcome feature that each area can make a distinctive and unique contribution to the study of human conditioning.

Psychophysiological research in conditioning occupies a small and neatly defined niche within the main development of conditioning research, and to some extent has been isolated from it. It is typically carried out with an electrodermal response as the dependent measure, though sometimes heart rate, peripheral vasomotor activity and (less often) salivation and pupillary responses are used. It traditionally excludes eyelid conditioning. The special nature of autonomic responses has determined in part the kind of experimental paradigm which it was convenient and appropriate to employ. These responses are, for example, of relatively long latency and slow recovery, too slow to occur within the (once) allegedly optimal CS–UCS interval of 500 msec. Autonomic responses occur readily to all kinds of stimuli, including 'neutral' CSs; yet they habituate with rapidity even to a reasonably intense and noxious UCS. The conditioning schedule has had to take account of these features; hence relatively long CS–UCS intervals tend to be used as well as differential schedules with CS + and CS − to permit assessment of CS–UCS pairing, and relatively short acquisition series.

During the 1940s and 1950s when psychophysiology was empirically working out its techniques and subject matter, and delineating its problem, conditioning included, eyelid-conditioning research was firmly placed within the theoretical deductive system espoused by Hull and Spence (1956). Autonomic conditioning was largely outside this theoretical framework, except for minor connections, e.g. with the generalization gradient (of Hovland, 1937). In many ways its behaviour was too irregular to be the measure of choice within an incremental habit-growth type theory. By-passed by conventional theory of the time, psychophysiologists adopted an empirical approach to the exploration of conditioning data. This kind of empiricism and the attention to the properties of the response which it entailed is to be contrasted with the strictly defined measures of eyelid conditioning which were made to suit theoretical requirements. Hull specified that all measures of conditioning index habit strength, and Spence (1956) was no doubt predisposed to see a general similarity between theoretical frequency curves and the empirical frequency curves of eyelid conditioning. The assessment of conditioning was largely based on presence or absence of a response, development and change in response shape being ignored.

The significance of human autonomic conditioning has only rarely been discussed in the mainstream of traditional (behavioural) conditioning theory. It is assumed that human emotion can be understood by employing the classical conditioning model, and that fear and anxiety are acquired via classical conditioning procedures. Analogies have been made between two-process avoidance theory and the development of fears and phobias in human beings, and techniques of extinction in clinical studies are often modelled on laboratory procedures. Yet direct experimental support of the theory is scanty. The goodwill and co-operation of the subject being necessary in most human conditioning experiments, it follows that painful or intense UCSs are very rarely employed. It is also the case that instrumental acts are included in very few SRR conditioning experiments. When they are it tends to be in a problem-solving capacity, i.e. the S has to evolve a strategy in order to avoid the UCS (Graham, Cohen & Shmavonian, 1964; Grings & Lockhart, 1966). While different from the massive escape–avoidance reactions of the traditional animal experiment, these instrumental acts do involve some small degree of interaction with the stimulus environment, and permit the subject some degree of control over the UCS.

Eyelid conditioning research has been largely guided in the past by hypotheses concerning the effects of emotional responses, particularly anxiety. Yet many researchers have questioned how far emotions like anxiety are aroused in the usual run of conditioning experiments. 'We believe that in order to examine this aspect of the CR the CS–US connection must be emotionally meaningful to the S. We have found that 'emotionally meaningful' can can be defined as a painful US—on average, about 10 per cent of our initial pool of Ss refuse to continue in an experiment after receiving one or two shocks ... ' (Mandel & Bridger, 1973). Intuitive evidence as well as formal observation suggest that when anxiety is really strongly aroused the concomitant activation of the autonomic nervous system is an unwelcome obtrusion in judgments, thinking and behaviour. If fear and anxiety are absent from the conditioning situation, however, what conceptual framework is applicable to human conditioning studies?

It seems plausible to suppose that the effects of cognitive factors become more dominant in those conditioning situations where emotions like fear and anger are relatively minimal. Historically, the role of cognitive factors has been regarded with ambivalence. Barely two decades ago, Spence (1956) scarcely entertained the role of cognitive–perceptual variables in conditioning, and would probably at that time have excluded them, restricting the term classical conditioning to those operations where perception of relations could be excluded. This attitude that cognitive factors could be swept aside naturally met with criticism from those whose main interest is human behaviour. How then 'do organisms, such as human organisms (still being careful to avoid the use of such a compromising term as *persons*) behave? Why, they are *conditioned* (meaning that learning is something they must have had done to them ... probably when they were not looking) ... ' (Bannister & Mair, 1968).

Contemporary views reflect doubts both as to whether traditional paradigms of conditioning hold any meaning, and as to how they should be classified. Razran (1955) chose to divide learning into two major classes, perceptual and non-perceptual: 'Conditioning with perceived relationship is neither "mere conditioning" nor "conditioning plus" but something else: it is relational or perceptual learning' (1955, p. 91; see also Grings' (1965) review of this controversy). At one extreme, it has recently been maintained that cognitive factors are the major determinants of human classical conditioning (Dawson, 1973), and at the other that cognitive activity correlates poorly with eyelid conditioning performance even though CS–UCS contingencies are apprehended by the subject (Grant, 1973).

Evidence for 'cognitive factors' (specifically verbalization of CS–UCS contingencies) as major determinants of human classical conditioning seems largely restricted to skin-resistance response (SRR) conditioning; the conclusions do not extend to eyelid conditioning, and it is debatable whether or not they extend to heart rate conditioning. Amplitude of CNVs, however, seem to relate to subjective 'certainty' of stimulus contingencies in a way which resembles SRR data. The CNV, like the SRR, can be modified by verbal statements. 'When the imperative stimulus was withdrawn without notice or warning the change in the pattern of physiological stimuli ultimately suppressed the CNV, but only after about 30 trials. In contrast, when the subject was told: "There will be no more flashes" the CNV disappeared immediately' (Walter, Cooper, Oldridge, McCallum & Winter, 1964.). These authors noted a differential effect depending on whether the experience of a stimulus is direct or based on verbal instruction, and suggest there may be qualitative as well as quantitative differences between the two effects.

Recent work has discussed the role of information processing of sensory events in eyelid conditioning, and their storage within the nervous system in some kind of neuronal model (Grant, 1972). Work on CNVs in very simple paradigms deals almost wholly in terms of attention, expectancies and the handling of informational input. Indeed, a wide range of studies is currently exploring this approach and its implications both for human conditioning and general theoretical formulations.

Laboratory studies of human conditioning should contribute abundantly to the re-evaluation of learning processes. At present they offer little in the way of a unified conceptual framework but they provide useful empirical evidence on many issues. In turning to this evidence we should be aware of the many ways in which human conditioning paradigms differ from typical animal procedures, and mindful that these deviations may help us to reconsider our conventional classification of conditioning paradigms.

15.1.1. CS–UCS components

A rigid, S–R, 'reflexological' interpretation of human conditioning is clearly not feasible. Environmental stimuli not only elicit physiological and behavioural responses: they elicit meanings, judgments, and interpretations. In the conditioning paradigm the CS is characteristically neutral, i.e. low in information and significance. The UCS, by contrast, is highly salient and produces stronger physiological and behavioural activity.

The UCS is no longer particularly regarded as eliciting a 'reflex' response. Indeed, in current writings on SRR conditioning as well as on the CNV there has been a tendency to refer to CS and UCS simply in terms of S_1 and S_2, the second stimulus being typically though not necessarily stronger in intensity or meaning than S_1. Razran (1957) has expressed this as a property of dominance. Research has concentrated on the types of response which occur in the $S_1 \rightarrow S_2$ situation when there is an interval of some seconds between the two stimuli, the characteristics of these responses in terms of amplitude, rise time, recovery etc., and the interaction which takes place between these adjacent responses.

The absence of theoretical constraints in autonomic conditioning and CNV studies meant that to some extent a more flexible attitude could be taken in the measurement of conditioned responsiveness. The 'irregularity' of responding which might disqualify autonomic data from representing a hypothetical growth function could reflect an extreme sensitivity to stimulus events and stimulus change. In the usual psychophysiological experiment simple sensory stimuli are used. These have specifiable physical properties (frequency, voltage, etc.) rise time and durations, and usually provide a sudden, sharp energy change on the receptors. The properties of the response are often reflected features of responding such as amplitude, duration, recovery, spontaneous activity. Thus response characteristics can in some instances be correlated fairly well with the properties of simple sensory stimuli; responding will reflect the onset of a stimulus, its intensity, its duration and its offset.

Adaptation quite commonly occurs to the stimuli of autonomic conditioning, and it seems well documented that different responses habituate to the same stimulus at different rates. Thus with repetition of the stimulus the pattern of observed activity will change. Some of the responses will cease, some diminish in amplitude, some lengthen in onset latency. Others (e.g., evoked responses) will tend to be more resistant to change though such change as there is may have been obscured in the past by averaging techniques. Introduce a novel stimulus and the original response pattern might well be reinstated. Pair the stimulus in a $S_1 \rightarrow S_2$ sequence and a different type of response will be developed. If therefore we want to know what impact a stimulus has on an individual we would gain a great deal of information from polygraph recordings, i.e. just those recordings which can be made from the surface of the body. This omits the range of interoceptive responding, the extent and significance of which are largely unknown at present. Apparently the impact of the stimulus is registered in multiple ways, and, presumably, stored in comparable complex ways. Indeed, recent work on the organization of memory (Norman, 1970) points strongly in this direction.

15.1.2. CS–UCS pairing: multiple responding

It has become apparent that there are several different types of response change which occur during $S_1 \rightarrow S_2$ pairing and which, when adequate controls have been incorporated, can qualify for the terms 'conditioned'. These include the response to CS onset, the anticipatory response which precedes the UCS, and the UCR-like response which occurs when the UCS is omitted as on test trials. These kinds of responses have been frequently described in the literature (Lockhart, 1966, 1973; Martin & Levey, 1969; Stern, 1972), mainly in relation to SRR conditioning. However, Lockhart (1966) has pointed out that similar types of responses occur in other autonomic modalities, and Levey & Martin (1974) have illustrated similar responses in eyelid conditioning.

These responses, which have been variously labelled (see Lockhart, 1973, and Stern, 1972) occur closely together in time, and it is not therefore surprising that several kinds of interaction between them have been observed. One interesting observation made early by Lykken (1959) was of a smaller UCR amplitude when the UCS is preceded by a CS compared with the UCR to UCS alone. The literature which has ensued on 'UCR diminution', as it came to be called, has spanned both eyelid conditioning (Kimble & Ost, 1961; Kimmel, 1965) and SRR conditioning (Grings & Schell, 1969; Kimmel, 1965; Martin, Slubicka & Levey, 1974), and animal studies (Lykken, 1962) as well as human. Unfortunately the literature on UCR diminution combines a range of studies some of which include the possible effect of CR on UCR and some of which exclude any CR effect by measuring UCR diminution only on trials where no CR occurred (e.g. Kimble & Ost, 1961). The provisional hypothesis which these diverse studies raise is that both CS (i.e., stimulus) and CR (i.e., response) effects occur on the UCR.

When CR and UCR both occur on a given trial the possibility of an interfering effect arises (Grings & Schell, 1969). Again, differences in measures and experimental schedules occur in the various reports on this topic. Prokasy & Ebel (1967) confined their analysis to unreinforced CS+ trials and concluded that the relationship between the conditioned anticipatory response (AR) and the UCR-like response in the SRR system is negative and essentially probabilistic. Martin, Slubicka & Levey (1974) measuring responses on reinforced trials reported a significant negative relationship between AR frequency and UCR frequency, and also between AR peak amplitude and UCR frequency. Results on unreinforced trials in this study, however, showed a positive relationship between the AR and the UCS-omitted response, suggesting a different kind of response interaction under partial reinforcement.

Various hypotheses have been put forward in connection with UCR diminution. Some writers emphasize that this is an inhibitory process which is under stimulus control. Kimble & Ost (1961) attributed the diminution of the UCR to an inhibitory effect through association; Dostalek & Krasna (1969) even when no conditioning occurs, attributed the diminution to induction, i.e. to specific cortical excitation ongoing at the time of S_2. Peeke & Grings (1968) favour an explanation in terms of a perceptual 'set' which develops most strongly when the time relations between CS and UCS are constant. Interestingly, the Pavlovian concept of 'induction' just mentioned is virtually analogous to that of 'set'.

An alternative hypothesis offered in the context of eyelid conditioning is that CR and UCR interact in an integrated fashion. It is postulated that S_1 and S_2 form an undifferentiated CS/UCS complex sharing the characteristics of both S_1 and S_2 and representing the entire current contents of immediate memory. From this it is argued that R_1 and R_2 form an undifferentiated CR/UCR complex which is a response developed to the CS/UCS complex (Levey & Martin, 1968). These CR/UCR complexes can take different forms, in part dependent upon the stage of conditioning which has been reached. examples of response types are illustrated in Figure 15.1. The development of the conditioned eyelid response was investigated by examining the response types illustrated in the figure on unreinforced trials. They were shown to occur in a predictable sequence, the CR alone or UCR alone occurring first, and the double CR/UCR and blend occurring later in the sequence. Levey & Martin (1974) explain this developmental sequence by assuming a comparator process by which the integrated response complex is gradually built up, operating on each trial by scanning a random subset of the information in the stimulus complex. On successive trials, further information would lead to progressive shaping and integration of the response model. Efficiency of responding is

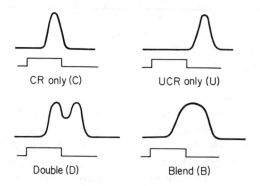

CR only (C) UCR only (U)

Double (D) Blend (B)

Figure 15.1. Types of eyelid response complexes occurring on acquisition test trials (UCS omitted). CR = anticipatory conditioned response occurring alone; UCR = UCS omitted response occurring alone; D = double response, i.e. CR and UCR; B = blended CR/UCR. (From Levey & Martin, *Journal of Experimental Psychology*, 1974, in press. Copyright 1974 by the American Psychological Association. Reprinted with permission.)

defined by the extent to which placing of the CR in relation to the UCR results in some or all of the 'work' of the UCR being accomplished before the UCS is administered. Thus the integration of the CR and UCR into a single blended response is regarded as an intrinsic part of the conditioning process.

It is interesting to compare these examples which are from eyelid conditioning with some from SRR conditioning studies by Grings, Lockhart & Dameron (1962). These are illustrated in Figure 15.2. Interestingly, these authors discuss 'efficiency' in terms of the extent to which the strength of CR approaches that of UCR as a result of training. Several authors have analysed CR topographical data showing that the peak latency of quite different CRs (the SRR and the nictitating membrane response of rabbits) moves toward the point of UCS application over the course of training. Gormezano (1972) postulates a temporal mechanism which must be available to the organism to permit the CR peak on test trials to be placed near the point in time where the UCS was delivered on reinforced trials, and offers this as an alternative to instrumental avoidance/reinforcement theories which seem inappropriate to these kinds of responses. Other evidence has been presented that blending of an anticipatory response with the S_2 response occurs, not only in the SRR (Gauthier, 1971) but in the penile plethysmographic response (Barr & McConaghy, 1972).

Another set of interesting findings is the relationship between spontaneous activity in a response system and reactivity to stimulation, including frequency

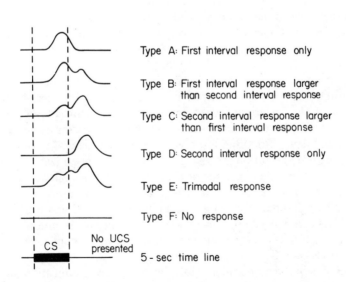

FIGURE 15.2. Types of GSR response complexes occurring on acquisition test trials (UCS omitted) (From Grings, Lockhart & Dameron, *Psychological Monographs*, 1962, **76,** No. 39. Copyright 1962 by the American Psychological Association. Reprinted by permission.)

and characteristics of CRs. Spontaneous activity is positively related to response frequency, negatively to base levels, and there is also evidence of a negative correlation with response latency (labile Ss producing shorter response latencies). The data have important implications in relation to the assessment of conditioning vs reactivity; many of the conditioning measures used may unduly reflect spontaneous activity rather than learning. Using a discrimination paradigm Ohman & Bohlin (1973) found very significant differences in level of skin conductance conditioning in sub-groups formed on the basis of amount of spontaneous activity. They raise the issue of a central vs a peripheral interpretation of the spontaneous activity/conditioning relationship, suggesting that while central factors undoubtedly contribute, the pronounced unresponsiveness of the low spontaneous activity group and its failure to discriminate between $CS+$ and $CS-$ might be attributable to some aspect of effector excitability. If this could be established, a good case might be made for excluding or separating some of the Ss on the grounds that they do not belong within the sample. Objective criteria for excluding deviant observations have long been used in the physical sciences though they have been discouraged in the biological sciences.

15.1.3. Informational content of CS

In most of the conditioning paradigms which have been discussed so far S_1 is the relatively neutral stimulus and S_2 the more intense or significant—in some sense salient to the organism's adaptive needs, either avoidant or adient. While the CS may typically be relatively low in information content, it nevertheless can serve as a signal which informs the subject of the appearance of the second stimulus. It is a possibility that SRR conditioning may represent a rather specific example of CS–UCS pairing, emphasizing the input in terms of perception rather than the output in terms of overt acts. Discussions about the nature of electrodermal conditioning emphasize concepts of perception, set and expectancy based on temporal contingencies operating in the individual's environment. 'The autonomic responses are seen as arousal correlates to the preparation and expectation process. This suggests the organization of concepts underlying such learning in terms of perceptual variables of at least two main types: perception of stimuli and perception of relations or contingencies' (Grings, 1973). Similar discussions occur in the CNV literature, except that emphasis has been placed not only on expectation but on attention, and experimental procedures have been designed to interfere with or enhance expectation of the occurrence of S_2.

When S_2 is still the more salient but when S_1 has communication or meaning added to the signalling property of the CS we have a relatively unusual conditioning paradigm. This is one which has recently been explored experimentally by Grant (1972). Most conditioning research has involved neutral CSs, e.g. lights, bells, buzzers. These neutral CSs require little information processing by the subject. Grant has introduced to the role of the CS an information carrying capacity. This may take one of several forms: verbal relatedness between CS+ and CS−; truth or falsity of the message conveyed by the verbal conditioned stimuli; information or misinformation conveyed by the CS regarding the CS/UCS contingency, and conflict or incongruity between the verbal and the sensory features of the CS. As an example, Grant has studied in a differential conditioning paradigm the effects of such CSs as the words BLUE and PINK, which may be presented in incongruous colours, i.e. BLUE in pink letters and PINK in blue letters; and the effects of the words 'DON'T BLINK' which were reinforced by a corneal puff and the word BLINK which was not reinforced. Grant has argued that when more complex, informational CSs are used the S has the double task of processing incoming information (from the CS) and also of response learning or shaping, and emission. Thus the frequency and topography of the S's conditioned response is likely to show characteristic progressive changes owing to the interrelationships between the CS, the CR and the UCS. Considerable response processing must occur in this situation, and this is said to operate on a 'trade-off' basis with input processing requirements.

The input processing requires that the CS can, over repeated training trials, be coded and stored in a stable, unambiguous way. This process takes up some of the central processing time, as does the development of conditioned response shaping. In Grant's view a critical determinant of the subsequent conditioning, learning and performance will depend on how much the demands for response shaping preempt the central processing capacity. If only a little central processing capacity is required for response shaping, a far larger proportion of processing capacity is available for more extensive and elaborate coding of the differential conditioned stimuli. Thus more complex verbal and semantic relationships can be elaborated in the CS codes. If, however, response shaping requirements place a heavy demand on the central processing capacity, only a little remains available for more general and complex processing of the conditioned stimuli. Smooth operation of the model requires the storing of stable, unambiguous codes in long-term memory stores, which is envisaged as that of a stable neuronal model of stimulus input following Sokolov's (1963) descriptions.

A different though not necessarily incompatible view of stimulus processing/response shaping is that the CS/UCS complex, held in immediate memory, is itself capable of producing unmediated responses (Martin & Levey, 1969). Response modification according to this view would occur directly as a result of the organization of stimulus input.

15.2. CSs AND UCSs—ORIENTING RESPONSES AND ANXIETY REACTIONS

15.2.1. Orienting and attention

A difficult question which is raised by autonomic conditioning is that of determining whether in the autonomic conditioning paradigm we are dealing with major differences between orienting and anxiety reactions, and if so what form they take. This is paralleled in the CNV literature by the interaction of attentional and arousal reactions (cf. Tecce, 1972). Earlier hypotheses placed emotional reactions at one end of an arousal continuum; more recent models have placed emphasis on perceptual input in terms of cognitions and information processing.

From the evidence referred to above it is clear that even in the simple CS/UCS $(S_1 \rightarrow S_2)$ paradigm a great deal of informational input must occur. Contingency learning has been mentioned, i.e. the fact that most Ss can verbalize the temporal connection between CS and UCS, and the expectancies of S_2 given that S_1 has occurred. There are presumably other perceptions which can be assessed through verbal report: undoubtedly each subject has a set of judgments, attitudes and evaluations concerning the stimuli. A UCS may be evaluated as liked or disliked, for example, and preliminary evidence suggests that this evaluation itself may be conditioned (Levey, 1974). Which of all these components is most relevant to learning and performance is not yet known.

In addition to this cognitive (i.e., verbalized) type of information there is the purely physiological registration of stimulus properties which has been so well described by Sokolov (1963) in connection with the orienting response. A configuration of expectancies occurs here, too, described in terms of a neuronal model which is formed on the basis of a repeated stimulus configuration. It may be noted that the term expectancy as used in this context is different from its usage in the context of conscious cognitions, although it may be related to it.

Pribram (1967) discusses the question of orienting and anxiety in terms of when incoming stimuli produce arousal which leads to registration, habituation and memory formation, and when arousal leads to a state of disruption more aptly described as emotional. Discounting the view that 'amount' of arousal can be conceived as amount of energy available to the neurobehavioural system, he suggests rather that it be viewed as amount of match and mismatch between expectancies and input. Amount of arousal is therefore to be conceived as a change in the uncertainty (and thus the information) of the system.

Tecce (1972) has reviewed the CNV literature and in a comparable way, has attempted to integrate the findings in terms of attention and arousal. He opts to retain the intensity aspect of arousal in a two-process explanation as follows:

(i) Attention hypothesis: the magnitude of CNV bears a positive monotonic relation to attention (see Figure 15.3).Attention is conceptualized as facilitating the selection of relevant stimuli from the environment: the selective processing of information is a key property of the attentional process.

(ii) Arousal hypothesis: the magnitude of CNV bears an inverted curvilinear relation to arousal level (see Figure 15.3). This is conceptualized as devoid of of the steering properties of attention, i.e. as a process that energizes behaviour

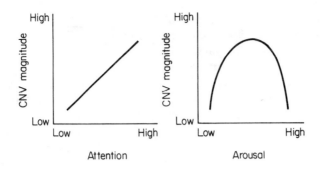

FIGURE 15.3. Schematic presentation of two-process theoretical model proposed to account for CNV changes (From Tecce, *Psychological Bulletin*, 1972, **77**, 73–108. Copyright 1972 by the American Psychological Association. Reprinted by permission.)

unselectively and affects only intensity of response. Tecce presents the evidence for and against these hypotheses, recognizing the problems which both attention and arousal present especially when considered as unitary concepts. They are offered, however, as a best fit for presently available findings.

Researches carried out in all the areas of human conditioning are converging in their interest in the perceptual properties of stimuli. It is the case, however, that some, albeit few, of human conditioning studies involve fear, anxiety, or other highly charged feelings. Some separate consideration therefore is necessary of the concepts of anxiety and fear.

15.2.2. Anxiety and fear

A desire for simplicity and the influence of operationalism have together led us to define anxiety in many and various ways, e.g. as a verbal report 'I feel anxious', as a physiological reaction (high autonomic arousal), and as a behavioural act (avoidance). It has to be recognized that the condition we want to refer to is all of these. They are all an aspect of the total, complicated response pattern we summarize under the label 'anxiety'. Our area of interest may lead us to emphasize the physiological aspects, but at least as far as understanding human behaviour is concerned they must be considered in conjunction with (and not separate from) perceptions, cognitions, verbal analyses and overt behaviour.

Lang's (1968) attempt to measure fear, for example, starts with the assumption that it is a response expressed in three main behavioural systems: verbal (cognitive), overt motor (behavioural) and somatic (physiological). Lazarus (1968) takes a similar view. What would an emotion be, he asks, without its motoric impulses, its causal appraisal as well as physiological change? This recognition of a multi-dimensional response pattern is evident not only in the difficult context of human emotional responses but increasingly in conditioning studies (cf. Dykman, Murphree & Ackerman, 1966; see also Lang 1971 for a discussion of the application of conditioning techniques to the different components of fear).

Apart from the measurement problems this view involves, there are problems posed by the use of operational definitions in this field. While under certain circumstances operational definitions may be acceptable, they may sometimes present more problems than they solve. One answer may lie in some form of construct validation, i.e. 'in the construction of a nomological network which serves to define the concept, and provides us with a system of hypothetico-deductive properties within which our attempts to measure emotion would have to fit' (Eysenck, 1973). All three types of responses—physiological, intro-spective, behavioural—can be taken as evidence of fear ånd can be made the basis of a system of measurement. At the same time, the multidimensional approach is able to cope with relative independence among measures, e.g. by forming composite measures which utilize all the information.

The low correlations obtained between measures in laboratory-type situations are probably due to the fact that the amount of emotion evoked is relatively small. 'This restriction of range is known, on simple psychometric grounds, to reduce the size of correlations drastically; we would be entitled to expect much higher correlations in truly fear producing situations ... ' (Eysenck, 1973). There are very few experimental studies which can claim to have produced extremely strong fear in their subjects. Campbell, Sanderson & Laverty (1964), however, working with human subjects, gave single-trial temporary inter-ruptions of respiration by means of 'Scoline' lasting for about 100 sec, an extremely harrowing experience which resulted in failure of the SRR to extinguish through many extinction trials.

Such strong autonomic reactions are presumably differentiated from orienting reactions in that they trigger adapting, avoiding or coping strategies to deal with the UCS. (The subjects of the Campbell et al. study described their (imagined) movements as 'part of a struggle to get away from the apparatus and to tear off the wires and electrodes'.) Lazarus (1968) and Pribram (1967) have both suggested that emotion leads to processes of environment evaluation resulting in thought or action which serves to exert some control of the environ-ment. Both analyses are couched in terms of the organism's capacity to process information; both emphasize cognitive appraisal mechanisms as antecedents of emotional and adaptive activities.

Lazarus (1968) is explicit in dealing with emotion as a response pattern—physiological, cognitive and behavioural—which is a complex, organized pattern of adaptive activity. In addition to the empirical argument concerning low correlations between measures Lazarus puts forward logical and theoretical reasons for expecting disagreements between the three response dimensions. 'The key point is that each response system from which inferences about emotional reactions are generally made has its own adaptive functions and, taken individually, communicates some special *transaction* taking place between the person and his environment. Thus, what the person reports to the observer, and to an extent his instrumental actions, reflects intentions concerning the social being with whom he is interacting. At the same time, the physiological state should also reflect the direct action tendencies which are mobilized for dealing in some fashion with the appraised threat'.

This notion of the response components having special transactional interactions with the environment is relevant to the problem of anxiety in conditioning situations. It would be difficult to say in the typical autonomic conditioning situation what 'transaction' the subject could have with his environment other than in terms of processing stimulus input. The matter of what he would really do if pain and fear were involved is intimated in the very few studies (Mandel & Bridger, Campbell *et al.*) mentioned above.

The same question can of course be raised concerning those eyelid conditioning studies which purport to relate conditioning to manifest anxiety. It is doubtful if subjects experience much in the way of general fear and anxiety and there can even be doubt that for many people the air-puff UCS is an unpleasant stimulus to the eye. Levey (1972) has reported that only 16 per cent of subjects describe the air-puff as unpleasant in a post-test questionnaire. Presumably these subjects feel the UCS as noxious though not a threat to the person as an individual. The eyelid response is such that there is a definite (albeit miniature) behavioural component inasmuch as blinking can modulate the incoming stimulus, i.e. the air-puff UCS. In a small but nevertheless significant way the subject can interact with the environment in a real 'transactional' way to minimize its unpleasantness. It is interesting to recall Grant's (1973) review of the evidence that factors of awareness do not markedly influence conditioning and performance of this response.

Thus in a situation where prompt instrumental acts are necessary to mitigate noxious stimulation the effects of cognitive factors may be relatively small. The relative contribution of cognitive and emotional factors in laboratory studies of human conditioning is difficult to assess. In the past, emphasis has been placed on the role of anxiety. Spence's theory, for example, was based on the motivating (drive) properties of anxiety as measured by the Taylor Manifest Anxiety scale. Eysenck (1967) has discussed the relationship of anxiety and inhibition to conditioning; his experimental paradigms have manipulated the inhibition factor to test the theory of introverted and extraverted conditioning behaviour. More recently Gray (1970) has further elaborated the role of anxiety in conditioning, suggesting that it is susceptibility to fear (or to express the same point differently, a heightened sensitivity to punishment and warnings of punishment) which leads to more rapid conditioning in aversive conditioning situations.

In spite of the emphasis on anxiety conditioning there is a gulf between human studies and theories of fear and avoidance conditioning which remains unbridged. According to the two-process theory of conditioning, the development and maintenance of an instrumental avoidance response depends upon the development of conditioned anxiety reactions which serve a motivating function. The classical conditioning component, i.e. the straight forward pairing of CS and UCS without avoidance, is assumed to be responsible for the appearance of emotional responses elicited by the CS. Some of the attributes of the original unconditioned response to the noxious stimulus are transferred to the once-neutral CS by this process of classical conditioning. It has been postulated that reinforcement of learned instrumental avoidance responses comes about through drive reduction. As is well known, avoidance is by and large a remarkably persistent behaviour. Animals will commonly respond for hundreds of trials without receiving the shock-UCS; indeed, experimenters have often given up trying to extinguish the animal before the animal has given up responding.

Difficulties with previous avoidance theories have been reviewed by Seligman & Johnston (1973) and a cognitive theory of avoidance learning put forward. This has two components, one cognitive and the other emotional. The cognitive component makes use of act–outcome expectancies and a corresponding preference between outcomes. The emotional component is based on classically conditioned fear as a response elicitor, and can be indexed by autonomic and skeletal responses elicited by the CS. The theory is labelled 'cognitive' since it attributes to an avoiding animal the capacity to store (in the form of expectancies) and use information about the relation of his actions to other events in the world. In an appendix to their chapter the authors elucidate on the logical status of their 'expectancies' and the ways in which the construct is used.

15.2.3. Cognitive/autonomic interactions

The problem of response interaction is, as has been seen in a previous context, an empirical one and has been rather extensively investigated in recent years. There are good reviews of this literature which deals (more often) with the effects of cognitions on autonomic responding and (less often) with the effects of altered autonomic responding on cognitions and perceptions. The following is a brief outline of the kind of work which has been carried out.

It is useful first to recall the findings of Mandler and his associates, namely that the perception of bodily change is not highly dependent upon actual bodily change (Mandler, Mandler & Uviller, 1958). It would seem that we are not always good judges of our own internal states.

The work of Lazarus (1968) has already been mentioned. By and large this research deals with cognitive effects on emotional states assessed by self-report or autonomic measures. Lazarus emphasizes that in his experimental situations, direct actions such as avoidance or attack were not feasible. The modes of coping emphasized and manipulated in these experiments were basically indirect, cognitive ones involving appraisals and reappraisals. His conclusion emphasizes the role of cognitive activity, either taking place before a harm is to be confronted or after it has been experienced, and its significance in lowering or raising the level of emotional disturbance.

The work of Schachter (1966) is perhaps the most widely quoted in the context of cognitions and labelling of physiological events. He has concluded that two factors are necessary to the production of emotional states: an un-differentiated state of arousal and the presence of cognitive labels that direct the state of arousal and its associated behaviour along emotional lines. These views have been widely and sometimes uncritically accepted. A careful criticism of Schachter's assumptions and experiments has been made by Lang (1971) who, again with reference to clinical problems, questions Schachter's view that a competing set easily overrides the emotional impetus of physiological arousal.

Lang's chapter also contains references to the direct training of autonomic responses through the use of exteroceptive feedback and operant training techniques. The possible limits of such autonomic control have been discussed in a recent review by Blanchard & Young (1973). These authors point out that the order of change in several cardiac functions (heart rate-level, heart rate variability, blood pressure and cardiac arrhythmias) as a result of operant training techniques is small, and though of sufficient magnitude to be statistically significant is of little clinical significance.

Valins (1970) has reported on the effect of providing false information about heart rate change on subjects' reactions to emotional stimuli. Slides of nudes were projected together with a (false) audible heart rate recording. Slides to which subjects heard their heart rates change, whether increased or decreased, were liked significantly more than nudes to which they heard no change. This result was interpreted in terms of individuals needing to evaluate and understand their bodily changes. Valins also raises the issue of individual differences in awareness of and reaction to internal bodily cues. Some individuals, for example, while 'experiencing' bodily changes 'ignore' them in the sense of not utilizing them as cues when evaluating emotional situations.

15.2.4. Autonomic/behavioural interactions

A curvilinear relation between arousal and performance has been frequently demonstated. In the conditioning situation it could be postulated that arousal would relate to overt behaviour in a curvilinear fashion, increasing to the point where overt instrumental acts are made and reducing when these latter are effective. There is some experimental evidence to support this view. Grings & Lockhart (1966) observed a rapid reduction in anticipatory SRR responding following the first correct avoidance trial. It was suggested that the results favoured an explanation in terms of reduced arousal once there is anticipation of avoidance rather than anticipation of shock. Similar results have been reported in a study where concomitant CNVs were recorded during classical eyelid conditioning. They are illustrated in Figure 15.4. During the establishment of the eyelid CR the CNV is prominent. In subsequent trials, when the eyelid CR is avoiding the airpuff, the CNV shrinks progressively, until after about 60 trials it is scarcely above the base-line and the eye is closed well before the air-puff (Walter et al. 1964).

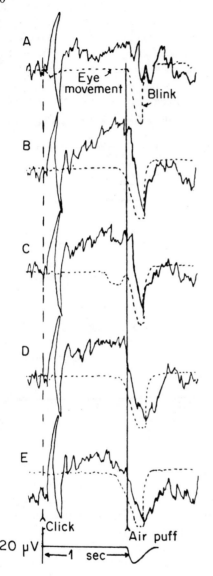

A
Eye movement
Blink

B

C

D

E

Click

Air puff

20 μV

← 1 sec →

FIGURE 15.4. Averages of 12 presentations; classical conditioning of involuntary blink, CS = click, UCS = airpuff to eye. A: first 12 trials show brain responses to both clicks and puffs; blink starts just after puff. B: second 12 trials. CNV appears, with conditioned blink just before puff which evokes no brain responses since eyelid is shut before corneal stimulus. C, D, E, progressive decline in CNV as eyelid CR is consolidated. (From Walter, Cooper, Aldridge, McCallum & Winter, *Nature*, 1964, **203**, 380–384. with permission.)

15.3. THE OVERALL RESPONSES: STRATEGIES AND PROGRAMMES

The studies discussed in the previous sections are given as examples of the type of autonomic/cognitive/behavioural interaction research which is currently ongoing. It far from exhausts the range of possible interactions: between cognitions and behaviour, autonomic reactions and perception, etc. The emotional response is conceived as being a pattern of many response systems, and most theorists have been wary of arranging the pattern in any hierarchical way, i.e. giving dominance to one system rather than another. Latter-day cognitivists, however, tend strongly to stress the role of cognitive factors. The conceptual framework which suggests that behaviour is a total overall pattern of responses must further imply that the pattern is meaningful in specifiable ways.

Various suggestions have been put forward in terms of strategies, plans, programmes and other complex central mediators (cf. Breger & McGaugh, 1975). These authors take issue with the behaviourist conception of neurosis as conditioned responses and habits, arguing that one of the major problems is the difficulty of explaining how *generality* of behaviour can result from specific learning experiences. They argue that within an S–R framework, with its narrow definition of generalization occurring along a dimension of physical stimulus similarity, it is difficult if not impossible to show how experiences can generalize without a great deal of mediational processing to 'carry the burden of generalization'.

As an alternative to traditional S–R theory Breger & McGaugh propose a view of learning (and the learning processes involved in therapy) which centres around the concepts of information storage and retrieval. This view is based on the idea that what is learned in a neurosis is a set of central strategies (or a programme) which guide the individual's adaptation to his environment. '"What is learned", then, is not a mechanical sequence of responses but rather, *what needs to be done in order to achieve some final event.*' Evidence is cited in terms of animal experiments in which the animals seem to be able to bypass the execution of specific responses in reaching an environmental achievement.

Even those responses which have been grossly defined as stable or stereotyped reveal, on examination, a highly complicated and adaptive method of responding. Levey (1966, 1972) has shown that the human conditioned eyelid response can be measured in a variety of ways to index the efficiency with which the developing CR approaches certain relatively stable end-points which are inferred from the S's behaviour. The underlying assumption of this approach is that whatever behaviour is optimized or maximized in the course of acquisition defines the S's self-selected goal. This affords a non-teleological definition of the adaptive function of the developing response. The general philosophy underlying this approach differs from those formulations (e.g., Skinner, 1938) which ask, for example, what stimuli in the environment are controlling the subject's behaviour. By contrast, it asks: what stimulus elements in the environment is the subject's behaviour bringing under control?

In the clinical situation we can make guesses about what the anxiety behaviour 'achieves' for the individual, in the sense that he may avoid unwanted situations, gain attention, in other words that he will interact with his environment in particular ways which are a function of his state of anxiety. The 'state' of anxiety experienced by an individual is the pattern of his perceptual/physiological/behavioural reactions, and it is both the overall pattern and the interactions of the parts which are amenable to study. The nature of the overall pattern is presumably of a highly idiosyncratic kind, presumably resulting from the interaction between individual predispositions, perceptual biases, and types of stimulus events ('reinforcement schedules') occurring in the person's life environment.

15.4. THE SHIFT IN PERSPECTIVE

As can be seen from almost all the studies discussed above, work with human subjects has resulted in a shift from concepts of SR reflexology to those which emphasize cognitions, expectancies, information processing and mediation concepts. The role of cognitions is heavily emphasized, yet it is far from clear exactly how the term is being used. Sometimes it seems restricted to a category of verbal reports of subjective CS–UCS contingencies; at other times it seems to be accepted that a 'cognitive view' can readily encompass the non-verbalizable, even the 'unconscious'. 'From our point of view'—i.e. the avowedly cognitive view of Breger & McGaugh—'there is no reason to assume that people can give accurate descriptions of the central strategies mediating much of their behaviour . . . .'

The conceptualization which seems to be implied by these and other writers is that of a representation of the stimulus input in terms of multiple internal 'models', some of them conscious and verbalizable, others at physiological, introspectively inaccessible levels. One might be an 'educated' model in terms of verbal assessments of subjective probability; another might be a stimulus model in the sense that Sokolov uses the term, i.e. a registration of the stimulus properties in a stable neuronal matrix on which basis both matches and mismatches of further input can be made. There is not necessarily a close correlation between the verbal report and the processing at physiological levels. That is to say, similarities and differences may be detected and verbally reported, but this process may not be identical to the detection of similarities and differences at a neuronal level. It is in this latter sense for example that Pribram (1967) discusses expectancies. Certainly Sokolov does not need to refer to 'cognitions' or 'cognitive appraisals'. All these writers, however, describe the process of organizing stimulus input as one of formulating models and handling redundancy, novelty and uncertainty.

There would seem to be little doubt that in the representation of the external world multiple models are formulated which overlap, interact and integrate in many and complex ways. Some part of these can be consciously accessed and verbally reported. Certainly in the case of simple habituation, or of the $S_1 \rightarrow S_2$ paradigm, the contingencies can be verbalized and this kind of knowledge may affect autonomic activity in the conditioning situation. In such a case it could be argued that this 'model' of the stimulus environment is important in influencing responsiveness. But equally it can be claimed (though the data may be clinical and anecdotal) that in a state of anxiety the autonomic 'model' of external events is the most powerful determinant of responsivity, and that verbalized representations of reality are not very effective in inhibiting excessive responsivity.

In this information processing approach to conditioning some of the old problems become viewed in a new light. The distinction between learning and performance seems important as well as the old problem of 'what is learned'. It is a puzzle that the literature on conditioning and memory of the past decades were virtually non-overlapping. Estes (1973) distinguishes a response-oriented tradition of learning research from a memory oriented view: ' ... even today we hear the results of a conditioning experiment almost universally described in terms of the conditioning of a response rather than in terms of the storage of information in memory.' Estes argues that neither an S–S nor an S–R association, nor any manageably simple way of chaining these together seems to provide a promising basis for explaining learning and conditioning performance. A basic difficulty appears to be that information concerning relations between events which results from an organism's experiences in a conditioning situation enters into a more complex organization than can be represented by linear chaining of associations.

Boundaries between conditioning, perception, memory and cognition are blurring, and there is a growing feeling that these distinctions may no longer be very useful. At the same time techniques and hypotheses have been developed which cut across these categories (Frith, 1973). Interaction between the different areas is much to be welcomed. Similarly, a freer interchange of ideas between CNV research, autonomic conditioning and traditional eyelid conditioning is likely to define more clearly the significance and issues of human conditioning studies.

However, it is already apparent that the walled-in paradigm of conditioning has lost its solid boundaries; it can be seen as participating in processes of perception and memory, storage and retrieval. In more applied situations, such as the persistent non-adaptive habits of neurosis, it has been argued that the terms stimulus and response are only remotely related to the traditional use of these terms in psychology.

In emphasizing specifically human attitudes to the conditioning situation, and in the shift of emphasis to information processing of input, it may yet be important to remember the essentially biological origins of conditioning work. Breland & Breland in 1961, and more recently Seligman and his co-workers (Seligman & Hager, 1973) have well documented the biological limitations of animal learning. In evolutionary terms, survival probably meant prompt action, possibly at the expense of finely discriminated perceptions. Conditioning in human subjects has lost in effector action and gained in elaboration of input. When all capacities are engaged in supporting overt muscular activities there may well be a narrowing of perception or a reduced utilization of perceptual cues. These latter conditions also seem applicable to states of high autonomic activation such as in emotion. When neither gross muscular action nor high autonomic activation is a factor in the situation there is time for the subject to make a more detailed and precise registration of input material.

Whether the modern concern with information processing will provide a useful model itself of brain and behaviour remains to be seen. Considerable sharpening of its hypotheses is required in human conditioning studies, for example in terms of the relevant dimensions along which information is constructed by subjects; on delineation of the functions of a 'central processing capacity', and on the probably increasing role of individual differences. Attention to the registration and storage of input should not neglect the actions which enable the individual to function effectively in his environment.

The recent exploration of cognitive factors in emotion and conditioning must be welcomed as a redress on previous neglect. But it does not replace earlier views on the contribution of physiological events: rather, it serves to enlarge them. It is essential to keep sight of the essentially biological, unmediated and organic modes of coping which comprise so large a part of behaviour. The problem before us is how these different components are integrated and organized into a response which provides meaningful interaction with the physical and social environment.

15.5. REFERENCES

Bannister, D. & Mair, J. M. M. *The evaluation of personal contructs*. London: Academic Press, 1968.

Barr, R. F. & McConaghy, N. A general factor of conditionability: A study of galvanic skin responses and penile responses. *Behaviour Research and Therapy*, 1972, **10**, 215–227.

Blanchard, E. B. & Young, L. D. Self-control of cardiac functioning: A promise as yet unfulfilled. *Psychological Bulletin*, 1973, **79**, 145–163.

Breger, L. & McGaugh, J. L. Critique and reformulation of 'learning theory' approaches to psychotherapy and neurosis. *Psychological Bulletin*, 1965, **63**, 338–358.

Breland, K. & Breland, M. The misbehaviour of organisms. *American Psychologist*, 1961, **16**, 681–684.

Campbell, D., Sanderson, R. E. & Laverty, S. G. Characteristics of a conditioned response in human subjects during extinction trials following a single traumatic conditioning trial. *Journal of Abnormal and Social Psychology*, 1964, **68**, 627–639.

Dawson, M. E. Can classical conditioning occur without contingency learning? A review and evaluation of the evidence. *Psychophysiology*, 1973, **10**, 82–86.

Dostalek, C. & Krasna, H. *The inductive effect of an accoustic stimulus upon the unconditioned eyelid reaction elicited by an optical stimulus*. Proceedings of the Czechoslovak Physiological Society, Czechoslovak Academy of Sciences, January, 1969.

Dykman, R. A., Murphree, O. D. & Ackerman, P. T. Litter patterns in the offspring of nervous and stable dogs. II. Autonomic and motor conditioning. *Journal of Nervous and Mental Disease*, 1966, **141**, 419–431.

Estes, W. K. Memory and Conditioning. In *Contemporary approaches to Conditioning and Learning*. F. J. McGuigan and D. Barry Lumsden (Eds.). Washington, D.C.: Winston, 1973.

Eysenck, H. J. A theory of the incubation of anxiety/fear responses. *Behaviour Research and Therapy*, 1963, **6**, 309–321.

Eysenck, H. J. *The Biological Basis of Personality*. Springfield, Illinois: Charles Thomas, 1967.

Eysenck, H. J. *The measurement of Emotion: Psychological parameters and methods*. Paper given at Conference on parameters of Emotion, Stockholm, Karolinska Institute, 1973.

Frith, C. D. Abnormalities of perception. In *Handbook of Abnormal Psychology*. H. J. Eysenck (Ed), London, Pitman, 1973.

Gauthier, R. J. E. The relationship between a pedophilic patient's GSR slope and anxiety under shock and non-shock conditions: A teleological approach. Alex. G. Brown Memorial Clinic, Department of Correctional Services, Ontario, 1971 (mimeo).

Gormezano, I. Investigations of defence and reward conditioning in the rabbit. In A. H. Black and W. F. Prokasy (Eds) *Classical Conditioning. II. Current theory and research.* New York: Appleton–Century–Crafts, 1972.

Graham, L., Cohen, S. I. & Shmavonian, B. M. Physiologic determination and behavioural relationships in human instrumental conditioning. *Psychosomatic Medicine*, 1964, **26**, 321–336.

Grant, D. A. A preliminary model for processing information conveyed by verbal conditioned stimuli in classical conditioning. In A. H. Black and W. F. Prokasy (Eds), *Classical Conditioning II: Current theory and research.* New York: Appleton–Century–Crofts, 1972.

Grant, D. A. Cognitive factors in eyelid conditioning. *Psychophysiology*, 1973, **10**, 75–81.

Gray, J. A. The psychophysiological basis of introversion–extraversion. *Behaviour Research and Therapy*, 1970, **8**, 249–266.

Grings, W. W. Verbal-perceptual factors in the conditioning of autonomic responses. In W. F. Prokasy (Ed), *Classical Conditioning.* New York: Appleton–Century–Crofts, 1965.

Grings, W. W. Cognitive factors in electrodermal conditioning. *Psychological Bulletin*, 1973, **79**, 200–210.

Grings, W. W. & Lockhart, R. A. & Dameron, L. E. Conditioning autonomic responses of mentally subnormal individuals. *Psychological Monographs*, 1962, **76**, No. 39.

Grings, W. W. & Lockhart, R. A. Galvanic Skin Response during avoidance learning. *Psychophysiology*, 1966, **3**, 29–34.

Grings, W. W. & Schell, A. M. Magnitude of electrodermal response to a standard stimulus as a function of intensity and proximity of a prior stimulus. *Journal of Comparative and Physiological Psychology*, **67**, 77–82.

Hovland, C. I. The generalization of conditioned responses. I. The sensory generalization of conditioned responses with varying frequencies of tone. *Journal of General Psychology*, 1937, **17**, 125–148.

Hull, C. L. *The principles of behaviour.* New York: Appleton–Century–Crofts. 1943.

Kimble, G. A. & Ost, J. W. P. A conditioned inhibitory process in eyelid conditioning. *Journal of Experimental Psychology*, 1961, **61**, 150–156.

Kimmel, H. D. Instrumental inhibitory factors in classical conditioning. In W. F. Prokasy (Ed), *Classical Conditioning. A symposium.* New York: Appleton–Century–Crofts, 1965.

Koestler, A. *The act of creation.* London: Hutchinson, 1964.

Lang, P. J. Fear reduction and fear behaviour: Problems in treating a construct. In J. M. Shlien (Ed), *Research in Psychotherapy*, Vol. 3. Washington: American Psychological Association, 1968.

Lang, P. J. The application of psychophysiological methods to the study of psychotherapy and behaviour modification. In A. E. Bergin and S. L. Garfield (Eds), *Handbook of Psychotherapy and Behaviour Change: An empirical analysis.* New York: Wiley, 1971.

Lazarus, R. S. Emotions and adaptation: conceptual and empirical relations. In W. J. Arnold (Ed), *Nebraska Symposium on Motivation.* Lincoln, Nebraska: University of Nebraska Press, 1968.

Levey, A. B. Some measures of response efficiency for the conditioned eyelid response. Paper read at the 4th World Congress of Psychiatry. Symposium on Higher Nervous Activity. Madrid: 1966.

Levey, A. B. Eyelid conditioning, extraversion and drive; an experimental test of two theories. Ph.D. thesis, University of London, 1972.

386

Levey, A. B. Classical conditioning of a human evaluative response. Unpublished manuscript, 1974.

Levey, A. B. & Martin, I. Shape of the conditioned eyelid response. *Psychological Review*, 1968, **75**, 398–408.

Levey, A. B. & Martin, I. The sequence of response development in human eyelid conditioning. *Journal of Experimental Psychology*, in press, 1974.

Lockhart, R. A. Comments regarding multiple response phenomena in long interstimulus interval conditioning. *Psychophysiology*, 1966, **3**, 103–114.

Lockhart, R. A. Cognitive processes and the multiple response phenomenon. *Psychophysiology*, 1973, **10**, 112–118.

Lykken, D. T. Preliminary observations on the preception phenomenon. *Psychophysiological Measurement Newsletter*, 1959, **5**, 2–4.

Lykken, D. T. Preception in the rat: autonomic response to shock as a function of length of warning interval. *Science*, 1962, **137**, 665–666.

Mandel, I. J. & Bridger, W. H. Is there classical conditioning without cognitive expectancy. *Psychophysiology*, 1973, **10**, 87–90.

Mandler, G., Mandler, J. M. & Uviller, E. T. Autonomic feedback: The perception of autonomic activity. *Journal of Abnormal and Social Psychology*, 1958, **56**, 367–373.

Martin, I. & Levey, A. B. *The genesis of the classical conditioned response*: International Series of Monographs in Experimental Psychology, No. 8. London: Pergamon Press, 1969.

Martin, I., Slubicka, B. & Levey, A. B. Response relationships in SRR conditioning. Unpublished manuscript. 1974.

McAllister, D. E. & McAllister, W. R. Incubation of fear: An examination of the concept. *Journal of Experimental Research in Personality*, 1967, **2**, 180–190.

Norman, D. A. (Ed) *Models of Human Memory*. London: Academic Press, 1970.

Öhman, A. and Bohlin, G. The relationship between spontaneous and stimulus-correlated electrodermal responses in simple and discriminative conditioning paradigms. *Psychophysiology*, 1973, **10**, 589–600.

Peeke, S. C. & Grings, W. W. Magnitude of UCR as a function of variability in the CS–UCS relationship. *Journal of Experimental Psychology*, 1968, **77**, 64–69.

Pribram, K. H. The new neurology and the biology of emotion: A structural approach. *American Psychologist*, 1967, **22**, 830–838.

Prokasy, W. F. & Ebel, H. C. Three components of the classically conditioned GSR in human subjects. *Journal of Experimental Psychology*, 1967, **73**, 247–256.

Razran, G. Conditioning and perception. *Psychological Review*, 1955, **62**, 83–95.

Razran, G. The dominance-contiguity theory of the acquisition of classical conditioning. *Psychological Bulletin*, 1957, **54**, 1–46.

Schachter, S. The interaction of cognitive and physiological determinants of emotional state. In C.D. Spielberger (Ed), *Anxiety and behaviour*. New York: Academic Press, 1966.

Seligman, M. E. P. & Hager J. (Eds). *Biological Boundaries of Learning*. New York: Appleton–Century–Crofts, 1973.

Seligman, M. E. P. & Johnston, J. C. A cognitive theory of avoidance learning. In F. J. McGuigan and D. B. Lumsden (Eds). *Contemporary Approaches to Conditioning and Learning*. Washington, D.C.: Winston, 1973.

Skinner B. F. *The Behaviour of organisms*. New York: Appleton–Century–Crofts, 1938.

Sokolov, E. N. Higher nervous functions: the orienting reflex. *Annual Review of Physiology*, 1963, **25**, 545–580.

Spence, K. W. *Behaviour Theory and Conditioning*. New Haven: Yale University Press, 1956.

Stern, J. A. Physiological response measures during classical conditioning. In N. S. Greenfield and R. S. Sternbach (Eds), *Handbook of Psychophysiology*. New York: Holt, Rinehart and Winston. 1972.

Tecce, J. J. Contingent negative variation (CNV) and psychological processes in man. *Psychological Bulletin*, 1972, **77**, 73–108.

Valins, S. The perception and labelling of bodily changes as determinants of emotional behaviour, Ch. II. In P. Black (Ed), *Physiological Correlates of Emotion*. New York: Academic Press, 1970.

Walter, W. G., Cooper, R., Aldridge, V. J., McCallum, W. C. & Winter, A. L. Contingent negative variation: An electric sign of sensori-motor association and expectancy in the human brain. *Nature*, 1964, **203**, 380–384.

Chapter 16

Psychophysiology and Human Memory

FERGUS I. M. CRAIK and KIRK R. BLANKSTEIN

Erindale College, University of Toronto, Canada

16.1. INTRODUCTION

In writing this chapter we were concerned entirely with studies of human memory and learning; animal studies were not reviewed. We surveyed the literature with a view to assessing the extent to which psychophysiological measures have helped in an understanding of the processes underlying memory and learning, and with an eye for the areas in which further collaboration between psychophysiologists and memory theorists might be particularly useful. The orginal experiments were carried out for a variety of reasons. Presumably the most basic was an attempt to specify the neural mechanisms which mediate memory; a more modest aim was to document the physiological changes which accompany particular memory phenomena. Although this type of research was started fairly recently, it is already extensive in the number of paradigms and techniques used. For the most part we will review and discuss studies on the following topics: autonomic and cortical indices of learning; the effects of arousal and activation on memory and learning; the relation between pupillary dilation and memory; the role of eye movements and of subvocal speech in memory processes; lastly, experiments on sleep and learning.

Theoretical notions about human memory have been changing rapidly over the last few years. Since these views are often contradictory and confusing, and since each new idea has typically been illustrated by a new empirical paradigm, we will first give a brief review of current theories and methods in human memory research.

16.2. THEORETICAL VIEWS OF HUMAN MEMORY

Since 1950, human memory has been viewed from two major theoretical standpoints: interference theory and information processing theory. Interference theory held an unchallenged position until the early 1960's but since then information-processing models of memory have become more dominant and probably are more generally accepted today.

Interference theory grew out of classical associationism and originally took the position that the basic thing to be explained in verbal learning is the acquisition and extinction of associative bonds between stimuli and responses. The paradigm devised to explore this idea was that of paired-associate (PA) learning. Typically a list of 12 pairs of items (words, digits or nonsense syllables) is presented on successive occasions until the stimulus terms reliably elicit the response terms. In the 1950's and 1960's it became increasingly clear that the PA paradigm was not only testing associative information, but that subjects also had to learn the subject of response items currently in use. Thus an important distinction must be made between memory for associations and memory for items. It seems likely that these different types of information are affected by different factors (Murdock, 1974), and apparently discrepant results may be due to the differential tapping of item and associative information in various experiments. A second major paradigm used by interference theorists is serial learning. In this case, a string of items is presented repeatedly until the subject can recite the items in their correct order. Although the distinction is rather arbitrary, an experiment may be thought of as testing 'memory' if the subject recalls or recognizes what he can after one presentation; 'learning' is measured by studying the rate of acquisition of the materials over several presentations. With the increasing interest in information processing theories, there has been an increased emphasis on memory as opposed to verbal learning (Tulving & Madigan, 1970). To some extent the psychophysiological literature is still reflecting the older emphasis on learning.

Information processing theory takes the view that information from the environment is perceived and assimilated by being processed through a number of qualitatively distinct stages; incoming information interacts with stored information from past learning to determine appropriate responses. Three main levels of memory function have been distinguished—sensory memory, short-term memory (STM) and long-term memory (LTM). At the sensory level, incoming stimuli are held very briefly in terms of their physical character-istics; visual, auditory and tactile qualities, for example. If the stimulus is attended to, it enters a limited-capacity short-term store where it stays as long as it is rehearsed. Information in STM may be lost by decay but it is more likely to be lost by being displaced by further incoming items. If STM items are rehearsed, information is transferred to a more commodious and permanent LTM (Atkinson & Shiffrin, 1968; Murdock, 1967).

The notion of 'short-term memory' has changed somewhat over the last 10 years. Originally the term implied both a short retention interval (30 sec, say) and a separate mechanism. Thus, if short-term retention was qualitatively different from retention over a longer interval, the difference was ascribed to recall from one or other mechanism. More recently, however, it has been suggested that retention interval is not synonymous with the mechanism utilized—on the one hand, meaningful items may enter LTM immediately, thus even immediate memory may draw on this store, and on the other hand items may have their stay in STM prolonged indefinitely by rehearsal. Thus, 'in STM' is coming to imply 'still being rehearsed' or even 'still in mind' (see for example, Craik & Lockhart, 1972).

Current issues in STM research concern the types of coding used (acoustic, articulatory, semantic, etc.), the capacity of the store and the characteristics and causes of forgetting. The paradigms used have included digit and word span, free recall, a variety of retrieval latency techniques (e.g., Sternberg, 1969) and the Brown–Peterson paradigm in which the subject engages in a distractor activity to prevent rehearsal. In LTM research, the issues concern the nature of organization within the system, differences between recall and recognition, the nature and interactions of encoding and retrieval processes. Many of the para-digms used to study LTM are similar to those used in STM research (free recall, recognition accuracy and latency, for example), while other methods are peculiar to LTM. Free recall learning (the same word list presented on several occasions) and the study of imagery and mnemonic techniques, are in this latter category.

From the point of view of memory theories generally, it may be hoped that psychophysiological indicators will be the bridge between observed changes in in memory and learning on the one hand and changes in brain states on the other. More specifically there are a number of important issues which might be clarified by psychophysiological measures: can central correlates of STM and LTM functions be found? can a stimulus be "tracked" as it is processed more deeply and elaborately? can the subject's utilization of different memory codes be indexed? are there consistent relationships between the level of arousal and encoding or retrieval processions? to what extent are the covert processes involved in rehearsal and imagery identical to those involved in speech and visual perception? After the findings from a number of research areas have been reviewed, we will assess the progress which has been made in bridging the gap between behaviour and neurophysiology.

16.3. AUTONOMIC AND CORTICAL INDICES OF LEARNING

In this section we shall examine some studies which have looked directly at the physiological changes accompanying memory and learning.

16.3.1. Autonomic measures

An early study by Brown (1937) failed to find consistent relations between the serial learning of a nonsense-syllable list and blood pressure or respiration. However, a strong correlation was obtained across subjects between the mean GSR response to a nonsense syllable and the speed with which it was learned— a large GSR response was associated with rapid learning. Since a typically bowed serial position effect was obtained, Brown suggested that more attention was paid to the first few and last few syllables, thereby giving rise to larger GSR responses and quicker learning. Brown also found larger GSR responses to each syllable before it was fully learned—an observation confirmed by Kintsch (1965).

Later studies have shown small or inconsistent relationships between learning and autonomic activities. Berry & Davis (1960) found that serial learning was positively related to the magnitude of jaw muscle tension. Furth & Terry (1961), using an index of arousal derived from two autonomic measures, found better learning in their low arousal subjects. Bearing in mind the large individual differences found in this area of research, Obrist (1962) investigated differences in learning efficiency in the same subjects at different times. The learning task was the serial learning of nonsense syllables and the autonomic measures were heart rate and skin resistance. The results were not clear cut, but in general an inverted U-shaped function was found in three subjects between learning performance and the autonomic measures (learning was best for intermediate levels of arousal), while linear functions (in some cases positive, in other cases negative) were found for the remaining two subjects. In line with this rather confusing picture, Mandler & Mandler (1962), in a study of the autonomic correlates of associative behaviour, concluded that individual differences in verbal behaviour were not related to differences in physiological response.

One possible source of the confusion has been documented by Kintsch (1965). He examined the relations between GSR and paired-associate learning and found that an overall analysis revealed only a rather noisy decline in GSR magnitude over successive learning trials. However, when the GSR to specific items was considered, it was found that the GSR reaction to each item increased until its paired response was correctly anticipated. On subsequent trials, these learned items were associated with lower GSR responses. Kintsch describes this finding in terms of increased attention (and greater GSR response) to an item while it is being learned, and then lessened attention (habituated GSR) after the association is in the learned state. There is an interesting parallel between Kintsch's results and the suggestion from Pribram's laboratory that the skin conductance response (GSR) indicates registration of an incoming signal in the 'neuronal store'. They comment: 'Tentatively the hypothesis may be entertained that the GSR is involved not in the production of orienting (or "attention") directly, but in its *registration*. Only when such registration has occurred can the nervous system perform its normal "tuning" or "coding" function and so allow the representations or neuronal models of experienced inputs to accrue' (Bagshaw, Kimble & Pribram, 1965). Their statement follows observation on monkeys with ablations of the amygdala—such animals continue to show behavioural orientation towards repeated signals but show decreased GSR responsivity. The suggestion is that previous presentations of the event were not registered, there was no build-up of a neuronal model and thus subsequent presentations are treated as novel events. In the intact animal, as the 'neuronal model' (or 'the association' in Kintsch's terms) is built up, there is at first partial recognition and an increased GSR. Once the neuronal model perfectly matches the input pattern (once the association is learned) habituation sets in and the GSR declines. Pribram's work, and its relations to input functions, memory and arousal, is discussed more fully by Mackworth (1969) and by Venables (1973).

Spence, Lugo & Youdin (1972) monitored heart rate while subjects listened to a 17-minute spoken passage. The subjects' task was to detect and remember phrases relating to a designated topic. In line with Lacey's (1967) work, the investigators found evidence for both tonic and phasic heart rate deceleration when target phrases occurred. Reasonably enough, no phasic changes occurred to phrases which the subject failed to recall or recognize later—presumably he did not detect them. A potentially more interesting observation was that phasic changes to recalled phrases were slightly different from phasic changes to targets which were later recognized but not recalled—the differences in the two heart rate profiles were apparently not significant, however. Although the authors suggest that a 'cubic change in rate is a good predictor of later recall' and that such changes are 'a sign that the stimulus is being coverted into long-term storage' (p. 1346), it may simply be that greater attention to the target phrases gave rise both to more heart rate deceleration and to better memory performance.

At a more cautious and less speculative level, it seems reasonable to conclude that such autonomic measures as heart rate and GSR largely reflect the amount of effort or degree of attention the subject is giving to the material being learned. Similar results have been obtained from pupillary dilation studies, to be reviewed later.

16.3.2. Cortical measures

Studies of changes in EEG activity during learning have generally revealed an increase in fast-wave activity during the active learning phase. For example, Thompson & Obrist (1964) found that both alpha desynchronization and beta augmentation (that is, increase in fast-wave activity) were greatest when the correct response was first elicited. This finding fits well with Kintsch's (1965) results. Thompson & Obrist conclude: 'It seems unlikely that the electrocortical changes represent a change in associative bonds, since such changes tend to diminish with practice. Rather, the results probably reflect variations in attention during the course of learning (p. 340).' In line with this suggestion, Thompson & Thompson (1965) found increased fast-wave activity and decreased alpha during learning of a nonsense-syllable list, but that overlearning was associated with a return to EEG resting levels. In a further study, Thompson & Wilson (1966) found that good learners tended to show more fast-wave activity (< 12-Hz) and less slow-wave activity (< 8-Hz) than poor learners. The EEG's were not recorded during learning but during a session of photic stimulation.

Since it seems generally agreed that beta (fast) activity is associated with attention and learning, Surwillo (1971) investigated the possibility that the dominant frequency of the EEG would increase as subjects held longer lists of digits in a short-term memory task. In fact, Surwillo found no relationship between list length and the dominant EEG frequency. Thus, it seems that the appearance of beta is associated with the necessity to pay attention to the material, but is not related quantitatively to the amount held in short-term memory.

A line of work just starting which might well dominate a similar chapter written in 1985, is the study of the evoked cortical response (ECR) (see also Chapter 14). The importance of the ECR in memory work was largely initiated and developed by John (1967). In recent work he has developed a 'statistical configuration theory' of memory, arguing that memories are mediated by common modes of activity in anatomically extensive regions of the brain (John, 1972). Studies specifically relating ECR to human learning include an experiment by Greenberg & Graham (1970) in which the authors investigated auditory evoked responses during the learning of syllables and tones. In general, they found increases in the 'largest amplitude spectral component' during the initial stages of learning and thereafter a decrease in this component. The authors speculatively suggest that the decrease in ECR may be related to arousal or may reflect the acquisition of meaning. Another interesting speculation relating ECR to memory was made by Wilkinson & Lee (1972). They suggested that the $N_1 - P_2$ component of the auditory evoked potential may be associated with the brief retention of auditory material in a sensory store.

Shucard & Horn (1972) reported small but significant correlations between the latency of positive peaks in the visual evoked potential and memory span. These correlations were significant only when the average evoked potentials were recorded under low arousal conditions. The interpretation of all these findings is still obscure, but the technique seems interesting and potentially useful as a bridge between neurophysiology and studies of cognitive behaviour.

In a recent important paper, Posner, Klein, Summers & Buggie (1973) suggest that the concept of attention can be usefully broken down into three components; namely, alertness, set and processing capacity. They claim that an increase in alertness does not affect the rate at which information builds up in the perceptual and memory systems but that a specific set does. To illustrate the effects of set, the authors presented a single letter for $\frac{1}{4}$ sec followed by a further letter after 1 sec. The subject responded 'same' or 'different' with regard to the letter pair. Posner *et al.* found that the P_3 wave of the visual ECR occurred earlier when the letters matched; they tentatively suggest that this wave may be released by the entry of the stimulus into a central limited-capacity mechanism associated with conscious awareness, and that the repetition of a letter speeds up the entry of the second letter into this mechanism. The possible identification of ECR components with stages of a general information-processing model of perception and memory (Broadbent, 1958) is an exciting prospect and we await further developments with interest.

16.4. AROUSAL AND MEMORY

Most of the studies reviewed in this section were carried out with the implicit assumption that arousal or activation may be considered unidimensional. Many psychophysiologists would now question this assumption, and it is more generally believed that there are several dimensions of arousal (e.g., electrocortical, autonomic and behavioural), each complex in itself. For example, Lacey (1967, p. 25) concluded that ' ... activational or arousal processes are not unidimensional but multidimensional and that the activation processes do not reflect just the intensive dimension of behaviour, but also the intended aim or goal of the behaviour'. Cases of 'directional fractionation' or 'situational stereotypy' in which two autonomic measures indicate apparently opposite trends in arousal, are now well documented. Thus, it is not just arousal, but arousal for a specific purpose, which must be studied. Increased attention to external stimuli appears to result in cardiac deceleration, but a higher level of mental work and attention to internal stimuli typically results in cardiac acceleration (Lacey, 1967; Elliot, 1972). This complexity is generally overlooked by those carrying out research on arousal and memory. A further distinction which is often disregarded is the difference between a tonic *arousal level* and a phasic *arousal increment* to some specific stimulus. We will attempt to disentangle these effects. Finally, arousal has been manipulated both by differences in the arousing qualities of the material to be remembered (by emotional words, for example) and it has also been manipulated independently of the material (e.g., by the presentation of white noise bursts). Again we will look at the effects of these techniques separately.

16.4.1. The effects of phasic arousal increments on retention

One of the most interesting and provocative results in the area linking psychophysiology and memory is Kleinsmith & Kaplan's (1963) finding that paired responses to 'high arousal' words like RAPE and VOMIT were poorly remembered in an immediate retention test, but well remembered by groups tested at longer intervals; further, that 'low arousal' responses were well remembered by the immediate group but poorly remembered by delayed retention groups. In greater detail, subjects were given one paired-associate learning trial in which the eight stimulus terms were words and the response terms were single digits from 2 to 9. The subjects were instructed to 'concentrate carefully' on the word-number pairs and also on colour slides interpolated between the pairs; no mention was made of a subsequent retention test. Skin resistance was measured during presentation, and the GSR deflections to the eight stimulus words were ranked for each subject. The three highest deflections for each subject were designated 'high arousal learning' and the three lowest were designated 'low arousal learning'. Different groups of subjects were given an unexpected retention test at 2, 20 and 45 min, 1 day and 1 week.

The results showed that responses to low arousal words were forgotten over time but that high arousal responses actually increased from a level which was lower than chance responding at 2 min, to over 40 per cent retention after 1 week. This is a very surprising result. The explanation offered by Kleinsmith & Kaplan (1963) is that the association is mediated at first by a reverberating circuit of neurons; under high arousal, this trace will reverberate at a greater rate, thus leading to better consolidation. While the trace is reverberating, however, it is unavailable to the organism since all neurons in the trace are occupied in the consolidation process.

The explanation is a curious one in several respects. First there is the highly speculative neurophysiology; the notion that short-term memory is mediated by reverating circuits of neurons is far from established, and the additional notion that under high arousal all possible neurons are working to their limit seems a little fanciful. At the psychological level the 'consolidation process' presumably must be an unconscious one, quite unlike conscious rehearsal, otherwise the consolidating items would be available in the short term as well as in the long term. More crucially, if a high arousal word gives rise to a non-specific arousal state, then that state can only last until the next low arousal word is presented—possibly in 16 second's time. Since each subject heard all eight words, the brain must alternate rather rapidly between high and low arousal following each word. At the time of immediate retention, the brain is most likely to be in a state of neutral arousal and there is thus no reason for the high arousal associations to be still inaccessible. There are two ways out of this logical dilemma. One is to suggest that when the stimulus word is given as a retrieval cue during the retention test, it reinstates the appropriate level of arousal. The second is to postulate trace-specific arousal levels, confined to the neurons in each trace, which perseverate for several minutes regardless of subsequent stimuli. With regard to the first point—this mechanism should operate at long as well as short retention intervals; also, Kaplan & Kaplan (1968a) reported that GSR levels at recall did not predict the effect. Second, the notion of trace-specific arousal systems is feasible but somewhat hard to maintain in the light of the general belief that memory traces are diffusely localized in the brain.

Whatever the deficiencies of the explanation, the empirical result is an interesting one. Kleinsmith & Kaplan (1964) replicated the finding using nonsense syllables as stimuli. A further replication was reported by Walker & Tarte (1963), using homogeneous and mixed lists of high- and low-arousal words as stimulus terms and again, single digits as response terms. In this case, high arousal words retained their high recall level at the 1-week retention interval, but did not actually increase over time. In fact Walker & Tarte found no differences between high and low arousal conditions in the 2-minute test. They invoke Walker's (1958) notions of action decrement to explain Kleinsmith & Kaplan's results—the idea is that an inhibitory process (action decrement) protects the memory trace during consolidation. The effect of this protection is to make the trace temporarily inaccessible. Again, however, action decrement must be thought of as trace-specific and as continuing throughout the presentation of subsequent low-arousal items, although Walker (1958, p. 139) describes the consolidating trace as being 'driven by nonspecific input'. A further replication of the Kleinsmith & Kaplan effect was reported by Butter (1970).

Other workers have reported related experiments using somewhat different paradigms. Kaplan & Sampson (1968) examined arousal effects on the intentional learning and subsequent immediate and delayed free recall of words and pictures. They found no relation between GSR and picture recall, but for words they found higher GSR scores (recorded during the learning session) for reminiscence items as opposed to forgotten items. A reminiscence item is one which was not recalled in the immediate test but which was recalled in the delayed (30 min) test; a forgotten item is one recalled in the first but not the second test. However, these results are put into question by a further study by Sampson (1969) in which the only significant relationship between GSR and word or picture recall was a *positive* one between GSR and immediate word recall—that is, high arousal words were best recalled.

Maltzman, Kantor & Langdon (1966) presented eight high-arousal and eight low-arousal words in an incidental learning paradigm. Their study thus deviates from Kleinsmith & Kaplan's technique in that the high- and low-arousal word were designated before the experiment; not on the basis of each subject's phasic arousal increments. They found that the high arousal words were better recalled than the low arousal words, both in immediate recall and in recall after 30 min. There was no interaction between arousal and retention interval. This result is thus opposed to Kleinsmith & Kaplan's theory and the authors prefer an explanation in terms of the orienting reflex. Emotional words simply elicit more attention and this leads to better learning. Kaplan & Kaplan (1968a) published a rejoinder to the Maltzman *et al.* paper, saying that while their own work had dealt with associative informaion, the Maltzman *et al.* study used free recall of items as the measure of learning. Kaplan & Kaplan also objected to the use by Maltzman *et al.* of words selected for their probably high or low emotional content; the Kaplans argued that for any subject, a word's arousal-inducing properties could change from time to time, and that the effects of emotionality on memory are not necessarily equivalent to the effects of arousal on memory.

Levonian (1967) recorded the skin resistance of subjects watching an instructional film and later gave them a yes-no recognition test about events in the films. The test was given to all subjects after retention intervals of 10 min and 1 week. He found an interaction between the arousal increment associated with the event's presentation and retention interval, in the direction predicted by Kleinsmith & Kaplan's work. However, the significant interaction is very largely due to low arousal items being forgotten. In what appears to be a second analysis of the same experiment, Levonian (1966) reported that a resistance decrement before a particular event in the film facilitated both immediate and long-term memory; while if the decrement followed the event, immediate retention was poor but long-term retention was good. In this study there were 56 forgotten events but 96 reminiscence events (Levonian, 1967); that is, performance was better after a week than after 10 min. Since it is universally acknowledged that recognition performance declines over time (see, for example, Kintsch, 1969), Levonian's study must be considered seriously atypical.

One final experiment will be described in this section: Corteen (1969) presented a list of words in an incidental learning/free recall paradigm. The words were presented very slowly (20–60 sec per word) to allow skin conductance to return to a baseline level. He then correlated log change in skin conductance with recall after either no-delay, 20 min or 2 weeks. Corteen found significant positive relationships between arousal and recall at all retention intervals, and that the size of the correlation increased with retention interval. He suggests that at short intervals, all traces are equally accessible, but at long intervals recall is predicted by trace strength which in turn is a function of arousal at input. This result is similar to the findings of Maltzman et al. (1966) and is consistent with several experiments in memory research (Glanzer, 1972) which have shown short-term retention to be insensitive to factors which affect long-term retention.

It has been suggested (Walker & Tarte, 1963; Bower, 1967) that the interaction between arousal and retention interval is at least contaminated by, and possibly caused by, a serial position artefact. It is known that the GSR response declines throughout the presentation list—in general the first item receives the largest response and the last item the smallest response (Walker & Tarte, 1963). Also, it has been shown that while the last items in a free recall or paired-associate list are the best recalled in an immediate memory test, these last-presented items are actually the least well remembered in a later test (Craik, 1970; Madigan & McCabe, 1971). When these two findings are combined, it follows that initial list items are most likely to be categorized as high arousal items and that these items will not be as well recalled as the low arousal (recency) items after a short retention interval. At longer intervals, however, the high arousal (primacy) items should be better recalled. This account of the effect handles the observed interaction and the cross-over quite nicely, but cannot handle any reminiscence effects. It also suggests that if high arousal items were selected before presentation (e.g., DEATH, RAPE compared with TABLE, WALK) rather than on the basis of GSR responses, the cross-over would not be found. This procedure was adopted by Walker & Tarte (1963), Maltzman *et al.* (1966) and by Kaplan & Kaplan (1970). When words were used, all three studies found no cross-over—high-arousal items were better remembered at all retention intervals; with nonsense syllables, a cross-over effect was still observed (Kaplan & Kaplan, 1970). There is thus some evidence that a serial position artefact can account for the original Kleinsmith & Kaplan effect. However, the point was directly examined by Kaplan & Kaplan (1968b) and rejected as a general explanation—two of the three studies re-analysed in terms of serial position yielded no systematic pattern at different retention intervals. Also, Butter (1970) in her replication of the Kleinsmith & Kaplan effect, reported finding no relationship between GSR and the item's serial position. It must be concluded, then, that while a serial position artefact may explain some of these studies and is certainly a factor to be aware of, it cannot account for all the available data.

16.4.2. The effects of differences in tonic arousal level on retention

Berry (1962) explored the effect of tonic arousal level on learning by correlating skin conductance level with performance on a paired-associate task. Berry used between-subject comparisons—the relative stability of an individual's arousal level was confirmed by the finding of a strong positive correlation (mean rho = +0.83) between skin conductance levels measured during the first minute of learning and the first minute of recall. The task was a 30-item paired associate list and the retention interval was 6 min. The data suggest that better learning performance is associated with moderate levels of skin conductance (and thus arousal) both during learning and recall. The finding of an inverted-U relation between arousal and learning conflicts with Kleinsmith & Kaplan's (1963) data which show that high-arousal items are the best learned. Thus Kleinsmith, Kaplan & Tarte (1963) suggested that Berry's results may apply only to short retention intervals. Accordingly, they repeated Berry's experiment with two groups of subjects—one tested after 6 min and the other tested after 1 week. They found an inverted-U relationship between GSR and recall in the 6-min group, but a positive linear relationship for the 1-week group. It is unclear, however, how stable the arousal levels were for the 1-week group and thus whether the 6-min results were due in part to arousal level differences at retrieval.

Is the relationship between arousal and short-term retention negative (Kleinsmith & Kaplan, 1963) or inverted-U (Berry, 1962; Kleinsmith, Kaplan & Tarte, 1963) in form? This contradiction was apparently resolved by Levonian (1968) who pointed out that Berry had used arousal *level* as an index of arousal and a between-subjects comparison, while Kleinsmith & Kaplan had measured arousal increment and a within-subjects design. Levonian found evidence for an inverted-U relationship in his data taking arousal level and between-subject comparisons, but a negative relationship between the arousing value of particular incidents and their subsequent recall within the same subjects.

Recent reports from some British investigators, however, have supported the notion of a negative relationship between arousal level and immediate recall. Blake (1967) found that digit span declined regularly from 10.30 a.m. to 9 p.m. He tested the same subjects at all times (on different days) and found that body temperature rose over the same time periods. He interpreted this second result as evidence for increasing arousal as the day progressed. If there is a positive relationship between arousal and long-term memory, then performance at LTM tasks should increase throughout the day. This proposition was ingeniously tested by Baddeley, Hatter, Scott & Snashall (1970). They gave subjects a series of 9-digit messages for immediate serial recall; some of the messages were repeated in the series and were thus better recalled. Recall of the nonrepeated messages was the STM measure, and the difference between the mean recalls of the repeated and nonrepeated items was the measure of learning or LTM performance. They found a significant decrease in STM performance from morning to afternoon; while the LTM measure increased, the difference was not significant. Similarly, Hockey, Davies & Gray (1972) reported superior STM performance for a group tested in the morning. It should be pointed out that these STM differences, while statistically reliable, are small—0·7 of a digit in Blake's study and 0·5 digits in the Baddeley et al. experiment.

The situation with regard to the effects of tonic arousal level on memory is thus a little confused. The one study which measured retention after a long time interval (Kleinsmith, Kaplan & Tarte, 1963) found that recall was a positive function of arousal. This result agrees with the findings from the arousal increment studies (Kleinsmith & Kaplan, 1963). With short retention intervals, there is something of an international split, since the American studies (Berry, 1962; Kleinsmith, Kaplan & Tarte, 1963; Levonian, (1968) find an inverted-U relationship, while the British studies (Blake, 1967; Baddeley et. al., 1970; Hockey et al., 1972) find that STM is negatively related to arousal (thereby agreeing with the American experiments in which arousal increment has been used). Since both the Baddeley et al. and the Hockey et al. experiments tested memory at only two points in the day (and thus at two levels of arousal), it remains possible that a third testing time might reveal an inverted-U relationship. Some support to this suggestion is given by Blake's (1967) finding that subjects tested at 8 a.m. had lower span scores than those tested at 10·30 a.m. A further ambiguous point about the short-term studies is the uncertainty as to whether arousal is affecting acquisition or retrieval processes.

The studies reviewed so far have dealt with differences in arousal level during learning; one study which attempted to manipulate arousal level at recall may be cited here. Uehling & Sprinkle (1968) had subjects learn a 10-item serial list to one perfect anticipation. Different groups of subjects were then tested immediately, after 24 h or after 1 week under one of three arousal conditions induced immediately prior to recall by (a) instructions to relax; (b) induction of muscle tension, or (c) presentation of 80-dB bursts of white noise. The number of trials required to relearn the list was measured. The authors found no differences for immediate recall (hardly surprising since all subjects had just learned the list, and performance was over 90 per cent correct), but found the white noise condition yielded better memory performance than the other two conditions (which did not differ) at both 24 h and 1 week. The result is interpreted as showing the beneficial effects of arousal on retrieval. The authors argue that previous results showing a relationship between arousal and memory may also be due to retrieval factors and thus it may be unnecessary to invoke differential effects of arousal on consolidation. This may be a plausible argument, but it should also be mentioned that Berlyne, Borsa, Craw, Gelman & Mandell (1965) failed to find an effect of white noise (72-dB) on the retrieval of paired associates at a 24-h interval.

16.4.3. The effects of induced arousal on retention

Most of the studies reviewed thus far have examined the effects of arousal changes which occurred spontaneously or as a reaction to the stimulus items. A few experiments have explicitly manipulated arousal by methods external to the learning task itself.

Berlyne *et al.* (1965) found that continuous white noise interfered with paired-associate learning in an immediate retention test but led to less forgetting after 24 h. That is, the white noise group was poorer in immediate retention but superior in the delayed test. The authors argue that since white noise heightens arousal, their results are consistent with Kleinsmith & Kaplan's findings. However, a subsequent experiment (Berlyne, Borsa, Hamacher & Koenig, 1966, Experiment II) found no difference due to white noise in an immediate test. The authors also reported better 24-h recall when the noise was presented during presentation of the stimulus-response pair; white noise after the response made no significant difference—a result which conflicts with Levonian's (1966) report that post-decrements yielded reminiscence. A further experiment in the same vein was described by McLean (1969). He found an interaction between the presence *vs* the absence of white noise during acquisition, and immediate *vs* delayed testing in both incidental and intentional paired-associate learning. However, the interactions appear to be caused largely by the superior performance of the 'no noise-immediate' group—all other groups have similarly low scores.

Hamilton, Hockey & Quinn (1972) further investigated the effects of white noise on free recall. In their first experiment they found that paired-associates learned under noisy conditions were poorly recalled in an immediate test (thereby supporting Kleinsmith & Kaplan), but only if the order of presentation of the pairs was randomized from trial to trial. When recall order was identical to presentation order, Hamilton *et al.* found that white noise enhanced recall. This effect was also found in a second experiment which showed better first-list learning, and also greater disruptive effects of a second list, when the list was presented with noise and under fixed-order conditions. They suggest Kleinsmith & Kaplan's results may be limited to the situation in which a randomized recall order is employed.

What direct evidence is there that white noise leads to an increase in arousal? Also, if arousal is raised, is the increase to be thought of as a transient arousal increment or as a shift in tonic arousal level? Both Berlyne *et al.* (1966) and McLean (1969) tackle the first question and present evidence that skin resistance drops significantly after the presentation of white noise. However, Berlyne *et al.* comment that skin resistance dropped over a period of 15–20 min, thus the technique is apparently not a good one for manipulating arousal precisely in time. It is unclear whether such shifts in arousal should be classed as phasic increments or changes in tonic level. A second source of difficulty with the white noise technique is the possibility that the noise burst might serve as a distractor which diverts the subject's attention from the learning material. Concurrent monitoring of heart rate might reveal the noise level at which a defensive rejection of the environment was observed (indicated by heart rate acceleration according to Lacey, 1967). Again the implication is that the complexities of the situation might be teased apart by the use of several physiological indices.

Other methods of manipulating arousal have included delayed auditory feedback and the use of drugs. King & Wolf (1965) found poorer immediate recall of a story when part of the story was read aloud under delayed auditory feedback conditions. However, at 24 h the differences in recall between the experimental and control groups had decreased or disappeared. The authors concluded that the information got into the central nervous system during the learning trial, but it was available only for delayed use. Surprisingly few studies have been reported which manipulated arousal by the use of drugs. Batten (1967) injected subjects either with dexedrine (10 mg) or phenobarbitol (100 mg) and tested retention of a paired-associate list after various intervals from 2 min to 1 week. The pattern of retention resembled Kleinsmith & Kaplan's data, but the differences were not statistically reliable.

16.4.4 Individual differences

The complex picture of relations between arousal and memory is complicated still further when individual differences are considered. One line of research stems from Eysenck's (1967) notion that introverts behave as if they are chronically aroused, while extraverts are chronically underaroused. When this notion is grafted onto Kleinsmith and Kaplan's results, it follows that extraverts should be superior at short-term retention tasks but inferior to introverts in long-term retention. This prediction was tested by Howarth & Eysenck (1968). Groups of extreme introverts and extraverts were given a learning task and tested for retention at intervals ranging from an immediate test to 24 h. Their procedure differed radically from Kleinsmith & Kaplan's method in that the learning task was performed under intentional conditions, subjects had several learning trials until learning was perfect and the recall score tapped both item and associative information. Specifically, subjects were asked to recall the seven stimulus members of the paired-associate list, then generate and correctly pair the seven response members; stimuli and responses were nonsense syllables of medium association value. In the immediate test, despite the fact that all subjects had just completed one correct recall, extraverts recalled about 85 per cent introverts only 50 per cent. For the group that recalled after 25 h these figures were approximately reversed. As the authors point out, "these findings offer strong support to Eysenck's latest theoretical position' (p. 116). Personally, we find the proposition that groups of introverts could show 100 per cent performance at the end of learning, 50 per cent retention seconds later but 80 per cent retention after 24 h, little short of incredible. Since the task involves a strong free recall component, the results of Howarth & Eysenck are actually in opposition to results reported by Maltzman *et al.* (1966) and by Kaplan & Kaplan (1968a). McLaughlin & Eysenck (1967) reported the more plausible result that extraverts learned a paired-associates list faster than introverts. This result was also found by McLaughlin (1968) but he obtained no differences between introverts and extraverts in later retention tests.

Osborne (1972) isolated extreme high- and low-arousal groups on the basis of their salivation response to lemon juice. The argument is that greater salivation is associated with high arousal and introversion (Osborne, 1972, p. 588). Osborne used the Kleinsmith & Kaplan paradigm and found a significant interaction between arousal level and retention interval ($2\frac{1}{2}$ min *vs* 24 h). The high-arousal group recalled 0·7 associates (out of 6) at $2\frac{1}{2}$ min, and 1·3 after 24 h; the low-arousal group recalled 1·3 and 0·7 associates respectively. It is difficult to accept the generality of this result; for one thing the average recall level for extraverts and introverts combined was identical at $2\frac{1}{2}$ minutes and 24 h—the lack of forgetting is quite surprising. Secondly, since introverts increased their recall from 0·7 to 1·3 items over 24 h, and since Osborne's experiment involved incidental learning, the result implies that introverts should remember *all* perceived stimuli better after 24 h than after a few minutes; this seems unlikely, to say the least. One final study in this area was carried out by Berlyne & Carey (1968). After a 24-h retention interval they found that paired-associate recall was superior for extravert subjects. This result is apparently opposed to the studies from Eysenck's laboratory, but the authors suggest that the usual result may reverse if difficult material is used. It is of course perfectly feasible that complex interactions exist between stimulus conditions, stimulus material, personality type and retention interval. The best we can say at the moment is that a start has been made in unravelling the complexities.

16.4.5. Conclusions concerning arousal and memory

It is difficult to summarize this body of literature in a few words. One result upon which all investigators seem agreed is that higher arousal at presentation leads to better long-term retention. This is true for both item and associative information and for both arousal increments and shifts in arousal level. With regard to short-term retention, the situation is complex or confused or possibly both. For associative information (that is, when the main memory task is to remember what goes with what) the modal finding is that arousal increments lead to a decrease in retention (Kleinsmith & Kaplan, 1963, 1964; Berlyne et al., 1965; McLean, 1969; Butter, 1970), but that an increase in arousal level is associated with an inverted-U relationship to STM (Berry, 1962; Kleinsmith, Kaplan & Tarte, 1963). When the task is primarily to remember items, arousal increments have usually been found to lead to an increase in STM (Maltzman et al., 1966; Kaplan & Kaplan, 1968a; Sampson, 1969; Corteen, 1969) while heightened arousal level leads either to a decrease in STM (Howartin & Eysenck, 1968; Baddeley et al., 1970; Hockey et al., 1972) or to an inverted-U relationship (Blake, 1967; Levonian, 1968). Since most of the studies consider only two groups (high and low arousal) the greater generality of an inverted-U relationship remains largely untested. In fact Berlyne et al. (1966) suggested that 'it seems likely ... that there is an optimum degree of arousal for immediate recall, the location of the optimum ranging widely with circumstances' (p. 5). This may be true although the proposition would be difficult to pin down experimentally, and almost impossible to falsify.

The area is plagued with difficulties of definition and with difficulties of integrating diverse theoretical approaches. For example, the distinction between item and associative information seems important, yet several paradigms involve both types of operation. Similarly, does a burst of white noise give rise to an arousal increment or a change in baseline arousal? 'Short-term memory' as the term is used by arousal theorists (retention up to 10 min) differs radically from the concept used by most current memory theorists (retention up to 10 sec, say). It seems at least possible that some arousal effects operate at retrieval, yet is often difficult and sometimes impossible (in the personality studies, for example) to separate acquisition and retrieval effects. Although presumably any final theory of psychology will have to find a place for individual differences, at present such studies tend to interpolate a further layer of uncertainty between memory and arousal variables. For the moment, it may be more profitable to study the relations between individual differences in arousal and memory *directly*, rather than via intervening constructs such as introversion and extraversion.

The main result of interest in this area has been the Kleinsmith & Kaplan finding and we would like to conclude this section with a few comments on the effect. First, it seems to us perfectly plausible that higher arousal should be associated with better long-term remembering, but it is not necessary to postulate a 'consolidation' mechanism for the effect to be observed. More simply, an arresting, emotional or interesting stimulus will receive greater attention—it is well known that learning is positively related to the amount of attention or processing the item received (Waugh & Norman, 1965). The finding of an interaction between arousal and retention interval is perfectly plausible since it implies merely that high-interest items are forgotten less rapidly than items which received less attention. The same comment may be made about the finding that reminiscence items tend to be high-arousal and forgotten items to be low-arousal events. The finding which is really hard for a memory theorist to accept is the progressively better performance over-time for high-arousal items. One major source of scepticism is the biological implausibility of the effect—it would be of little comfort to an organism seized by a predator, to reflect that although it had forgotten about the predator's approach for the moment, it would have remembered a day later!

16.5. STUDIES OF COGNITIVE LOAD

Hess (1965) reported the intriguing finding that subjects exhibited pupillary dilation when presented with interesting or pleasurable visual stimuli. Also, Hess & Polt (1964) observed pupillary dilation during the solution of arithmetic problems followed by constriction of the pupil when the answer was reported. Since Hess & Polt found no constriction of the pupil while the solution was still retained by the subject, Kahneman & Beatty (1966) speculated that pupillary dilation might also provide an index of the amount held in STM. The hypothesis was confirmed: the amount of pupillary dilation was related to the number of items held in memory. Kahneman & Beatty also demonstrated a loading phase during which the pupil constricts with each item reported. Thus, pupil diameter provides a very sensitive measure of the momentary load on the subject as he performs the task. Other findings reported by Kahneman & Beatty include the observation that loading functions were steeper when more difficult material was used, and that when complex sentences were presented rapidly no dilations occurred during the listening phase, but a very large dilation occurred at the end of presentation. This last finding is particularly interesting as it implies that pupillary dilation is not affected by sensory or echoic storage, but only by active verbal processing or storage in primary memory. The result provides further justification for Neisser's (1967) suggestion that echoic memory does not require active processing—it is 'preattentive'.

Further results by Kahneman and his colleagues include the finding of pupillary dilation when material is retrieved from LTM (Beatty & Kahneman, 1966). Again the dilation effect appears to index the amount currently 'in mind'. It might be interesting to determine whether it is the amount retrieved or the difficulty of retrieval which is more closely related to the dilation observed. The amount of effort expended on the task has been explored by Kahneman & Peavler (1969). When incentives were provided, subjects showed better learning and greater pupillary dilation for highly rewarded items although, within an incentive condition, the amount of pupillary dilation to each item did not predict its later recall. Pupillary responses were greater during the retrieval phase than during the presentation phase, a finding which may either reflect greater effort or more anxiety (Kahneman & Peavler, 1969). A final result of interest is the observation that initial items in the learning list gave rise to the largest dilations and were also best remembered. This finding fits well with the suggestion that the primacy effect observed in both PA learning and free recall is due to greater effort or more attention being given to the first item in the list.

To the memory theorist one of the main uses of the pupillary dilation technique may be to provide some insights into the rehearsal process. The construct of rehearsal is universally invoked but poorly understood. Kahneman, Onuska & Wolman (1968) found differences in pupillary responses depending on how digit strings were presented and, presumably, rehearsed. In a later study, Kahneman & Wright (1971) hypothesized that total serial recall of a list of items should lead to more rehearsal than partial recall when only four of the 12 items were requested. The argument is plausible, since in the total recall condition the subject must remember the first items in order to start his recall, while in the partial recall condition the experimenter may request the first, middle or last block of four items. It was found that pupillary dilation was greater under the total recall condition, thereby supporting the prediction. The authors make the point that subjects' introspective reports of their rehearsal processes are very confused—the main contribution of the pupillary dilation technique may be the provision of an objective, observable method for the study of such covert processes as rehearsal. A recent study by Stanners & Headley (1972) found greater dilation when subjects were instructed to recall a group of digits as well as recognize whether a test digit had been a member of the group. This finding may contribute to evidence on different types of processing for recall and recognition, but it may also simply reflect more intensive rehearsal when the subject had both tasks to perform.

It has recently been established that imagery is one of the most powerful factors in human memory. As part of a larger body of work on this variable, Paivio (1971b) has reported a series of experiments exploring the physiological correlates of imagery. In general, pupillary dilation appears to be related to image formation. Pavio & Simpson (1966) showed that relative to concrete words, dilation was greater when subjects were instructed to form images from abstract words. Also, maximum pupillary dilation occurred longer after presentation of abstract words—4 sec as opposed to 3 sec for concrete words. These findings are in agreement with the notion that images are more difficult to form from abstract words; this in turn may be the reason for the superior retention of concrete words (Paivio, 1971a). Further work from Paivio's laboratory has shown that the concrete/abstract differences in pupillary response are attenuated when the subject does not indicate overtly (e.g., by pressing a key) that he has formed an image. Paivio (1971b) concludes that the pupillary response may be heightened by such factors as the necessity to make an explicit decision, and the mild anxiety associated with making a public response.

A further application of the pupillary dilation phenomenon has been to the study of sentence processing. Wright & Kahneman (1971) investigated the differences in pupillary response when subjects were asked either to repeat the sentence or to answer a question about it. Pupil dilations were larger for the repetition condition during presentation of the sentence and throughout a short retention interval. This finding probably reflects the greater effort necessary to keep all words in mind for verbatim repetition as opposed to the easier task of abstracting the meaning. During the response phase, pupil dilations were larger for the question group—it is possible that framing an answer to the question was more difficult than passive repetition of the words. In a third condition, the question was asked before sentence presentation, and in this case pupil dilations were lower during the retention and response phases—presumably because now only the answer to the question was retained. In a similar experiment, Stanners, Headley & Clark (1972) found that when short sentences were presented either for repetition or for the subjects to paraphrase, the decrease in pupil size following sentence presentation was more gradual in the 'paraphrase' condition. The authors suggest that more effort is required to put the sentence into the subjects' own words. It would be more satisfactory if both the Wright & Kahneman (1971) and the Stanners *et al.* (1972) studies had found greater pupillary dilation when 'deeper', more semantic structures were involved, but this was not so—Wright & Kahneman observed greater dilations when sentences were held for verbatim reproduction. Thus it may be tentatively concluded that it is the amount of cognitive effort which is indexed by the pupillary response and that this effort may be greater when surface structure is held or greater when deep structures are accessed, depending on the precise details of the task. It may be noted, finally, that although Kahneman & Beatty (1966) reported no dilation until the end of sentence presentation, both Wright & Kahneman (1971) and Stanners *et al.* (1972) reported increasing dilation during presentation. This discrepancy probably depends on such factors as the rate of presentation and complexity of the sentence—subjects must necessarily start processing slow or complex sentences during presentation.

A final example of how the pupillary dilation technique can be used to gain insight into memory processes is provided by Johnson (1971). He found that a signal to forget prior list items during presentation of a 5-word list gave rise to momentary dilation followed by steady constriction of the pupil. This finding ties in neatly with previous observations that 'forget signals' can reduce proactive interference from early list items.

What exactly do pupillary dilations indicate? The initial work of Hess suggested that interest or arousal was being measured but the later work of Kahneman and others suggests that congnitive load or effort may be a better description. It seems likely that both affective and cognitive load factors may be represented in the response. Both Bradshaw (1968) and Stanners *et al.* (1972) have reported a decrease in the magnitude of pupillary dilations over trials. It is possible to argue that the subject learns how to perform the task, thereby reducing cognitive load, but it seems at least as plausible that the subject's mild anxiety reduces throughout the experiment. Despite a number of ambiguities in the interpretation of the measure, the pupillary dilation response should prove a useful tool in the refining of such concepts as rehearsal, primary memory capacity, depth of processing and the transformations between surface structure and deep structure in sentence processing.

Although the pupillary dilation studies have made an interesting contribution, it seems unfortunate that only a few studies have been reported in which further autonomic indices of cognitive load have been recorded. Goldwater (1972) commented that 'there seem to be few if any rigorous studies in which the pupil and other autonomic responses are systematically correlated and compared as to their power to discriminate among different stimulus conditions'. One such study (Kahneman, Tursky, Shapiro & Crider, 1969) recorded heart rate and skin resistance in addition to pupil size during a digit transformation task; they found highly similar changes in all three autonomic systems. Since the pupillary response has been reported as one of the components of the orienting reflex (Goldwater, 1972), future work might profitably examine the relations between pupillary dilation on the one hand and such measures as heart rate deceleration and contingent negative variation on the other (Lacey & Lacey, 1970). Finally, heart rate variability has also been related to mental load (see Chapter 5).

16.6. EYE MOVEMENTS IN VISUAL AND VERBAL PROCESSING

One of the consequences of the information processing approach has been a more exploratory attitude to memory research and an interest in a wider range of materials and phenomena. For example, Paivio (1971a) has reported an extensive series of studies on the effects of imagery on memory and learning. An interesting question in this context is whether the physiological changes underlying image formation are similar to those observed in normal perception. Are eye movements necessary for imagery to occur? Some studies of dreaming suggested an affirmative answer to this question. Roffwarg, Dement, Muzio & Fisher (1962) found a good correspondence between the sleeper's recorded eye movements and his subsequent description of the dream. Also, Antrobus, Antrobus & Singer (1964) reported an increase in eye movements when subjects were asked to imagine active scenes such as a tennis match. However, further research has shown that while eye movements may sometimes accompany imagery and dreaming, they are not a necessary component of such mental states; eye movements may reflect the scanning of a generated image (Paivio, 1971b). More directly, Hale & Simpson (1971) found that the vividness of experienced imagery was not affected by asking subjects to make or refrain from making eye movements. Bower (1972) also reports a study in which subjects were asked either to scan their images or to maintain a steady gaze. The experiment found no recall differences between the two eye-movement conditions.

Consistent relationships between EEG indices and imagery have been equally hard to find. While early results appeared to show that habitual visualizers exhibited attenuated alpha rhythms relative to habitual verbalizers, these results have not been replicated by later investigators. The early results may have been due to the rather casual methodology employed (Paivio, 1971b).

In general, it seems that alpha blocking may indicate cognitive activities but (like pupillary dilation) the measure does not discriminate between different types of mental activity.

Eye movements have also been used by McCormack to check predictions from interference theory. In a series of studies (e.g., McCormack & Moore, 1969) he investigated the notion that paired-associate learning is a two-stage process—response consolidation, followed by the formation of the S–R bond. If this is so, subjects should pay more attention to the response terms in the early stages of learning, and switch to the stimulus terms as learning progresses. By monitoring eye movements McCormack has obtained support for the two-stage model. Further work has demonstrated how low meaningfulness the response terms can delay the crossover of attention to the stimulus (McCormack & Moore, 1969). Although not strictly memory research, some very interesting work has recently been initiated by Kinsbourne (1972). He has found that when right-handed subjects solve verbal problems, they usually turn their head and eyes to the right, whereas with numerical and spatial problems, subjects look up and left. Kinsbourne suggests that the differences in eye movements may reflect the cerebral lateralization of the mental activities. It would not be difficult to extend this technique to studies of visual and verbal memory—questions concerning the cerebral localization of postulated imagery and verbal codes (Paivio, 1971a) might receive an answer through this eye movement technique.

The work of Gould (e.g., Gould & Peeples, 1970) suggests that more eye-fixations occurred to visual targets than nontargets and that the duration of fixations was greater for targets. The eye-fixation pattern may be taken as an objective measure of the amount of attention paid to particular visual events. This work has been extended to memory in an impressive paper by Loftus (1972). In one experiment, pairs of pictures were presented for the subject to study; each picture was allocated a value corresponding to the payoff for later recognition. It was found that high value pictures received a greater number of fixations and were recognized better in the subsequent memory test. For a given number of fixations, however, variations in fixation time did not affect recognition. It is the number of different fixations, not the total fixation duration, which gives rise to good recognition performance. This conclusion was confirmed in further experiments. Loftus suggests that for visual processing, the number of fixations may be analogous to rehearsal of verbal material. In general, rehearsal may be of two types—simple repetition and further elaboration of the stimulus trace. Although Loftus' data do not distinguish between these possible functions of eye fixations he suggests that subsequent fixations may correspond to the abstraction of more visual features from the picture, thereby leading to a qualitatively richer memory trace. In fact, if the duration of fixations is analogous to simple repetition and the number of fixations is analogous to trace enrichment, Loftus' results are in accordance with Craik & Lockhart's (1972) suggestion that repetitions maintain but do not strengthen the memory trace; only further, elaborative processing leads to improved performance. The observations of Loftus also fit well with Gaarder's (1968) suggestion that visual information is transmitted to the brain in discrete packages linked to saccadic eye movements and to evoked cortical responses. Thus the study of eye-fixation patterns may yield important convergent evidence for both memory theory and psychophysiology.

16.7. SUBVOCAL SPEECH

One question raised by the behaviourist school in the 1920's and 30's was whether such mental activities as thinking and imagery were covert manifestations of more overt behaviours—subvocal speech and eye movements, for example. In its most extreme form the behaviourist view postulated that no mental activities could exist in the absence of their overt counterparts (see Boring, 1950, pp. 643–644.). While this point of view is generally discounted today, the involvement of motor-output processes in receptive and central functions is still considered probable; it is a central notion in the influential analysis-by-synthesis theory of speech perception (Neisser, 1967). Again, a literal peripheralist view is impossible to maintain—for example, we can still perceive speech when the laryngeal muscles are paralyzed (Neisser, 1967, p. 192)—but it may be important for theories of memory to specify the degree to which speech muscles are involved in subvocal speech and rehearsal. Electrophysiological techniques are an obvious aid to these investigations.

In a series of studies, Locke & Fehr have shown that the subvocal rehearsal used by subjects in verbal recall experiments is a form of speech. Their technique consisted of recording electromyographic (EMG) activity during the presentation and rehearsal of labial and nonlabial words. Greater EMG activity was observed for the former class of words, thereby indicating phonetic involvement (Locke & Fehr, 1970). In a later study (Locke & Fehr, 1972) they found greater phonetic activity when the stimulus mode differed from the response mode (visual presentation to spoken response or auditory presentation to written response). The authors suggest that covert phonetic activity may be maximized by the need to translate the code from stimulus to response.

Subvocal speech may typically accompany reading and memorizing, and indeed there is evidence that learning is accelerated when the subject is permitted to whisper or speak the material (Murray, 1965). However, subvocal speech is not necessary for comprehension of the material: Hardyck, Petrinovich & Ellsworth (1966) extinguished subvocal speech by a feedback technique in which an auditory cue sounded when the laryngeal EMG rose above the relaxation level. Subjects showed no decrease in the comprehension of light reading material. In a further study, Hardyck & Petrinovich (1970) found greater EMG changes when subjects read a difficult essay as opposed to easier material. The feedback-suppression technique was again used; subjects who suppressed their subvocal speech were no poorer than control subjects in a subsequent comprehension test for the easy material, but suppressed subjects were considerably poorer than controls on the difficult essay. The authors suggest that speech sounds and muscle movements are generated to the visual symbols when a child learns to read. These mediators are gradually eliminated, but reappear when a high degree of stimulus redundancy is required. The comprehension of difficult written material provides such a case. Thus, EMG information has been helpful in analysing cognitive processes. An interesting related question concerns the extent to which subvocal activity is necessary to maintain covert verbal rehearsal—are speech muscles necessarily involved in keeping verbal items in primary memory?

A recent study by Glassman (1972) provides a final example of how EMG techniques have been useful in analysing memory problems. Control (1964) showed that many errors in the short-term retention of verbal material were acoustic in nature; subsequent research has attempted to ascertain whether such errors were genuinely 'acoustic' or were more properly 'articulatory.' Glassman found poorer recall of word triads when the words were acoustically similar to each other, but also found no further decrement for subjects who had been trained to minimize their subvocal articulations. The number of 'acoustic errors' was greatly influenced by the minimizing manipulation however—minimizers made fewer such errors. This study provides further evidence that acoustic confusions are actually products of the articulatory system; also, since subjects who suppressed their subvocalizations were no poorer at recall, it suggests that primary memory storage is flexible—if one mode of storage is not available, subjects switch to an alternative mode.

16.8. THE EFFECTS OF SLEEP ON MEMORY AND LEARNING

Over the last 20 years, some reports have suggested the possibility of learning during sleep—this is an interesting and exciting possibility and obviously one in which psychophysiological indices could play an important part. However, later investigations have yielded the notion that learning takes place only to the extent that subjects awaken briefly during presentation of the materials. For example, Simon & Emmons (1956) used very precise EEG control and were unable to find any evidence for the learning of complex verbal material as long as the EEG pattern was representative of sleep. Similarly Koukkou & Lehmann (1968) presented sentences to subjects during Stage 2 and 3 sleep (relatively slow-wave, non-REM) and found that unless approximately 25 sec of EEG activation (indicative of wakening) followed stimulus presentation, the stimulus was not recalled later. They also found that better recall was associated with higher EEG frequencies during learning—a result in line with Thompson & Obrist's (1964) findings.

It seems that perception and memory are better if stimuli are presented during REM episodes, but it is possible that such enhancement is due to transient wakenings rather than to the REM state itself (Synder & Scott, 1972). Goodenough, Sapan, Cohen, Portnoff & Shapiro (1971) have proposed that the consolidation of memory traces is impaired during non-REM sleep. They cite such phenomena as the reduced likelihood of recalling a dream after the subject has returned to non-REM sleep—although this observation might be better described as forgetting caused by the loss of context from consciousness, in the same way as it may be more difficult to remember a point made in conversation once the topic has changed. In a series of studies, Goodenough *et al.* confirmed Koukkou & Lehmann's finding that, for subjects permitted to return to sleep immediately, memory was positively related to the time before falling asleep. The authors describe their findings in terms of the effects of arousal on consolidation.

Three final experiments are mentioned which contradict the idea that memory is impaired by non-REM sleep. Both Yaroush, Sullivan & Ekstrand (1971) and Hockey *et al.* (1972) found that retention was better during the first half of a night's sleep. In both studies, the learning material was presented and tested while the subject was awake. Since the first half of sleep is characterized by slow-wave non-REM sleep, it seems that non-REM sleep *favours* rather than impairs retention. An alternative explanation may be that the dreaming activities during the second half of sleep, acts as interference to disrupt the memory.

In a further well-controlled experiment from Ekstrand's laboratory, Barrett & Ekstrand (1972) controlled for possible time-of-day artefacts by testing three groups of subjects [first half of sleep (F); second half of sleep (S); and awake (A)] over the same retention interval 2.50 a.m.–6.50 a.m. They report a clear superiority in retention of a paired-associate list for the two sleep groups and also that group F was superior to group S. Monitoring of EEG, EOG and EMG was carried out; there were no differences between F and S subjects in proportions of stages I, II or III sleep, but F subjects spent much longer in stage IV sleep (29 per cent compared to 7 per cent) while S subjects spent longer in REM sleep (23 per cent compared to 11 per cent). This seems clear evidence that non-REM sleep is associated with less forgetting but it is still unclear whether stage IV sleep helps memory by facilitating consolidation or whether REM sleep disrupts memory—perhaps by acting as general interpolated interference. The work relating learning to sleep is interesting and full of potential, but obviously still in an early stage.

16.9. CONCLUSIONS

This review has concentrated on a few areas where the interaction between psychophysiology and memory appeared to be most interesting and fruitful. No attempt has been made to catalogue every experiment and no mention has been made of some complete areas of research. For example, work stemming from Sokolov's (1963) concepts of habituation, neural models and the orienting response has not been reviewed although these ideas may provide a further important area in which psychophysiologists and learning theorists can collaborate.

To what extent have psychophysiological techniques helped to unravel the complex problems of learning and memory? Although a promising start

412

has been made, it seems properly cautious to conclude that psychophysiological measures have not yet provided deep insights into learning processes. At the moment many indices yield information on the extent to which the subject is paying attention to the material he is memorizing, but few psychophysiological measures yield measures which relate to qualitatively different stages of learning and recall. Perhaps the most promising measure in this regard is the evoked cortical response. If Wilkinson & Lee's (1972) and Posner *et al.*'s (1973) tentative identification of ECR components with information processing stages can be validated, we shall at last be 'inside' cognitive processes rather than on the periphery.

The relative shortage of really good work linking psychophysiological research to human memory is not too surprising when the imposing technological demands of current psychophysiological research are considered. Apart from a good background in general physiology, it is necessary to be competent in electronics and computer techniques. Also, it is now obvious that a clear picture of neurophysiological functioning can only be obtained by considering several psychophysiological indices recorded concurrently— it is not sufficient to monitor cortical or autonomic activities independently. These technical difficulties are compounded by the rapid evolution of theoretical ideas in both psychophysiology and human memory research. A pious (if somewhat hackneyed) plea for interdisciplinary collaboration would seem to be in order.

It is interesting to note the extent to which the concepts of arousal and consolidation still dominate work on the psychophysiology of memory. It seems to us unfortunate that a number of studies we have reviewed have been conducted to confirm theoretical positons constructed from these very loosely formulated concepts. This precedence of theory over observation can very often lead to conflicting reports about empirical effects. Naturally enough, theorists are keen to document their ideas with evidence but if the evidence itself is disputed, the theory obviously has limited value. The literature relating memory and arousal provides an example of the difficulties and dangers related to this method of conducting science. In our view it is preferable to start with a number of robust phenomena and gradually evolve a theoretical description which fits the agreed empirical facts. The work on the pupillary response has proceeded in this direction and has generated a less contentious literature.

Sermonizing aside, although the gap between neurophysiology and behavioural studies of memory is still immense, a start has been made to connect the two areas. Psychophysiological observations form the obvious materials from which the bridge must be constructed.

16.10. ACKNOWLEDGMENTS

We are grateful to a number of our colleagues at Toronto and at neighbouring universities for providing materials and suggestions which proved most helpful in writing this chapter. We are especially grateful to Bill Glassman, Morris Moscovitch and Karalyn Patterson for their extremely useful comments on an earlier draft.

16.11. REFERENCES

Antrobus, J. S., Antrobus, J. S. & Singer, J. L. Eye movements accompanying daydreaming, visual imagery, and thought suppression. *Journal of Abnormal and Social Psychology*, 1964, **69**, 244–252.

Atkinson, R. C. & Shiffrin, R. M. Human memory: A proposed system and its control processes. In K.W. Spence & J. T. Spence (Eds), *The psychology of learning and motivation*, Vol. 2. New York: Academic Press, 1968.

Baddeley, A. D., Hatter, J. E., Scott, D. & Snashall, A. Memory and time of day. *Quarterly Journal of Experimental Psychology*, 1970, **22**, 605–609.

Bagshaw, M. H., Kimble, D. P. & Pribram, K. H. The GSR of monkeys during orientation and habituation and after ablation of the amygdala, hippocampus, and inferotemporal cortex. *Neuropsychologia*, 1965, **3**, 111–119.

Barrett, T. R. & Ekstrand, B. R. Effect of sleep on memory. III. Controlling for time-of-day effects. *Journal of Experimental Psychology*, 1972, **96**, 321–327.

Batten, D. E. Recall of paired-associates as a function of arousal and recall interval. *Perceptual and Motor Skills*, 1967, **24**, 1055–1058.

Beatty, J. & Kahneman, D. Pupillary changes in two memory tasks. *Psychonomic Science*, 1966, **5**, 371–372.

Berlyne, D. E., Borsa, D. M., Craw, M. A., Gelman, R. S. & Mandell, E. E. Effects of stimulus complexity and induced arousal on P-A learning. *Journal of Verbal Learning and Verbal Behaviour*, 1965, **4**, 291–299.

Berlyne, D. E., Borsa, D. M., Hamacher, J. H. & Koenig, I. D. V. Paired-associate learning and the timing of arousal. *Journal of Experimental Psychology*, 1966, **72**, 1–6.

Berlyne, D. E. & Carey, S. T. Incidental learning and the timing of arousal. *Psychonomic Science*, 1968, **13**, 103–104.

Berry, R. N. Skin conductance levels and verbal recall. *Journal of Experimental Psychology*, 1962, **63**, 275–277.

Berry, R. N. & Davis, R. C. The somatic background of rote learning. *Journal of Experimental Psychology*, 1960, **59**, 27–34.

Blake, M. J. F. Time of day effects on performance in a range of tasks. *Psychonomic Science*, 1967, **9**, 349–350.

Boring, E. G. *A history of experimental psychology*. New York: Appleton–Century–Crofts, 1950.

Bower, G. H. Comments on Walker's paper. In D. P. Kimble (Ed), *The organization of recall*. New York: New York Academy of Sciences, 1967, pp. 210–214.

Bower, G. H. Mental imagery and associative learning. In L. W. Gregg (Ed), *Cognition in learning and memory*. New York: Wiley, 1972.

Bradshaw, J. L. Load and pupillary changes in continuous processing tasks. *British Journal of Psychology*, 1968, **59**, 265–271.

Broadbent, D. E. *Perception and communication*. London: Pergamon Press, 1958.

Brown, C. H. The relation of magnitude of GSRs and resistance levels to the rate of learning. *Journal of Experimental Psychology*, 1937, **20**, 262–278.

Butter, M. J. Differential recall of paired-associates as a function of arousal and concreteness-imagery levels. *Journal of Experimental Psychology*, 1970, **84**, 252–256.

Conrad, R. Acoustic confusions in immediate memory. *British Journal of Psychology*, 1964, **55**, 75–84.

Corteen, R. S. Skin conductance changes and word recall. *British Journal of Psychology*, 1969, **60**, 81–84.

Craik, F. I. M. The fate of primary memory items in free recall. *Journal of Verbal Learning and Verbal Behaviour*, 1970, **9**, 143–148.

Craik, F. I. M. & Lockhart, R. S. Levels of processing: A framework for memory research. *Journal of Verbal Learning and Verbal Behaviour*, 1972, **11**, 671–684.

Elliott, R. The significance of heart rate for behaviour: A critique of Lacey's hypothesis. *Journal of Personality and Social Psychology*, 1972, **22**, 398–409.

Eysenck, H. J. *The biological basis of personality*. Springfield: Thomas, 1967.

Furth, H. G. & Terry, R. A. Autonomic responses and serial learning. *Journal of Comparative and Physiological Psychology*, 1961, **54**, 139–142.

Gaarder, K. Interpretive study of evoked responses elicited by gross saccadic eye movements. *Perceptual and Motor Skills*, 1968, **27**, 683–703.

Glanzer, M. Storage mechanisms in recall. In G. H. Bower (Ed.), *The psychology of learning and motivation*, Vol. 5. New York: Academic Press, 1972.

Glassman, W. E. Subvocal activity and acoustic confusion in short-term memory. *Journal of Experimental Psychology*, 1972, **96**, 164–169.

Goldwater, B. C. Psychological significance of pupillary movements. *Psychological Bulletin*, 1972, **77**, 340–355.

Goodenough, D. R., Sapan, J., Cohen, H., Portnoff, G. & Shapiro, A. Some experiments concerning the effects of sleep on memory. *Psychophysiology*, 1971, **8**, 749–762.

Gould, J. D. & Peeples, D. R. Eye movements during visual search and discrimination of meaningless, symbol and object patterns. *Journal of Experimental Psychology*, 1970, **85**, 51–55.

Greenberg, H. J. & Graham, J. T. Electroencephalographic changes during learning of speech and nonspeech stimuli. *Journal of Verbal Learning and Verbal Behavior*, 1970, **9**, 274–281.

Hale, S. M. & Simpson, H. M. Effects of eye movements on the rate of discovery and the vividness of visual images. *Perception and Psychophysics*, 1971, **9**, 242–246.

Hamilton, P., Hockey, G. R. J. & Quinn, J. G. Information selection, arousal and memory. *British Journal of Psychology*, 1972, **63**, 181–189.

Hardyck, C. D. & Petrinovich, L. F. Subvocal speech and comprehension level as a function of the difficulty level of reading material. *Journal of Verbal Learning and Verbal Behavior*, 1970, **9**, 647–652.

Hardyck, C. D., Petrinovich, L. F. & Ellsworth, D. W. Feedback on speech muscle activity during silent reading: Rapid extinction. *Science*, 1966, **154**, 1467–1468.

Hess, E. H. Attitude and pupil size. *Scientific American*, 1965, **212**, 46–54.

Hess E. H. & Polt, J. M. Pupil size in relation to mental activity during simple problem-solving. *Science*, 1964, **143**, 1190–1192.

Hockey, G. R. J., Davies, S. & Gray, M. M. Forgetting as a function of sleep at different times of day. *Quarterly Journal of Experimental Psychology*, 1972, **24**, 386–393.

Howarth, E. & Eysenck, H. J. Extraversion, arousal, and paired-associate recall. *Journal of Experimental Research in Personality*, 1968, **3**, 114–116.

John, E. R. *Mechanisms of memory*. New York: Academic Press, 1967.

John, E. R. Switchboard versus statistical theories of learning and memory. *Science*, 1972, **177**, 850–864.

Johnson, D. A. Pupillary responses during a short-term memory task: cognitive processing, arousal, or both? *Journal of Experimental Psychology*, 1971, **90**, 311–318.

Kahneman, D. & Beatty, J. Pupil diameter and load on memory. *Science*, 1966, **154**, 1583–1585.

Kahneman, D., Onuska, L. & Wolman, R. Effects of grouping on the pupillary response in a short-term memory task. *Quarterly Journal of Experimental Psychology*, 1968, **20**, 309–311.

Kahneman, D. & Peavler, W. Incentive effects and pupillary changes in association learning. *Journal of Experimental Psychology*, 1969, **79**, 312–318.

Kahneman, D., Tursky, B., Shapiro, D. & Crider, A. Pupillary, heart rate, and skin resistance changes during a mental task. *Journal of Experimental Psychology*, 1969, **79**, 164–167.

Kahneman, D. & Wright, P. Changes of pupil size and rehearsal strategies in a short-term memory task. *Quarterly Journal of Experimental Psychology*, 1971, **23**, 187–196.

Kaplan, S. & Laplan, R. Arousal and memory: A comment. *Psychonomic Science*, 1968, **10**, 291–292(a).

Kaplan, S. & Kaplan, R. Human memory and consolidation. Unpublished progress report on Grant MH 111599, 1968(b).

Kaplan, S. & Kaplan, R. The interaction of arousal and retention interval: Within-subject versus normative GSR. *Psychonomic Science*, 1970, **19**, 115–117.

Kaplan, S., Kaplan, R. & Sampson, J. R. Encoding and arousal factors in free recall of verbal and visual material. *Psychonomic Science*, 1968, **12**, 73–74.

King, D. J. & Wolf, S. The influence of delayed auditory feedback on immediate and delayed memory. *Journal of Psychology*, 1965, **59**, 131–139.

Kinsbourne, M. Eye and head turning indicates cerebral lateralization. *Science*, 1972, **176**, 539–541.

Kintsch, W. Habituation of the GSR component of the orienting reflex during paired-associate learning before and after learning has taken place. *Journal of Mathematical Psychology*, 1965, **2**, 330–341.

Kintsch, W. *Learning, memory and conceptual processes.* New York: Wiley, 1969.

Kleinsmith, L. J. & Kaplan, S. Paired-associate learning as a function of arousal and interpolated activity. *Journal of Experimental Psychology*, 1963, **65**, 190–193.

Kleinsmith, L. J. & Kaplan, S. Interaction of arousal and recall interval in nonsense syllable paired-associate learning. *Journal of Experimental Psychology*, 1964, **67**, 124–126.

Kleinsmith, L. J., Kaplan, S. & Tarte, R. D. The relationship of arousal to short- and long-term verbal recall. *Canadian Journal of Psychology*, 1963, **17**, 393–397.

Koukkou, M. & Lehmann, D. EEG and memory storage in sleep experiments with humans. *Electroencephalography and Clinical Neurophysiology*, 1968, **25**, 455–462.

Lacey, J. I. Somatic response patterning and stress: Some revisions of activation theory. In M. M. Appley and R. Trumbull (Eds), *Psychological stress.* New York: Appleton-Century–Crofts, 1967.

Lacey, J. I. & Lacey, B. C. Some autonomic-central nervous system interrelationships. In P. Black (Ed), *Physiological correlates of emotion.* New York: Academic Press, 1970.

Levonian, E. Attention and consolidation as factors in retention. *Psychonomic Science*, 1966, **6**, 275–276.

Levonian. E. Retention of information in relation to arousal during continuously-presented material. *American Educational Research Journal*, 1967, **4**, 103–116.

Levonian, E. Short-term retention in relation to arousal. *Psychophysiology*, 1968, **4**, 284–293.

Locke, J. L. & Fehr, F. S. Subvocal rehearsal as a form of speech. *Journal of Verbal Learning and Verbal Behavior*, 1970, **9**, 495–498.

Locke, J. L. & Fehr, F. S. Subvocalization of heard or seen words prior to spoken or written recall. *American Journal of Psychology*, 1972, **85**, 63–68.

Loftus, G. R. Eye fixations and recognition memory for pictures. *Cognitive Psychology*, 1972, **3**, 525–551.

Mackworth, J. F. *Vigilance and habituation.* Harmondsworth: Penguin Books, 1969.

Madigan, S. A. & McCabe, L. Perfect recall and total forgetting: A problem for models of short-term memory. *Journal of Verbal Learning and Verbal Behaviour*, 1971, **10**, 101–106.

Maltzman, I., Kantor, W. & Langdon, B. Immediate and delayed retention, arousal and defensive reflexes. *Psychonomic Science*, 1966, **6**, 445–446.

Mandler, G. & Mandler, J. M. Associative behaviour and somatic response. *Canadian Journal of Psychology*, 1962, **16**, 331–343.

416

McCormack, P. D. & Moore, T. E. Monitoring eye movements during the learning of low-high and high-low meaningfulness paired-associate lists. *Journal of Experimental Psychology*, 1969, **79**, 18–21.

McLaughlin, R. J. Retention in paired-associate learning related to extroversion and neuroticism. *Psychonomic Science*, 1968, **13**, 333–334.

McLaughlin, R. J. & Eysenck, H. J. Extraversion, neuroticism, and paired-associate learning. *Journal of Experimental Research in Personality*, 1967, **2**, 128–132.

McLean, P. D. Induced arousal and time of recall as determinants of paired-associate recall. *British Journal of Psychology*, 1969, **60**, 57–62.

Murdock, B. B., Jr. Recent developments in short-term memory. *British Journal of Psychology*, 1967, **58**, 421–433.

Murdock, B. B., Jr. *Human memory: theory and data*. Potomac, Md.: Lawrence Erlbaum Associates, 1974.

Murray, D. L. Vocalization-at-presentation and immediate recall, with varying presentation rates. *Quarterly Journal of Experimental Psychology*, 1965, **17**, 47–56.

Neisser, U. *Cognitive Psychology*. New York: Appleton–Century–Crofts, 1967,

Obrist, P. A. Some autonomic correlates of serial learning. *Journal of Verbal Learning and Verbal Behaviour*, 1962, **1**, 100–104.

Osborne, J. W. Short- and long-term memory as a function of individual differences in arousal. *Perceptual and Motor Skills*, 1972, **34**, 587–593.

Paivio, A. *Imagery and verbal processes*, New York: Holt, Rinehart & Winston, 1971(a).

Paivio, A. Psychophysiological correlates of imagery. Department of Psychology, University of Western Ontario, Research Bulletin No. 215, 1971(b).

Paivio, A. & Simpson, H. The effect of word abstractness and pleasantness on pupil size during an imagery task. *Psychonomic Science*, 1966, **5**, 55–56.

Posner, M. I., Klein, R. M., Summers, J. & Buggie, S. On the selection of signals. *Memory and Cognition*, 1973, **1**, 2–12.

Roffwarg, H. P., Dement, W. C., Muzio, J. N. & Fisher, C. Dream imagery: Relationship to rapid eye movements of sleep. *Archives of General Psychiatry*, 1962, **7**, 235–258.

Sampson, J. R. Further study of encoding and arousal factors in free recall of verbal and visual material. *Psychonomic Science*, 1969, **16**, 221–222.

Shucard, D. W. & Horn, J. L. Evoked cortical potentials and measurement of human abilities. *Journal of Comparative and Physiological Psychology*, 1972, **78**, 59–68.

Simon, C. W. & Emmons, W. H. Responses to material presented during various levels of sleep. *Journal of Experimental Psychology*, 1956, **51**, 89–97.

Snyder, F. & Scott, J. The psychophysiology of sleep. In N. S. Greenfield and R. A. Sternbach (Eds), *Handbook of Psychophysiology*. New York: Holt, Rinehart & Winston, 1972.

Sokolov, E. N. *Perception and the conditioned reflex*. New York: Macmillan, 1963.

Spence, D. P., Lugo, M. & Youdin, R. Cardiac change as a function of attention to and awareness of, continuous verbal text. *Science*, 1972, **176**, 1344–1346.

Stanners, R. F. & Headley, D. B. Pupil size and instructional set in recognition and recall. *Psychophysiology*, 1972, **9**, 505–511.

Stanners, R. F., Headley, D. B. & Clark, W. R. The pupillary response to sentences: Influences of listening set and deep structure. *Journal of Verbal Learning and Verbal Behaviour*, 1972, **11**, 257–263.

Sternberg, S. Memory scanning: Mental processes revealed by reaction-time experiments. *American Scientist*, 1969, **57**, 421–457.

Surwillo, W. W. Frequency of the EEG during acquisition in short-term memory. *Psychophysiology*, 1971, **8**, 588–593.

Thompson, L. W. & Obrist, W. D. EEG correlates of verbal learning and overlearning. *Electroencephalography and Clinical Neurophysiology*, 1964, **16**, 332–342.

Thompson, L. W. & Thompson, V. D. Comparison of EEG changes in learning and over-learning of nonsense syllables. *Psychological Reports*, 1965, **16**, 339–344.

Thompson, L. W. & Wilson, S. Electrocortical reactivity and learning in the elderly. *Journal of Gerontology*, 1966, **21**, 45–51.

Tulving, E. & Madigan, S. A. Memory and verbal learning. *Annual Review of Psychology*, 1970, **21**, 437–484.

Uehling, B. S. & Sprinkle, R. Recall of a serial list as a function of arousal and retention interval. *Journal of Experimental Psychology*, 1968, **78**, 103–106.

Venables, P. H. Input regulation and psychopathology. In M. Hammer, K. Salzinger, & S. Sutton (Eds) *Psychopathology*. New York: Wiley, 1973.

Walker, E. L. Action decrement and its relation to learning. *Psychological Review*, 1958, **65**, 129–142.

Walker, E. L. & Tarte, R. D. Memory storage as a function of arousal and time with homogeneous and heterogeneous lists. *Journal of Verbal Learning and Verbal Behaviour*, 1963, **2**, 113–119.

Waugh, N. C. & Norman, D. A. Primary memory. *Psychological Review*, 1965, **72**, 89–104.

Wilkinson, R. T. & Lee, M. V. Auditory evoked potentials and selective attention. *Electroencephalography and Clinical Neurophysiology*, 1972, **33**, 411–418.

Wright, P. & Kahneman, D. Evidence of alternative strategies of sentence retention. *Quarterly Journal of Experimental Psychology*, 1971, **23**, 197–213.

Yaroush, R., Sullivan, M. J. & Ekstrand, B. R. Effects of sleep on memory. II. Differential effect of the first and second half of the night. *Journal of Experimental Psychology*, 1971, **88**, 361–366.

Chapter 17

Progress in Psychophysiology: Some Applications in a Field of Abnormal Psychology

PETER H. VENABLES

Department of Psychology,
University of York,
Heslington, York YO1 5DD,
England

17.1. INTRODUCTION

It was stated in the preface that it was the aim of the editors of this book to compile a set of chapters which would give to psychologists in general a flavour of the work being carried out in psychophysiology, and to present particularly in the chapters in this final section, examples of ways in which workers in other areas might benefit from the integration of psychophysiological facts and ways of thinking with those which are the current substance of their own work.

It is perhaps worthwhile to examine in this final chapter some of the features of the sub-discipline of psychophysiology and to present a point of view, however idiosyncratic, of some of the characteristics of its practitioners. Later as an example, and for purposes of illustration, material will be presented which arises in the course of carrying out work in the area of the 'high risk' studies which were mentioned in the final section of Chapter 12. From consideration of this material ideas have arisen which relate psychophysiology to physiological psychology, behaviour genetics, psychometrics etc., and these illustrate further ways in which psychophysiology may be related to other aspects of general psychological knowledge.

17.2. PSYCHOPHYSIOLOGY

It is now 10 years since the most formal type of recognition of the sub-discipline was made by the publication of the journal, *Psychophysiology*. This did more than provide a unified forum where workers in this field might publish their material and hope to see a concentration of the material in which they were primarily interested; it also set a seal on an area of research with some 70 years of background, but a background which was not originally viewed as particularly separate from the rest of work in psychology. Thus, for example, some of the earliest work in one of the presently most fashionable areas of psychophysiology, the perceptual and attentional concomitants of heart rate deceleration, had its orgins in Wundt's laboratory, that traditional heartland of experimental psychology. Ax, by his first editorial (1964), and Stern (1964) by his definitional paper, outlined the differences between psychophysiology and physiological psychology. In staking out its territory in this way the sub-discipline gained strength to grow in power and status, but unfortunately there was a sense in which, by concentrating on what it could do uniquely well, it has built up a set of special ideas and forms of communication that have in a way tended to cut it off from other psychologists. With equal force it could of course be said that each sectional interest within psychology has tended to concentrate on communication among its own adherents and with consequent loss of interchange between areas.

It is hoped, therefore, that this book, which maybe will be read by psychologists in general and not solely by psychophysiologists, will have gone some way to break down barriers.

17.3. THE CHARACTERISTICS OF PSYCHOPHYSIOLOGISTS

It can probably be held that among psychophysiologists there is a belief that 'the proper study of mankind is man' and that ultimately the understanding of human behaviour cannot be achieved through work on animals but should be concerned with the physiology and psychology of the 'intact human organism'. The second characteristic of the psychophysiologist would appear to be an inability to stop at an overt behavioural level of explanation in attempts to understand behaviour. Thus, the psychophysiologist is at least a partial reductionist. Thirdly, although perhaps less obviously, the psychophysiologist is implicitly or explicitly concerned with individual differences. An example may clarify these last two points. The more behaviourally oriented psychologist, studying, for example, the effects of noise on performance, presents a noise during a task, and shows that in comparison with a control trial in quite, there is a change in performance. This is all right if he leaves it there. If, however, he then hypothesizes that this change is brought about by a change in 'arousal' this tends to bring about an orienting—or even a defensive—response in the psychophysiologist. The psychophysiologist would wish to know how the behavioural psychologist can presume there has been a change in 'arousal' and that this change has been the same in all experimental subjects other than as a derivation from the fact that there has been a change in performance.

The use of the term 'arousal' would also probably be questioned by many psychophysiologists. While it is possible that arousal may have been a useful explanatory concept in the same way perhaps that intelligence is a useful concept, the fact that measures of change of physiological indices which might purport to measure 'arousal' correlate less well together than those which purport to tap the concept 'intelligence' places the two concepts on a rather different footing. The psychophysiologist, in 1975, would thus probably not allow himself the luxury of such an easily intellectually-manipulable concept as arousal but would recognize that the indices which in the past have been said to measure it have particular biological functions of their own which need to be fully understood before they can be related to more behavioural concepts.

Within psychophysiology there are, of course, many points of view. It is possible at one end of a sort of continuum merely to use psychophysiological techniques and to view, for instance, the skin conductance response as no different from any other single piece of behaviour save that it is 'covert' until the polygraph makes it 'overt'. It is, of course, 'covert' as far as the ordinary observer is concerned and is thus not directly, potentially, productive of behaviour in others as is a skeletal movement or a speech act. From a transactional point of view at this level the SCR is thus asymmetrical.

If, on the other hand, a point of view is taken that the SCR, as part, perhaps, of the totality of the orienting response, is at one level an index of central processes, for instance, following Koepke & Pribram (1966) an index of registration of an external stimulus in a Sokolovian (1963) neural model, or at another is a direct indication of a part of orientation concerned with movement and manipulation (Edelberg, 1973a), then clearly the level of explanation has moved another discrete step. The contrast between a behavioural and a biological approach is nicely made by Obrist, Sutterer & Howard (1972) in their discussion of the function of cardiac change.

17.4. PSYCHOPHYSIOLOGY AND PHYSIOLOGICAL PSYCHOLOGY

It is perhaps the relational, indicative aspect of psychophysiological research which makes it somewhat unacceptable to some more hard-core experimental psychologists (apologies are due for these undefined sub-classifications of groups of psychologists). At its worst, a claim that psychophysiologists indulge in 'neurophysiologizing' is on occasion justified. It is really no more permissible to say that, for instance, a skin conductance response represents the activity of the reticular formation than a change in 'arousal' is shown by a change in performance. There exists a continuous danger of an unwarranted interchange between the function of a 'real' aspect of brain structure and an hypothetical construct given, for convenience, the same name. It would seem to be the case that physiological psychologists (to be discriminated from psychophysiologists by the order of their independent and dependent variables) are more acceptably included in the experimental tradition. This is undoubtedly because their scientific method of clearly manipulating a variable (e.g., ablating part of the cortex), examining a piece of behaviour, and analysing the results (e.g., by analysis of variance) is entirely acceptable.

However, (a) this can only be done using animals as subjects, and (b) it tends to assume that ablating a piece of the brain (or stimulating it) is clearly manipulating a single variable. The multiple consequences and non-biological nature of ablation or stimulation would seem to place physiological psychology in just as an uncertain and dubious a position as psychophysiology.

However, the purpose here is not to make scoring points and suggest that one aspect of experimental research with psychology and physiology in the title is right and the other with its terms the other way round is wrong. It is more important to recognize that each has its strengths and weaknesses and more will be gained by working in conjunction than has tended to be the case so far. No branch of psychology can do more than make tentative approaches to the solution of problems, but the chances of convergence by iteration are increased if every opportunity to incorporate data from all sources is seized.

The remainder of the chapter is an attempt to set this theoretical discussion in the context of a topic which has general psychological importance but where a psychophysiological measure of special interest is very specific and with an underlying mechanism or mechanisms which are largely not understood. In contrast to the other three chapters in this final section, the attempt is thus made to see how far by taking a rather particular point as a springboard it may be used as an illustration of one example of psychophysiological thinking and characteristic methodology. Also unlike the other three chapters the material presented starts from work in the area of abnormal psychology.

17.5. SOME EXAMPLES OF GROWING POINTS AND AREAS OF CO-OPERATION RESULTING FROM 'HIGH RISK' RESEARCH

17.5.1. Introduction

In Section 4 of Chapter 12 work on high risk samples was introduced. One of the findings of Mednick & Schulsinger's work in Copenhagen on children of schizophrenic mothers (Mednick & Schulsinger, 1968; Mednick, 1970) was that of the measurements taken in the pre-morbid state, one that was predictive of later breakdown was electrodermal activity, and within that classification the recovery limb of the skin conductance response appeared to be of particular importance. Those children of schizophrenic mothers who suffered later breakdown exhibited shorter half-times of recovery of the SCR than those who did not. Short half-recovery times ($t/2$) of the SCR have also been shown to be characteristic of adult schizophrenics (Ax & Bamford, 1970; Gruzelier & Venables, 1972, 1973).

On the other hand, a long $t/2$ appears to be associated with criminal and psychopathic types of behaviour. Of Mednick & Schulsinger's original 1962 normal control sample of 104 children, seven subsequently exhibited recidivistic criminality. These seven had longer half-recovery times than seven normal subjects with whom they were closely matched (Mednick & Loeb, unpublished). Similar data are reported by Siddle, Nicol & Foggitt in a reanalysis (unpublished) of their 1973 data. These authors had reported on the skin conductance orienting responses of three groups of Borstal boys showing three levels of antisocial behaviour, in the reanalysis of the data in which half-recovery times were measured, the group with the highest level of antisocial behaviour exhibited the longest $t/2$.

These findings of two types of clinical abnormality associated with abnormally fast or abnormally slow recovery of the skin conductance response are repeated in the same context in a preliminary report (unpublished) of a re-analysis of Mednick & Schulsinger's data collected in 1962 resulting from a complete psychiatric re-assesssment of the original subjects in 1972–9173. If from the original 207 subjects at high risk because of the schizophrenic status of their mothers, those with diagnoses of 'schizoid and paranoid personalities', 'borderline schizophrenia' and 'schizophrenia', are selected a group of 85 results. Of these, 35 had a rating of moderately severe, severe, or extremely severe, level of illness. This group of 35 was divided into those with criminality' and those 'without criminality'. In those 'with criminality' nine had criminal records and six without criminal records had criminal parents. Of the 15 'with criminality' 12 have a slower rate of recovery (i.e., a longer $t/2$) than the median of the high risk group, of the 20 'without criminality' 16 have a faster rate of recovery than the median.

This very preliminary presentation of yet unpublished data and that provided earlier suggests the value of analysing in greater detail what the recovery limb of the skin conductance response represents and what its mechanism might be.

In discussing this topic it is hoped that some of the ways in which this psycho-physiological data interact with other aspects of psychology may be thrown into relief and thus illuminate some of the more theoretical discussion in the first section of the chapter. It is hoped also that the work which seems to arise from an analysis of the mechanism of the SCR recovery limb will point to some further areas in which advances in psychophysiological techniques may be made.

17.5.2. The problems

Given that an empirical finding has been established the problems which appear to be involved in making progress in understanding it may be drawn up in a preliminary and by no means exhaustive list.

(a) What is the optimal method of measuring rate or speed of recovery so that the method of measurement does not itself introduce error?
(b) How reliable is the measure and how far does it remain characteristic of a person?
(c) How soon in his life is it characteristic of a person, assuming that it is a fairly stable individual characteristic?
(d) How far, and in what ways, is it modified by the situation in which it is measured?
(e) What are its peripheral physiological mechanisms?
(f) What are its hormonal concomitants?
(g) What are its central physiological mechanisms?
(h) What is its central conceptual basis?
(i) What are its behavioural concomitants?
(j) What are its psychophysiological concomitants?
(k) Is it inherited?

This list clearly extends what is the investigation of a small specific area of psychophysiology into a much more extensive field, but one which needs the co-operation of ranges of expertise outside psychophysiology for the solution. In so far as the elucidation of the mechanism of the recovery of the SCR requires an examination of other ares of psychophysiology the problem immediately becomes widened again and illustrative material will not, therefore, necessarily be confined to this small aspect of the area.

17.5.3. Measurement of the recovery limb of the skin conductance response

17.5.3.1. Choice of metric

The recovery limb was first described by Darrow in 1932, and he concluded in 1937 that it was exponential in form. The exponential form of the recovery limb was generally supported by the work of Edelberg (1970). If the supposition of exponentiality is correct then recovery rate is theoretically independent of the amplitude of the response peak from which it starts. The time constant t_c) of the decay of an exponential function is that time which is taken by that function to decay to 37 per cent of its peak value. The reciprocal of the time constant is called the rate constant (r_c). Rather than measuring the time taken for the conductance to decay to 37 per cent of its original value it is more convenient to measure the time taken to decay to half peak value, i.e. the half recovery time $(t/2) = 0.7\ t_c$. Use of r_c, t_c or $t/2$ gives a measure which is thus independent of amplitude, provided that mathematically the recovery function remains exponential. In discussing a curve matching technique for measuring t_c Edelberg (1970) says, 'The curve matching method is somewhat ... difficult, *it soon becomes clear that many* (recovery limbs) *depart from the exponential shape and matching is ambiguous*' (reviewers italics). Independence of recovery from amplitude cannot, therefore, it would seem, be measured by the choice of a method on mathematical grounds if the mathematical assumptions cannot be upheld. However, as long as there is approximation to exponentiality, then the convenient half-time $t/2$ method may be the best to use.

Empirical data, however, show that $t/2$ is correlated to SCR amplitude—and in a variety of ways. Edelberg (1970) presents within subjects amplitude—$t/2$ correlations of 0.21, -0.20, 0.28, 0.62, 0.74 and 0.19 for six subjects. Independence of the two measures is thus shown differently by different subjects, it is also shown differently by different groups. Gruzelier & Venables' (1972) data provides correlations between amplitude and $t/2$ for non-patients of -0.08 and for schizophrenic patients of -0.64. Lockhart (1972) shows a similar low amplitude $t/2$ correlation of -0.06 for normal subjects, in responses to standard shocks. However, in 'disparity' conditions when a UCS is presented after a CS^- the correlation between amplitude and $t/2$ was $+0.44$.

The overall $t/2$–amplitude correlation found in Mednick's data collected in 1962 was -0.45 and this led him to reconsider the form of measurement and to employ what is intuitively a more independent measure but one which mathematically should be related to amplitude. Mednick's measure is half recovery *rate* that is virtually the linear slope of recovery up to half recovery time and measured in micromhos per second. In the 1962 sample this slope measure was more independent of amplitude than $t/2$ having a correlation with amplitude of only -0.11. While mathematical considerations suggest that there should be a relationship of a particular kind between half-recovery time and amplitude of response, these considerations cannot necessarily have force in the relation between $t/2$ and other aspects of electrodermal activity. Data suggests (Darrow, 1932, 1964) Patterson (personal communication) that $t/2$ is related to skin conductance level (SCL), faster $t/2$ values being found in conjunction with higher SCLs. Bundy (1973) provides data which suggest that faster recovery times occur when the response on which the recovery is measured is preceded at a short temporal interval by another response. On this basis short $t/2$ values should occur when there are many spontaneous responses and as a high level of spontaneous responding is usually found in conjunction with a high SCL then Darrow and Patterson's data receive additional support.

Such considerations lead to doubts about the nature of the time of recovery as an independent index. Physiological data presented in Section 17.5.6.1, however, can be used to suggest that an empirical analysis of relationships as presented above does not provide the whole answer. Furthermore, data presented in Section 17.5.8, suggest that the degree of heritability of the recovery function is different from that of other aspects of electrodermal activity again reinforcing ideas of its independence.

The material presented in this section suggests that the principles involved in psychophysiological measurement, the attempts to measure a unitary function, having a 'valid' relation to something else, are in many ways no different from those facing workers employing other forms of measurement in psychology. Where perhaps there is a difference from some other areas, is that there is in this instance at least a hope that there is a second level of reference available in an analysis of the physiological basis of the more superficial aspects of the phenomena.

17.5.3.2. Choice of method of electrodermal measurement

Full consideration of methods of electrodermal measurement is provided in Venables & Christie (1973) where a constant voltage method of measurement using silver–silver chloride electrodes and 0·5 per cent KCl in agar jelly electrolyte is advocated. The extent to which this electrolyte may by hydrating the skin surface have a major effect on the recovery limb is called into question by the work of Fowles & Rosenberry (1973). These workers showed that in comparison to a glycol medium the hydration produced by 0·5 per cent KCl produced a marked diminution in the positive wave of the skin potential response. This has relevance in the present discussion in so far as the positive wave of the SPR tends to be a relatively constant accompaniment of short recovery of the SCR.

Thus, although the empirical results reported in Section 17.5.1 were achieved using a variety of methods e.g. zinc–zinc sulphate electrodes and electrolyte and a constant-current method of measuring the skin resistance response in the original Mednick data, and the method advocated by Venables & Christie (1973) above, in the Gruzelier & Venables data, it is probably necessary to investigate further the methods of measurement which may be optimal for the measurement of the recovery of the SCR.

17.5.4. Reliability of measurement

In the strict use of the term reliability, there would appear to be no published data which would bear on the problem of 'test-retest' reliability. There are, however, two sources of data which are in the course of analysis. On a long term basis—over about 10 years—the subjects of the original study carried out in 1962 by Mednick & Schulsinger were retested using similar but more up-to-date methods in 1972–73; these data will be available shortly. On a shorter term basis 200 children on the island of Mauritius were tested as part of a large sample of 1800 when they were 3 years of age. They have since been retested, using identical methods, at age 3½ years and will be retested at age 4 and 5 years. This substantial body of data will become available within the next 2 years.

On a basis analogous to a 'split-half' measure of reliability there would appear to be a degree of consistency from the $t/2$ of the SCR to one stimulus and the $t/2$ of the SCR to other similar stimuli; no formal figures of this kind are, however, published. From another point of view the fact that a $t/2$ of an SCR measured in 1962 should be characteristic of breakdown in 1972 is a measure of the predictive validity and as a necessary consequence an indication of the reliability of the earlier measure. It should, however, be noted that this is a form of reliability from mean age 15 to mean age 25; from one state of fairly mature physiology to another. How far the above mentioned Mauritian data starting from 3-year-old children will manifest high reliability is a matter of some conjecture. By re-testing on a yearly basis, however, the point of stabilization of this measure as one characteristic of the individual (if this is so) will become apparent. It is perhaps interesting that a necessary feature of research which psychometrists have faced many years ago (e.g., constancy of the IQ) now becomes a point of issue for psychophysiologists. This requires establishment of the reliability of methods, by eliminating unnecessary error variance, and the analysis of within-subject variance over time of the particular measures of interest; techniques where psychophysiologists might well learn from the principles laid down earlier by the psychometricians.

17.5.5. Situational modification

Edelberg (1970) reports mean figures of 7·9 and 7·8 sec for the $t/2$ of SCRs to neutral tones and flashes. Gruzelier & Venables (1972) provide a mean figure of 8·7 secs for $t/2$ of SCRs to neutral tones, while Gruzelier (1973) gives a mean figure of 10·3 sec for the right hand and 8·3 sec for the left hand for $t/2$ of SCRs to neutral tones. These data are from normal subjects, under similar conditions $t/2$ of SCRs for non-institutionalized schizophrenics have a mean figure of 4·6 sec and for institutionalized schizophrenics 6·8 sec.

In a context where neutral and signal stimuli (i.e., stimuli to which reaction is required) are presented randomly, half recovery times are approximately halved for both schizophrenic and normal groups (Gruzelier & Venables, 1973). Edelberg (1970) also reports faster half recovery times in an RT situation ($t/2 = 3·4$ sec). There is thus a suggestion of a shorting of recovery times in situations where there is task involvement. On the other hand, where stimuli are unpleasant, e.g. the cold pressor test (Edelberg, 1972a) in spite of a higher general level of skin conductance activity, recovery times are long. Similarly, Furedy (1972) reports longer recovery limbs with responses to stimuli which signal unpleasant shocks. In a study of responses to auditory stimuli of 70, 85 and 100-dB, Lobstein (1974) showed the longest half recovery times for both normals and schizophrenics to 100-dB tones. At 70-dB recovery times were shorter than with 100-dB tones, but markedly shorter among schizophrenics and it was only at this intensity that schizophrenics' $t/2$ values were significantly different from those of normals. Conversely, as far as SCR amplitudes were concerned these increased in a more or less linear fashion with intensity in normal subjects, however, in a manner similar to that shown by Gruzelier, Lykken & Venables (1972) the amplitude of SCR response to high intensity stimuli showed a decrease in schizophrenics to a value less than given to 85-dB stimuli.

There is ample evidence that although subject differences are on the whole maintained over different stimulus and task parameters there is paramount need to take these into account in work where the main emphasis is on individual differences. Edelberg (1972a), over a wide range of tasks and using normal subjects, reports a highly significant task × subjects interaction term; he suggests, however, that over the range of tasks he used, fast recovery Ss are consistently fast and slow recovery Ss consistently slow. He used only normal subjects, however, and future work needs to examine how far overlap may occur when a wider range of subject groups is studied. This section perhaps shows in some detail the preoccupation of the psychophysiologist with individual differences while at the same time attempting to look at effects of stimulus variables (see Section 17.3).

17.5.6. Mechanisms of the SCR recovery limb

From what has already been said it will be recognized that it is important to bear in mind in the consideration of any proposals for the mechanisms of the recovery limb that they must take into account not only the finding that the length of recovery time reflects individual differences but also that 'the recovery limb could indeed change markedly from one wave to the next, as a function of stimulus change, even though response amplitude, conductance level and potential level were the same' (Edelberg, 1973a). While it is possible to suggest that consistency of individual differences might reflect something relatively permanent, such as a consistent hormonal level which determines a peripheral sweat reabsorption process, it must also be borne in mind that consistency of an individual's response may reflect consistency of perceptual attentional factors or learned approaches to a task. Thus, it is not by any means possible to equate individual differences with peripheral determinants and task differences with central determinants of recovery.

17.5.6.1. Peripheral factors

One fundamental piece of evidence is the relation of the recovery limb of the SCR to the presence of components of the SPR. Darrow (1932, 1964) showed an association between rapid recovery SCRs, the presence of the positive component of the SPR, high initial SCL, and surface sweating. Edelberg (1970) similarly showed that rapid recovery SCRs were accompanied by positive SPRs in contrast to slower recovery SCRs which were accompanied by monophasic negative SPRs. Edelberg (1966) showed that positive SPRs accompanied reabsorption of surface moisture and (1970) that SCRs associated with a reabsorption reflex showed a more rapid recovery than those not accompanied by reabsorption. Fowles (1973) provides further evidence for the association of rapid recovery SCRs and the positive component of SPR. Underlying these findings is the two component theory of phasic electrodermal activity (Edelberg, 1971, 1972b, 1973a; Fowles, 1973; Venables & Christie, 1973) suggesting that both the activity of duct filling and the passage of current through an epidermal membrane may be involved in SCRs. It is suggested that in the slow recovery SCR evidence of the duct filling component is seen while in the rapid recovery SCR there is reflection of the activity of an epidermal membrane probably situated in the sweat duct wall at the level of the germinating layer. This does not rule out the idea of a similar membrane on the duct wall at dermal level; however, the possibility is that the dermal mechanism is concerned mainly with selective reabsorption of NaCl from sweat and is not very permeable to water. At the epidermal level, however, both water and NaCl are absorbed and the consequent greater conductivity of the epidermal mechanism makes it a more important candidate as an underlying mechanism for SCR. It is important, therefore, to consider mechanisms which may be involved in the activation of an epidermal ductal mechanism and hence the modification of components of the SCR. From this consideration of the mechanisms involved it is possible to see how far the ideas put forward in Section 17.5.3.1 on a mainly mathematical choice of an independent metric for measuring $t/2$ of SCR maybe subject to modification.

One initial factor is that the level of sweat in the duct must reach the epidermal mechanism. Mild stimulation at resting levels of activity produces minimal SCRs with long recovery limbs at low SCLs. This would be expected and is found when ducts do not fill and no surface sweat is visible. Once surface sweating takes place and sweat is at the level of the epidermal membrane in the duct wall where reabsorption may take place then we should possibly expect larger SCRs with shorter $t/2$ values, starting from higher SCLs. Bundy's (1973) data showing short $t/2$ after closely preceding stimuli is consistent with this statement. Once reabsorption *may* take place then two factors may come into play. One would be the triggering of the reabsorption mechanism, the second would be the capacity of that mechanism for reabsorption. Factors which can possibly trigger the reabsorption mechanism are (1) sodium concentration in sweat, (2) ductal hydrostatic pressure. Several possibilities are available to trigger reabsorption by this second mechanism they are (2a) increase in pressure due to increased sweating when there is poral restriction due to hydration of the skin surface; (2b) ductal myoepithelial contraction (Bligh, 1967) which has been suggested to be adrenergically innervated and hence provides the possibility of sympathetic innervation independent of the cholinergically mediated secretory activity; (2c) pressure on the sweat glands by underlying vasomotor activity; again offering the possibility that a mechanism to trigger reabsorption is one of direct innervation, a possibility considered by Edelberg (1971) as a by-product of the arrival of efferent neural impulses serving to sensitize peripheral receptors.

The idea of a mechanical triggering of the reabsorption mechanism is supported by the work of Edelberg (1973b) who examined the concomitants of the local electrodermal response of Ebbecke. This response was elicited by the use of small bladders placed on the skin to give a standard mechanical stimulus. It was found that the amplitude of the Ebbecke response was significantly but not strongly correlated with the $t/2$ of SCRs collected on the same occasion but not to mechanical stimuli.

Given that the reabsorption mechanism is triggered by one of the means suggested above, then the extent of reabsorption of sodium is probably under the control of mineralocorticoid activity such as that of aldosterone, cortisol, or cortisone. While it is possible that the extent of sodium reabsorption affects speed of recovery of the SCR it should be pointed out that no direct experimental work appears to have been carried out to verify whether this is so.

In summary, at least three factors may influence control over the recovery function of the SCR at the periphery; these are, the extent of the secretory activity, the triggering of the epidermal ductal reabsorption mechanism and the momentary capacity of that mechanism dependent on the modulation by hormonal control. Such multifactorial determination allows for the momentary changes in recovery rate elicited by changes in task demands and also allows for longer term differences due to the stressful nature of a task situation while also permitting the possibility of more permanent characteristics such as the elevated levels of adrenal cortical steroids as found in schizophrenic patients (e.g., Oken, 1967) having an influence in shortening recovery. Thus, task demands, by having stimuli close together in time will lead to shorter $t/2$ as shown by Bundy (1973) by maintaining the relative fullness of the ducts. Additionally, the difficulty of the task, by raising general electrodermal activity, will raise SCL and increase the number of spontaneous fluctuations having a similar effect to that of close proximity of elicited responses.

It should be noted that the analysis presented leads to expectations about the relations between SCL, SCR amplitude and the $t/2$ of SCRs. On the one hand, small amplitude non-duct filling SCRs have long recoveries, and little correlation between SCL, SCR amplitude and SCR $t/2$ should be expected when the subject remains at a resting level and low intensities of stimuli are used. On the other hand, if the subject is highly aroused and all stimuli are intense there will equally be minimal correlation between SCR amplitude and SCR $t/2$ as all responses will be of the high amplitude short recovery type. Only where a range of SCR activity can be expected bridging secretory duct filling and membrane reabsorption aspects of the SCR might a negative intra-individual correlation be expected. As far as the interindividual correlations are concerned similar considerations apply, although with individual differences in reabsorption in the duct filling state it is difficult to predict the relative direction in relation due to this factor.

Consideration of the peripheral mechanisms which might be of importance in the control of recovery does at best have the function of providing a meaningful background to the measurement problems considered earlier in the paper, and points to some of the parameters which need to be emphasized in using the index for task-oriented or individual difference-oriented measurement. Routine application of psychophysiological techniques by those who merely want an index or an indicator without attempting to understand the biological nature of the mechanism which they are measuring is, as this example has possible suggested, likely to lead to uninterpretable results.

17.5.6.2. Central physiological factors

Little direct evidence is available in the literature on possible central physiological control of the recovery of the skin conductance response. Happily, however, the evidence that is available nicely illustrates a cooperative enterprise between physiological psychologists and psychophysiologists, which is one of the aspects of work in this area which it is the aim of the chapter to demonstrate.

In 1965, Bagshaw, Kimble and Pribram published a paper on the skin resistance orienting response in monkeys with ablation of the amygdala and hippocampus. The data were particularly relevant to the theoretical positions of Mednick (1970) and Venables (1972, 1973) concerned with the involvement of the limbic system in schizophrenia, both from the point of view of SCR $t/2$ and the finding of an equal distribution of SC responders and non-responders in a schizophrenic population (see Chapter 12; and Gruzelier and Venables, 1972, 1973, 1974)

The original Bagshaw, Kimble and Pribram data were not analysed for the rate of recovery of the SRR, and additionally were presented in the form of mean SRRs of 10 trial blocks. Bagshaw agreed to reanalyse the data with particular respect to the recovery limb of the SRR and to represent the data on an individual response basis (Bagshaw & Kimble, 1972). Bagshaw divided responses into those between 1 and 2 KΩ and those between 2 and 4 KΩ. Stimuli were 1000 Hz, 77-dB and presented for 2 sec. For control animals $t/2$ values for small responses had a mean value of 2·45 sec and for large responses 3·68 sec. For hippocampectomized animals $t/2$ values for small responses were 1·72 sec and for large response 2·20 sec. The mean overall size of resposes for the hippocampectomized animals was significantly larger than for the control animals. Thus, although as expected between groups of animals faster recovery was found with large responses, nevertheless, the recovery time for the small responses in the hippocampectomized monkeys was shorter than the recovery time of the large responses for the control group. It would thus appear that hippocampectomy has an effect of shortening recovery time which may be independent of the size of response given. Of the six amygdalectomimed animals two were hyper-responsive and had very short values of $t/2$ the other four animals were under-responsive or gave no responses. If responses were given they had large values of $t/2$.

Thus, ablation of parts of the limbic system known to have major effects on orienting, attentional and avoidance behaviour produce changes in the recovery limb of the SCR. Lesions of the hippocampus produce chronic increases in levels of ACTH (e.g., Knigge, 1961) and hence elevated levels of adrenal cortical steroids. The mechanism by which hippocampectomy leads to shorter SCR $t/2$ may thus be the function of increased adrenal cortical activity leading to faster sodium reabsorption of secreted sweat. Conversely, lesions of the amygdala (e.g., Mason, Nauta, Brady, Robinson & Sachar, 1961) lead to depression of steroid output and consequently, by the function of a slower rate of sodium reabsorption to a longer SCR $t/2$. The fruitful cooperation which gave rise to these findings was only possible, of course, because Dr Bagshaw and her colleagues were already measuring electrodermal activity and using monkeys as subjects. It is to be hoped that other physiological psychologists having carried out lesion work on primates and hence producing extermely valuable types of subjects may in the future take the opportunity to carry out psychophysiological studies on them. Unfortunately for work on SCR recovery, much work on animals, electrodermal activity has used the cat as a subject—an animal lacking an epidermal ductal reabsorption mechanism, as evidenced, for instance, by the lack of a true positive component of the SPR (see Venables & Christie, 1973).

It is possible that future work in this area may be carried out on rodents whose footpads do have epidermal ductal reabsorption mechanisms. The difficulty in this instance lies in the evolution of suitable techniques for measurement; SCRs may be measured from rats under restraint, however, the effects of restraint may effectively overlay the characteristics of the animal or the stimulus situation which it is required to study. Recent work by Marcy and Quermonne (1974) has pioneered a method of measurement of electrodermal activity in mice in an unrestrained situation which clearly should receive further investigation and extension to see whether it can also be used with rats.

17.5.7. Concomitants of the SCR recovery limb

In the absence of extensive knowledge of the physiological mechanisms which control the extent of recovery of the SCR further insight into its determinants may be gained by consideration of situations producing, and concomitants of, SCRs with different values of $t/2$.

Edelberg (1970) suggests that although the length of recovery time may distinguish between a rest and a task state and hence should possibly be considered as yet another measure of arousal, more specifically, the speed of recovery reflects the extent of mobilization for goal directed behaviour. In 1972 he extended this hypothesis by examining a wide range of tasks, and showed, for instance, that although levels of tonic arousal measured by SCL and frequency of spontaneous fluctuations of SC were similar for a mirror tracing task and for a cold pressor test, that SCR recovery time was markedly different in the two situations. In the mirror tracing task $t/2$ was short and decreased with better performance and increasing task complexity. In the cold pressor test recovery was long and suggests that enhanced electrodermal activity with retarded recovery may signal a defensive reaction. The interpretation of short recovery as an accompaniment of goal oriented performance is, according to Edelberg, difficult to fit with the finding of short recovery in schizophrenics. It is also not easy to envisage a dimension from 'goal orientation' to 'defensiveness' which can accompany a range of recovery from short to long.

One speculative possibility is to suggest that the behaviour accompanying different lengths of recovery is akin to the notion of 'openness vs closedness' to the environment and is thus in some ways akin to the type of dimension of activity that might be considered to accompany heart rate deceleration or acceleration (Lacey, 1967). This point of view cannot be supported directly but requires the martialling of several pieces of disparate material. Data has already been cited which shows that short recovery times are characteristic of schizophrenics. Venables (1973) reviewing data on 'input regulation' in schizophrenia suggested that these patients characteristically as a primary part of the disease process exhibit an openness to the environment. Recent work by Lobstein (1974) has shown that under stimulus presentation conditions where startle is not produced (e.g., by the use of auditory stimuli with controlled rise time) large heart rate deceleration may be observed in schizophrenics even when very loud stimuli are presented suggesting an abnormal 'openness' to the environment. In the same context Lobstein (1974) showed that it was with the least intense stimuli that he used (75 dB) that he obtained the shortest values of SCR $t/2$ which differed significantly from those shown by normals. However, with more intense 85 and 100-dB stimuli SCR $t/2$ values were more similar to those shown by normal subjects (see Section 17.5.5). Most striking in this area are preliminary results by Patterson (personal communication) showing that schizophrenics having mean values of SCR $t/2$ which are short (4·1 sec in an orienting situation) (*cf.* 4·6 sec, Gruzelier & Venables data cited in Section 17.5.5) had a significantly lower mean absolute auditory threshold than another group of schizophrenics having a long (13·9 sec) value of SCR $t/2$.

Conversely, as shown in Section 17.5.1 tendencies to psychopathy or criminality are associated with large values of SCR $t/2$. Hare (1972) reports a tendency for psychopaths to give marked heart rate acceleration to simple stimuli, a response characteristic which could be thought of as being 'defensive'. It could be suggested that one of the characteristics of psychopaths is that they are not open to the nuances of the environment which might otherwise lead to socially acceptable behaviour. These facts, seen alongside Edelberg's (1972) suggestion that 'retarded recovery' may signal a 'defensive reaction' and

Furedy's (1972) finding that signals indicating the presence of noxious stimulation (and hence requiring a defensive posture) give responses with long recovery limbs; provide some credence to the notion that long SCR $t/2$ values signal a 'closed' gate to the environment.

It is worthwhile recalling at this point that short times of recovery are found in hippocampectomized animals (Section 17.5.6.2) and that the Douglas–Pribram (1966) model of attentional behaviour postulates that it is the function of the hippocampus to 'exclude stimulus patterns from attention through a process of efferent control of sensory reception known as gating'. Hippocampectomy would thus lead to a breakdown in this 'gating' and consequent openness to the environment. It thus seems not unreasonable to paraphrase Edelberg's (1972) notion of goal-orientation as the concomitant of short recovery by the term 'open attention'; the paradox posed by Edelberg that the short recovery characteristic of schizophrenics suggests that they are highly goal oriented thus disappears.

Other speculations may be made concerning the relation of the recovery of the SCR to aspects of behaviours—again via involvement of the limbic system. It is known for instance (e.g., Olton & Isaacson, 1968) that rats with hippocampal lesions are superior at two-way active avoidance tasks, while animals with amygdalectomies (Goddard, 1964) show impaired active avoidance. On this basis, taking into account Bagshaw's results reviewed earlier, it might be expected that active avoidance would be an accompaniment of short recovery; while where any responses are shown at all in amygdalectomized animals whose active avoidance is impaired then these tend to have long recovery times.

This association of short recovery with good active avoidance fits well with the theories of Mednick (1958) and Mednick & Schulsinger (1973), which suggest that schizophrenics exhibit superior active avoidance behaviour. It is, however, suggested that this is because the speed of SCR recovery reflects functions of the limbic and the adrenal cortical systems, rather than that it reflects speed of recovery from general fear arousal. This latter notion would seem to be negated by the suggestion made earlier that stimuli producing short $t/2$ values of SCRs in schizophrenics are also those which produce deceleratory behaviour of the heart, a cardiovascular activity that does not seem to be characteristic of fear. Moreover, recent work (Patterson, personal communication) suggests that although schizophrenics with fast recovery SCRs show greater pupillary dilatation in the first second after stimulation they also show a greater constriction and one which takes longer to reach its maximum than those with long recovery SCRs. Neither of these findings points to a simple explanation which relates recovery of the SCR to recovery from fear arousal.

Much of this last section has involved pure speculation, however, enough of a skeleton of facts is available to suggest that the speculation is not entirely wild. Clearly, advance in understanding the factors underlying skin conductance recovery must be made by research which involves not only the psychophysiologists, more particular province of peripheral physiology but also physiology and a very clear analysis of the behavioural states which result in characteristic changes in SCR half recovery time.

17.5.8. Genetics of the SCR recovery limb

One of the nagging doubts that underlies work centring on such a particular piece of behaviour as the recovery limb of the skin conductance response is that in fact it is so related to other aspects of electrodermal activity that it has no status in its own right. Data reviewed so far, while suggesting an independent status, are not definitive in their answers at the present state of knowledge.

The fact that the speed of recovery exhibited by a subject does seem to be related to the pathological state of his parents (see Section 17.5.1) suggest that it has a heritable basis. However, preliminary data (Bell, Gottesman & Mednick, unpublished) from a twin study, suggest firstly that SCR $t/2$ has a high degree of heritability ($H = 0.89$, $r_{mz} = 0.89$, $r_{dz} = 0.46$) but also that no other aspects of skin conductance activity measured, SCL, SCR amp. SCR lat numbers of responses showed any significant value of H or even approached it. These figures, if replicated, suggest an independent status for SCR $t/2$ and also reinforce its usefulness in genetically based studies. A similarly discriminating finding is also available in a study by Herrman (unpublished). In this work the effect of early separation from parents in children from genetically high and low risk for schizophrenia groups was studied. While SCR $t/2$ significantly discriminated the risk groups, effects of separation were seen only in the variables of SCR amp. and SCR lat .

It is evident that much more work needs to be done on the genetic factors affecting aspects of electrodermal activity if the very provocative evidence presented above is to be firmly established. While undoubtedly much of this could readily proceed with the use of established twin samples, progress in psychophysiological techniques using animals, particularly rodents as subjects could enable insights to be gained more quickly. In addition the psychophysiological parameters of established genetic strains of rats such as the Roman High and Low avoidance strains (Bignami, 1965) could enable the testing of some of the suggestions of the pathology of schizophrenia to be examined in in relation to those aspects of electrodermal activity such as SCR $t/2$ which appear to be so characteristic of breakdown.

17.6. EPILOGUE

There is one moral to be learned from work on SCR $t/2$. With the exception of that ubiquitously foreseeing pioneer CW. Darrow virtually nobody had bothered to measure the rate of recovery of the 'GSR' before the 1960s, and even now it is not regularly measured. Some at least of the findings reported in this chapter are the results of analysis of existing data. There are undoubtedly other instances where psychophysiologists could do more to wring out from their data more than they do at present—perhaps there are more seams of gold still untapped which exist in yards of well collected data. From a general viewpoint, however, it is hoped that the rather detailed description concentrating on work using a particular component of a particular psychophysiological response will not have led the reader too far away from the original purpose of this chapter.

It has been seen that work using SCR $t/2$ in problems in abnormal psychology appears to be only capable of being fully understood if much of the armanentarium of other aspects of psychology is brought to bear. Undoubtedly work in this area would be immensely facilitated by co-operation with physiological physiologists. A soundly and widely based increase in animal psychophysiology, particularly using rodents where cardiovascular work has received most emphasis, would enable some problems to be answered in an economical fashion. Primarily, however, a very clear understanding of the behavioural concomitants of SCR $t/2$ are likely to produce the greatest insights and hopefully lead to a more successful application of such measurement to an area of prime importance.

17.7. ACKNOWLEDGMENTS

This chapter was prepared while the author was in receipt of grants from the Medical Research Council and while in the Department of Psychology, Birkbeck College, London.

17.8. REFERENCES

Ax, A. F. Editorial. *Psychophysiology*, 1964, **1**, 1–3.

Ax, A. F. & Bamford, J. L. The GSR recovery limb in chronic schizophrenia. *Psychophysiology*, 1970, **7**, 145–147.

Bagshaw, M. H. & Kimble, D. Bimodal EDR orienting response characteristics in limbic lesioned monkeys: correlates with schizophrenic patients. Paper presented to a meeting of the Society for Psychophysiological Research, Boston, Massachusetts, 1972.

Bagshaw, M. H., Kimble, D. P. & Pribram, K. H. The GSR of monkeys during orienting and habituation and after ablation of the amygdala, hippocampus, and inferotemporal cortex. *Neuropsychologia*, 1965, **3**, 111–119.

Bignami, G. Selection for high rates and low rates of conditioning in the rat. *Annual Behaviour*, 1965, **13**, 221–227.

Bligh, J. A. A thesis concerning the processes of secretion and discharge of sweat. *Environmental Research*, 1967, **1**, 28–45.

Bundy, R. S. The effect of previous responses on the skin conductance recovery limb. Paper presented to a meeting of the Society for Psychophysiological Research, Galveston, Texas, 1973.

Darrow, C. W. The relation of the GSR recovery curve to reactivity, resistance level, and perspiration *Journal of General Psychology*, 1932, **7**, 261–273.

Darrow, C. W. The equation of the galvanic skin reflex curve. I. The dynamics of reaction in relation to excitation "background". *Journal of General Psychology*, 1937, **10**, 285–309.

Darrow, C. W. The rationale for treating the change in the galvanic skin response as a change in conductance. *Psychophysiology*, 1964, **1**, 31–38.

Douglas, R. J. & Pribram, K. H. Learning and limbic lesions. *Neuropsychologia*, 1966, **4**, 197–220.

Edelberg, R. Response of cutaneous water barrier to ideational stimuli. *Journal of Comparative and Physiological Psychology*, 1966, **61**, 28–33.

Edelberg, R. The information content of the recovery limb of the electrodermal response. *Psychophysiology*, 1970, **6**, 527–539.

Edelberg, R. Electrical properties of the skin. In H. R. Elden (Ed), *A treatise on the skin.* Vol. 1. New York: Wiley, 1971.

Edelberg, R. Electrodermal recovery rate, goal-orientation, and aversion. *Psychophysiology*, 1972, **9**, 512–520(a).

Edelberg R. The electrodermal system. In N. S. Greenfield & R. A. Sternbach (Eds), *Handbook of psychophysiology.* New York: Holt, 1972(b).

Edelberg, R. Mechanisms of electrodermal adaptations for locomotor manipulation or defense. In E. Steller and J. M. Sprague (Eds), *Progress in Physiological Psychology.* Vol. 6, New York: Academic Press, 1973(a).

Edelberg, R. The role of an epidermal component in control of electrodermal recovery rate. Paper presented to a meeting of the Society for Psychophysiological Research, Galveston, Texas, 1973(b).

Fowles, D. C. Mechanisms of electrodermal activity. In R. F. Thompson & M. M. Petterson (Eds), Methods in physiological psychology. Vol. 1, *Bioelectric recording techniques. Part C. Receptor and effector processes.* New York: Academic Press, 1973.

Fowles, D. C. & Rosenberry, R. Effects of epidermal hydration on skin potential responses and levels. *Psychophysiology*, 1973 **10**, 601–610.

Furedy, J. J. Electrodermal recovery time as a supra-sensitive autonomic index of anticipated intensity of threatened shock. *Psychophysiology*, 1972, **9**, 281–282.

Goddard, G. V. Functions of the amygdala. *Psychological Bulletin*, 1964, **62**, 89–109.

Gruzelier, J. H. Bilateral asymmetry of skin conductance orienting activity and levels in schizophrenics. *Biological Psychology*, 1973, **1**, 21–42.

Gruzelier, J. H., Lykken, D. T. & Venables, P. H. Schizophrenia and arousal revisited. Two flash thresholds and electrodermal activity in activated and non-activated conditions. *Archives of General Psychiatry*, 1972,

Gruzelier, J. H. & Venables, P. H. Skin conductance orienting activity in a heterogenous sample of schizophrenics. *Journal of Nervous and Mental Disease*, 1972, **155**, 277–287.

Gruzelier, J. H. & Venables, P. H. Skin conductance responses to tones with and without attentional significance in schizophrenic and non-schizophrenic psychiatric patients. *Neuropsychologia*, 1973, **11**, 221–230.

Gruzelier, J. H. & Venables, P. H. Bimodality and lateral asymmetry of skin conductance orienting activity in schizophrenics: Replication and evidence of lateral asymmetry in patients with depression and disorders of personality. *Biological Psychiatry*, 1974, **8**, 55–73.

Hare, R. D. Dissociation of conditioned electrodermal and cardiovascular responses in psychopathy. Paper presented to Society for Psychophysiological Research, Boston, Massachusetts, 1972.

Knigge, K. M. Adrenocortical response to stress in rats with lesions of the hippocampus and amygdala. *Proceedings of the Society for Experimental Biology and Medicine*, 1961, **108**, 17–21.

Koepke, J. E. & Pribram, K. H. Habituation of GSR as a function of stimulus duration and spontaneous activity. *Journal of Comparative and Physiological Psychology*, 1966, **61**, 442–448.

Lacey, J. I. Somatic response patterning and stress: Some revisions of activation theory. In M. H. Appley & R. Trumbull (Eds), *Psychological Stress.* New York: Appleton–Century–Crofts, 1967.

Lobstein, T. J. Heart rate and skin conductance activity in schizophrenia. Unpublished Ph.D. thesis, University of London, 1974.

Lockhart, R. A. Interrelations between amplitude, latency, rise time and the Edelberg recovery measure of the galvanic skin response. *Psychophysiology*, 1972, **9**, 437–442.

Marcy, R. & Quermonne, M. A. An improved method for studying the psychogalvanic reaction in mice and its inhibition by psycholeptic drugs. Comparison with effects of other pharmacological agents. *Psychopharmacologia* (Berl.), 1974, **34**, 335–349.

Mason, J. W., Nauta, J. H. W., Brady, J. V., Robinson, J. A. & Sachar, E. T. The role of limbic structures in the regulation of ACTH secretion. *Acta Neurovegetativa*, 1961, **23**, 4–14.

Mednick, S. A. A learning theory approach to research in schizophrenia. *Psychological Bulletin*, 1958, **55**, 316–327.

Mednick, S. A. Breakdown in individuals at high risk for schizophrenia: Possible predispositional perinatal factors. *Mental Hygiene*, 1970, **54**, 50–63.

Mednick, S. A. & Schulsinger, F. Some premorbid characteristics related to breakdown in children with schizophrenic mothers. In Rosenthal, D. & Kety, S. S. *The transmission of schizophrenia*. Oxford: Pergamon, 1968, Chapter.

Mednick, S. A. & Schulsinger, F. A learning theory of schizophrenia thirteen years later. In Hammer, M., Salzinger, K. & Sutton, S. (Eds), *Psychopathology*. New York: Wiley, 1973, Chapter 18.

Obrist, P. A., Sutterer, J. R. & Howard, J. L. Preparatory cardiac changes: A psychobiological approach. In A. H. Black & W. F. Prokasy (Eds), *Classical Conditioning II. Current Research and Theory*. New York: Appleton-Century-Crofts, 1972, Chapter 13.

Olton, D. S. & Isaacson, R. L. Hippocampal lesions and active avoidance. *Physiology and Behaviour*, 1968, **3**, 719–724.

Oken, D. The psychophysiology and psychoendocrinology of stress and emotion. In M. H. Appley & R. Trumbull (Eds), *Psychological stress*. New York: Appleton–Century–Crofts, 1967.

Siddle, D. A. T., Nicol, A. R. & Foggitt, R. H. Habituation and overextinction of the GSR component of the orienting response in anti-social adolescents. *British Journal of Social and Clinical Psychology*, 1973, **12**, 303–308.

Stern, J. A. Toward a definition of psychophysiology. *Psychophysiology*, 1964, **1**, 90–91.

Sokolov, E. N. *Perception and the conditioned reflex*. New York: Macmillan, 1963.

Venables, P. H. Psychophysiological research in schizophrenia. Paper presented at symposium Applications of Psychophysiology to Clinical Psychology, Iowa, 1972.

Venables, P. H. Input regulation in psychopathology. In M. Hammer, K. Salzinger, & S. Sutton (Eds), *Psychopathology*, New York: Wiley, 1973, Chapter 14.

Venables, P. H. & Christie, M. J. Mechanisms, instrumentation, recording techniques and quantification of responses. In W. F. Prokasy & D. C. Raskin (Eds), *Electrodermal Activity in Psychological Research*, New York: Academic Press, 1973, Chapter 1.

Index